Sixth Edition

Appleton & Lange's Review of

PHARMACY

Sixth Edition

Appleton & Lange's Review of
PHARMACY

Gary D. Hall, MS
Professor of Pharmaceutics

Barry S. Reiss, PhD
Professor of Pharmaceutics
Albany College of Pharmacy
Union University
Albany, New York

Appleton & Lange
Stamford, Connecticut

Notice: The author(s) and the publisher of this volume have taken care to make certain that the doses of drugs and schedules of treatment are correct and compatible with the standards generally accepted at the time of publication. Nevertheless, as new information becomes available, changes in treatment and in the use of drugs become necessary. The reader is advised to carefully consult the instruction and information material included in the package insert of each drug or therapeutic agent before administration. This advice is especially important when using new or infrequently used drugs. The publisher disclaims any liability, loss, injury, or damage incurred as a consequence, directly or indirectly, of the use and application of any of the contents of this volume.

Copyright © 1997 by Appleton & Lange
Copyright © 1993 by Appleton & Lange
Copyright © 1990, 1985 by Appleton & Lange
A Publishing Division of Prentice Hall
Copyright © 1980, 1976 by Arco Publishing, Inc.

97 / 10 9 8 7 6 5 4 3 2 1

Prentice Hall International (UK) Limited, *London*
Prentice Hall of Australia Pty. Limited, *Sydney*
Prentice Hall Canada, Inc., *Toronto*
Prentice Hall Hispanoamericana, S.A., *Mexico*
Prentice Hall of India Private Limited, *New Delhi*
Prentice Hall of Japan, Inc., *Tokyo*
Simon & Schuster Asia Pte. Ltd., *Singapore*
Editora Prentice Hall do Brasil Ltda., *Rio de Janeiro*
Prentice Hall, *Englewood Cliffs, New Jersey*

Library of Congress Cataloging in Publication Data

Hall, Gary D.
    Appleton & Lange's review of pharmacy / Gary D. Hall, Barry S. Reiss. — 6th ed.
        p.   cm.
    Includes bibliographical references.
    ISBN 0-8385-0281-4 (pbk. : alk. paper)
    1. Pharmacy—Examinations, questions, etc.   I. Reiss, Barry S., 1944–   . II. Title.
    [DNLM: 1. Pharmacy—examination questions.   QV 18.2 H176a 1997]
RS97.H35   1997
615′.1′076—dc21
DNLM/DLC   97-12352
for Library of Congress   CIP

Acquisitions Editor: Marinita Timban
Associate Editor: Amy Schermerhorn
Production Editor: Eileen L. Pendagast

PRINTED IN THE UNITED STATES OF AMERICA

ISBN 0-8385-0281-4

90000

9 780838 502815

Appleton & Lange Review Titles for Health Professions

A&L/PREP REVIEW SERIES

Appleton & Lange's Review of Cardiovascular-Interventional Technology
Vitanza
1995, ISBN 0-8385-0248-2, A0248-3

Appleton & Lange's Review for the Chiropractic National Boards, Part I
Shanks
1992, ISBN 0-8385-0224-5, A0224-4

Appleton & Lange's Review for the Dental Assistant, 3/e
Andujo
1992, ISBN 0-8385-0135-4, A0135-2

Appleton & Lange's Review for the Dental Hygiene National Board Review, 4/e
Barnes and Waring
1995, ISBN 0-8385-0230-X, A0230-1

Appleton & Lange's Review for the Medical Assistant, 5/e
Palko and Palko
1997, ISBN 0-8385-0285-7, A0285-5

Appleton & Lange's Review of Pharmacy, 6/e
Hall and Reiss
1997, ISBN 0-8385-0281-4, A0281-4

Appleton & Lange's Review for the Physician Assistant, 3/e
Cafferty
1997, ISBN 0-8385-0279-2, A0279-8

Appleton & Lange's Review for the Radiography Examination, 3/e
Saia
1997, ISBN 0-8385-0280-6, A0280-6

Appleton & Lange's Review for the Surgical Technology Examination, 4/e
Allmers and Verderame
1996, ISBN 0-8385-0270-9, A0270-7

Appleton & Lange's Review for the Ultrasonography Examination, 2/e
Odwin
1993, ISBN 0-8385-9073-X, A9073-6

Essentials of Advanced Cardiac Life Support: Program Review & Exam Preparation (PREP)
Brainard
1997, ISBN 0-8385-0259-8, A0259-0

Radiography: Program Review & Exam Preparation (PREP)
Saia
1996, ISBN 0-8385-8244-3, A8244-4

More on reverse →

Appleton & Lange Review Titles for Health Professions

MEPC/A&L QUICK REVIEW SERIES

Appleton & Lange's Quick Review: Dental Assistant
Andujo
1997, ISBN 0-8385-1526-6, A1526-1

Appleton & Lange's Quick Review: Massage Therapy
Garofano
1997, ISBN 0-8385-0307-1, A0307-7

Appleton & Lange's Quick Review: Pharmacy, 11/e
Generali
1997, ISBN 0-8385-6342-2, A6342-8

Appleton & Lange's Quick Review: Physician Assistant, 3/e
Rahr and Niebuhr
1996, ISBN 0-8385-8094-7, A8094-3

Dental Assistant: Program Review & Exam Preparation (PREP)
Andujo
1997, ISBN 0-8385-1513-4, A1513-9

Medical Assistant: Program Review & Exam Preparation (PREP)
Hurlbut
1997, ISBN 0-8385-6266-3, A6266-9

MEPC: Medical Assistant
Examination Review, 4/e
Dreizen and Audet
1989, ISBN 0-8385-5772-4, A5772-7

MEPC: Medical Record,
Examination Review, 6/e
Bailey
1994, ISBN 0-8385-6192-0, A6192-7

MEPC: Obstetrics & Gynecology
Ross
1997, ISBN 0-8385-6328-7, A6328-7

MEPC: Occupational Therapy
Examination Review, 5/e
Dundon
1988, ISBN 0-8385-7204-9, A7204-9

MEPC: Optometry
Examination Review, 4/e
Casser et al.
1994, ISBN 0-8385-7449-1, A7449-0

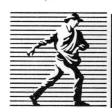

To order or for more information,
visit your local health science bookstore
or call Appleton & Lange toll free at
1-800-423-1359.

Contents

Acknowledgments

We would like to thank Marinita Timban, Editor, and Amy Schermerhorn, Associate Editor, at Appleton & Lange for their editorial guidance throughout the development of this newly revised edition. We would also like to thank all pharmacy students, past, present, and future, who aspire to excel in their chosen profession.

Gary D. Hall, MS
Barry S. Reiss, PhD

Preface

Pharmacy licensing examinations are designed to determine whether a candidate has the requisite ability to enter and then carry out the responsibilities of the profession. A candidate preparing for the licensing examination must be prepared to demonstrate competence in many areas, any one of which may be the subject for in-depth questioning.

This book is designed as a self-testing tool for the pharmacy student to identify individual areas of strength and weakness, to suggest areas for further review, and to impart new concepts and other information useful to both the student and the practicing pharmacist. The book consists of three major sections: Chapters 1 through 6 concentrate on specific disciplines in order to improve the student's competence in each. Within each chapter, some questions dealing with related subject matter have been grouped together, whereas others have intentionally not been categorized, necessitating a return to certain areas of study in later questions to reinforce prior learning. In each chapter, questions are followed by an Answers and Explanations section, which we think is the keystone of our book. Some comments are quite extensive and represent miniature reviews, whereas others are limited to brief specifics. In every instance, the cited references offer a way for more extensive review.

Chapter 7 consists of patient profiles, each accompanied by a series of related questions. Information obtained from the questions and commentaries in Chapters 1 through 6 will probably aid in answering questions in Chapter 7.

The final section, Chapter 8, is a practice examination to test the reader who has faithfully completed all of the previous material.

A self-assessment disk is new to the Sixth Edition and helps in preparing you for the computerized format of the NAPLEX. A description of the computer-based examination is provided on page xv. The study disk includes the following key features:

- diagnostic feedback of strengths and weaknesses
- ability to create multiple customized practice tests
- an electronic notebook to save comments while studying
- a digital timer to show elapsed study/test-taking time

There are also two appendices: the first lists more than 200 drugs by generic names that the authors consider most likely to be dispensed by pharmacists. Included in the table are trade or brand names, manufacturing companies, a brief description of therapeutic uses, and common dosage forms and strengths. It is NOT necessary to memorize the name of the company manufacturing a certain product, especially with the numerous company name changes. However, many individuals find it easier to relate a trade name to a company. To complete the cycle, the second appendix serves as a cross-reference of trade names with generic names.

We trust that this book will not be viewed as simply a means to review material for the licensing examination. Passing this examination does not guarantee continued competence throughout a long professional career. Practicing pharmacists must not only retain their previously acquired knowledge and skill, but must remain up to date on contemporary modes of practice. We hope that this book will serve both as a means for self-assessment of competence to practice as well as a valuable guided review. A statement listing professional competency in pharmacy originally prepared by the California State Board of Pharmacy appears on the next page. Many of the test items in this book relate to these competencies.

Professional Competence in Pharmacy

A competent pharmacist is one who is able to confer with a physician about the care and treatment of his or her patient. The pharmacist should appreciate the essentials of the clinical diagnosis and understand the medical management of the patient. He or she should also be informed about the drugs that may be used in the treatment of the patient—their mechanism of action; their combinations and dosage forms; the fate and disposition of the drugs (if known); the factors that may influence the physiological availability and biological activity of the drugs from their dosage forms; how age, sex, or secondary disease states might influence the course of treatment; and how other drugs, foods, and diagnostic procedures may interact to modify the activity of the drug.

A competent pharmacist is one whose overall function is to ensure optimum drug therapy. He or she should know the appropriate indications and dosage regimen for the drug therapy being undertaken as well as the contraindications and potential untoward reactions that may result during therapy. He or she should also be informed as to the proprietary products that might interact adversely with or be useful adjuncts to drug therapy, facilitating administration or improving overall patient care.

A competent pharmacist must be aware of the proposed therapeutic actions of proprietary medications, their composition, and any unique applications or potential limitations of their dosage forms. He or she should be able to objectively appraise advertising claims. At the patient's request, he or she should be able to ascertain the probable therapeutic usefulness of a certain drug in resolving the patient's complaints.

A competent pharmacist should be able to review a scientific publication and summarize the practical implications of the findings as they may relate to the clinical use of drugs. He or she should be able to analyze a published report of a clinical trial in terms of the appropriateness of the study design and the validity of the statistical analysis, and should be able to prepare an objective summary of the significance of the data and the authors' conclusions.

A competent pharmacist is a specialist as to the stability characteristics and storage requirements of drugs and drug products, the factors that influence the release of drugs from dosage forms, and the effect of the site of administration or its environment within the body on the absorption of a drug from the administered dosage form. Most importantly, the pharmacist understands the effect of the interaction of all these factors on the onset, intensity, or duration of therapeutic action.

A competent pharmacist should be precisely informed as to the legal limitations on procurement, storage, distribution, and sale of drugs; the approved use of a drug as specified by federal authorities and acceptable medical practice; and his or her legal responsibilities to the patient when drugs are used in experimental therapeutic procedures.

A competent pharmacist should be able to recommend the drug and dosage form that are most likely to fulfill a particular therapeutic need, supporting his or her choice objectively with appropriate source material. In addition, he or she should be capable of identifying a drug, within a reasonable period of time, on the basis of its color, shape, and proposed use, as described in reference books or other sources.

On the basis of symptoms described in an interview with the patient, a competent pharmacist should know what additional information he or she must obtain from the patient. Based on this information, he or she should be able to refer the patient to the proper medical practitioner, specialist, or agency that would be of most help.

A competent pharmacist should be aware of drug toxicities, as well as the most effective means of treatment for them.

A competent pharmacist should be able to instruct patients on the proper administration of prescription and proprietary drugs. He or she should know which restrictions should be placed on food intake, other medication, and physical activity.

A competent pharmacist should be able to communicate with other healthcare professionals or laymen on appropriate subjects, ensuring that the recipient understands the contents of the message being communicated.

A competent pharmacist should be capable of compounding appropriate drugs or drug combinations in acceptable dosage forms.

Finally, a competent pharmacist is a person who takes appropriate measures to maintain his or her level of competency in each of the areas described above.

Computer-Based Examinations

Following the lead of the nursing profession, many professions have reorganized their entry level professional examinations to a computer-adaptive format. Candidates have an open-window time period, usually 1 or 2 weeks, several times a year during which they may take the licensing exam. The actual exam format is similar to previous examinations. For pharmacy, this involves the use of patient profiles followed by a series of questions that may or may not require reviewing the patient's profile. Using the computer keyboard or mouse, the candidate can scroll back to the profile for any needed information to answer a specific question. The questions will be presented one at a time and must be answered in sequence—that is, one may not skip or skim questions with the intention of returning to them later. Also, once the candidate has selected an answer and entered it into the computer, it is NOT possible to retrieve the answer and make changes. Be sure that you are satisfied with your answer before entering it into the computer. Once entered, forget about that question even if later questions lead you to believe that you gave a wrong answer.

Remember that no one is expected to answer all questions correctly. Instead, the examining body has set reasonable goals based on both easy and more difficult questions or concepts. The examination is designated as a "computer-adaptive" test because the system evaluates each individual candidate by varying the question difficulty depending on the candidate's response to previous questions. Thus, different candidates at the same testing site may be answering different questions of varying difficulty. The scoring will be based at least partially on the number of questions answered correctly and the relative level of question difficulty.

When preparing for computer-based exams, the candidate should review material in the exact manner as for any other examination. It is suggested that the candidate participate in any tutorial session offered at the exam site just prior to the actual examination. These sessions will include instruction in the mechanics of operating the computer system being used. However, any anxiety about the use of the computer will soon be overcome once the exam has started. In addition, you are likely to benefit by receiving your grade and pharmacist license much earlier!

Helpful Hints

There are several ways to maximize learning from this review book. For example, the reader could answer a short series of questions before looking for the answers at the end of each chapter. Keeping score will make these chapters function as miniature tests. Unfortunately, when challenged by multiple-choice questions, even in the nonthreatening environment of a self-learning program, our behavioral response is often predictable. When more than 75% of the questions are answered correctly, satisfaction and confidence dominate. As the percentage of missed questions increases, frustration and even panic develop. Such reactions lead to a self-limiting response: namely, the quick memorization of answers. Keep in mind, however, that although you may have increased your knowledge by one fact, you may not have maximized your learning experience. Do you really expect to see the same question on another examination? Do you realize why the other answer choices are not correct? Have you read the explanations of all the questions, even those you answered correctly? Hopefully, these explanations will contain additional tidbits of information that will increase your knowledge base. If the question mentions a drug with which you are not familiar, be sure to look up the drug in one of the reference sources at your disposal. The next time you see that drug may be when it is the subject of a question. Some questions may concern topics with which you are not familiar. This is a perfect opportunity for learning!

Rather than blindly guessing at the answers, seek information in the cited reference or other sources and then attempt to answer the question. If your answer does not agree with the one given in this book, check further in another source. Keep digging—learning cannot be passive. Recognize that a question stating "which of these does NOT" or "all of these EXCEPT" gives you four positive facts or statements. These, in themselves, have expanded your knowledge base.

References

The references listed represent a small collection of source material that can be found in most pharmacy libraries or represent a collection that any pharmacist or pharmacy student could accumulate during a career in pharmacy. Because of the increasing costs and frequent issuing of new editions, the authors of *Appleton & Lange's Review of Pharmacy* have attempted to limit the total number of books but realize that there are many other textbooks containing similar material. To maintain an up-to-date personal library, the reader should obtain at least a general pharmaceutical science book (eg, Ref. 1 or 24), a pharmacology book (Ref. 6 being the classic), a book with a clinical pharmacy orientation (Ref. 11 or 19), and a book devoted to discussions of drug therapy in managing certain disease states (Ref. 16). To keep current with new drugs, drug products, and recent developments in drug therapy, it is necessary to have publications that are updated periodically (monthly for Ref. 3 and yearly for Refs. 9 and 25.)

Notice that the last line of each explanation of answers includes a number identifying the reference source used for each question. The first number in the cited reference indicates the reference source used and usually the second number provides the exact page. For example, (1:825; 23:84) refers to page 825 in Ref. 1, *Remington: The Science and Practice of Pharmacy*, and page 84 in Ref. 23, Ansel's *Pharmaceutical Calculations*. The *USP/DI* has been cited as three sources (18a, 18b, and 18c), reflecting the three volumes that make up this series. Citations for Koda-Kimble's *Applied Therapeutics* include the chapter number followed by the page reference (example: 40–14 refers to page 14 of Chapter 40).

1. Gennaro AR. *Remington: The Science and Practice of Pharmacy.* 19th ed. Easton, PA: Mack Publishing Co., 1995.
2a. American Pharmaceutical Association. *Handbook of Nonprescription Drugs.* 11th ed. Washington DC: American Pharmaceutical Association, 1996.
2b. American Pharmaceutical Association. *Nonprescription Products: Formulations & Features '96–97.* Washington DC: American Pharmaceutical Association, 1996.
3. Kastrup EK, Olin BR. *Facts and Comparisons.* Philadelphia, PA: Facts and Comparisons Division, JB Lippincott Co, 1996.
4. AMA Division of Drugs. *Drug Evaluations Annual.* Chicago, IL: American Medical Association, 1995.
5. Dipiro JT, et al. *Pharmacotherapy.* 3rd ed. Stamford, CT: Appleton & Lange, 1996.
6. Hardman JG, Limbird LE. *Goodman and Gilman's Pharmacological Basis of Therapeutics.* 9th ed. New York, NY: McGraw-Hill, 1996.
7. Katzung BG. *Basic & Clinical Pharmacology.* 6th ed. Norwalk, CT: Appleton & Lange, 1995.
8. Hansten PD, Horn JR. *Drug Interactions and Updates.* Vancouver, WA: Applied Therapeutics, 1996.
9. AHFS Drug Information 96. Bethesda, MD: American Society of Health-System Pharmacists, 1996.
10. Product literature drug package inserts current in 1996.
11. Herfindal ET, Gourley DR. *Textbook of Therapeutics.* 6th ed. Baltimore, MD: Williams & Wilkins, 1996.

12. Martin A. *Physical Pharmacy.* 4th ed. Philadelphia, PA: Lea & Febiger, 1993.

13. Turco SJ. *Sterile Dosage Forms.* 4th ed. Philadelphia, PA: Lea & Febiger, 1994.

14. Schumacher GE. *Therapeutic Drug Monitoring.* Norwalk, CT: Appleton & Lange, 1995.

15. Rowland M, Tozer TN. *Clinical Pharmacokinetics.* 3rd ed. Baltimore, MD: Williams & Wilkins, 1995.

16. Isselbacher KJ, et al. *Harrison's Principles of Internal Medicine.* 13th ed. New York, NY: McGraw-Hill, 1994.

17. Shargel L, Yu ABC. *Applied Biopharmaceutics and Pharmacokinetics.* 3rd ed. Norwalk, CT: Appleton & Lange, 1993.

18a. USP Convention Inc. *USP DI Volume I—Drug Information for the Health Care Professional.* 16th ed. Rockville, MD: USPC Inc., 1996.

18b. USP Convention Inc. *USP DI Volume II—Advice for the Patient.* 16th ed. Rockville, MD: USPC Inc., 1996.

18c. USP Convention Inc. *USP DI Volume III—Approved Drug Products and Legal Requirements.* 16th ed. Rockville, MD: USPC Inc., 1996.

19. Young LY, Koda-Kimble MA. *Applied Therapeutics: The Clinical Use of Drugs.* 6th ed. Vancouver, WA: Applied Therapeutics, Inc., 1995.

20. Trissel LA. *Stability of Compounded Formulations.* Washington DC: American Pharmaceutical Association, 1996.

21. Trissel LA. *Handbook on Injectable Drugs.* 9th ed. Bethesda, MD: American Society of Health-System Pharmacists, 1996.

22. Catania PN, Rosner M. *Home Health Care Practice.* 2nd ed. Palo Alto, CA: Health Market Research, 1994.

23. Stoklosa MJ, Ansel HC. *Pharmaceutical Calculations.* 10th ed. Baltimore, MD: Williams & Wilkins, 1996.

24. Ansel HC, Popovich NG, Allen LV. *Pharmaceutical Dosage Forms and Drug Delivery Systems.* 6th ed. Baltimore, MD: Williams & Wilkins, 1995.

25. *Physician's Desk Reference.* 50th ed. Montvale, NJ: Medical Economics Co., 1996.

26. Morris M. *The American Heritage Dictionary.* 3rd ed. Houghton Mifflin Co., 1992.

27. *Stedman's Medical Dictionary.* 26th ed. Baltimore, MD: Williams & Wilkins, 1995.

CHAPTER 1

Pharmacology

Since 1940, the first edition of the book cited in the references as reference 6 has been known to successive classes of pharmacy students as simply *Goodman and Gilman*. On page 1 of the current edition, the following statement can be found: "In its entirety, pharmacology embraces the knowledge of the history, source, physical and chemical properties, compounding, biochemical and physiological effects, mechanisms of action, absorption, distribution, biotransformation and excretion, and therapeutic and other uses of drugs. Since a drug is broadly defined as any chemical agent that affects processes of living, the subject of pharmacology is obviously quite extensive."

The test items in this chapter deal with some of these areas of pharmacology. Related questions may be found in chapters on biopharmaceutics and pharmacokinetics and on clinical pharmacy.

Questions

DIRECTIONS (Questions 1 through 180): Each of the numbered items or incomplete statements in this section is followed by answers or by completions of the statement. Select the ONE lettered answer or completion that is BEST in each case.

1. An adverse effect commonly associated with the use of theophylline products is

   (A) crystaluria
   (B) skin rash
   ✓ (C) syncope
   (D) ptosis
   (E) insomnia

2. Which of the following statements is (are) true of epinephrine?

   I. May be administered by inhalation
   II. Reduces arterial blood pressure
   III. Peripheral vasodilator

   (A) I only
   (B) III only
   (C) I and II only
   (D) II and III only
   ✓ (E) I, II, and III

3. Which of the following statements is (are) true of finasteride?

   I. Pregnancy category X
   II. Employed in the treatment of BPH
   III. Administered parenterally

   (A) I only
   (B) III only
   ✓ (C) I and II only
   (D) II and III only
   (E) I, II, and III

4. Dipivefrin (Propine) can best be described as a (an)

   (A) cholinesterase inhibitor
   (B) osmotic diuretic
   (C) beta-adrenergic blocking agent
   (D) prodrug
   (E) chelating agent

5. Which of the following statements is (are) true of ticlopidine HCl (Ticlid)?

   I. Only administered parenterally
   II. Dissolves blood clots
   III. Inhibits platelet aggregation

   (A) I only
   (B) III only
   (C) I and II only
   (D) II and III only
   (E) I, II, and III

6. Nicardipine HCl is used for the treatment of

   I. angina pectoris
   II. hypertension
   III. atrial fibrillation

   (A) I only
   (B) III only
   (C) I and II only
   (D) II and III only
   (E) I, II, and III

7. Which of the following statements is (are) true of alteplase (Activase)?

   I. Produced by recombinant DNA technology
   II. Stimulates erythrocyte production

III. Administered orally

(A) I only
(B) III only
(C) I and II only
(D) II and III only
(E) I, II, and III

8. Which of the following agents has (have) been found useful in the treatment of rheumatoid arthritis?

   I. Ergotamine tartrate (Ergostat)
   II. Loperamide (Imodium)
   III. Auranofin (Ridaura)

(A) I only
(B) III only
(C) I and II only
(D) II and III only
(E) I, II, and III

9. As an antiarrhythmic drug, procainamide is most similar in action to which one of the following agents?

(A) Amiodarone
(B) Propranolol
(C) Digoxin
(D) Verapamil
(E) Quinidine

10. The antiarrhythmic action of tocainide (Tonocard) and mexiletine (Mexitil) most closely resembles that of

(A) acebutolol
(B) verapamil
(C) quinidine
(D) lidocaine
(E) disopyramide

11. Which of the following statements is (are) true of acetylcysteine?

   I. Mast cell stabilizer
   II. Acetaminophen antidote
   III. Mucolytic

(A) I only
(B) III only

(C) I and II only
(D) II and III only
(E) I, II, and III

12. Which one of the following agents may be added to local injections of Xylocaine in order to prolong its effect?

(A) Succinylcholine chloride
(B) Sodium carboxymethylcellulose
(C) Atropine sulfate
(D) Polyethylene glycol
(E) Epinephrine

13. Colestipol HCl is most commonly employed as a (an)

(A) antidote for atropine overdosage
(B) hypoglycemic agent
(C) bile acid sequestrant
(D) fat substitute
(E) bronchodilator

14. Which of the following is (are) true of pravastatin?

   I. Antihypertensive agent
   II. Pregnancy category X
   III. HMG-CoA reductase inhibitor

(A) I only
(B) III only
(C) I and II only
(D) II and III only
(E) I, II, and III

15. Which one of the following drugs does NOT lower plasma lipoprotein concentrations?

(A) Simvastatin
(B) Clofibrate
(C) Probucol
(D) Cholestyramine
(E) Nicotinamide ✗

16. A drug that has been shown to have a strong antagonism for both histamine and serotonin is

    (A) chlorpheniramine (Chlor-Trimeton)
    (B) triprolidine (Actidil)
    (C) cyproheptadine (Periactin)
    (D) loratidine (Claritin)
    (E) promethazine (Phenergan)

17. Idoxuridine (Herplex) is an effective treatment for dendritic keratitis, which is caused by

    (A) *Escherichia coli*
    (B) *Pseudomonas aeruginosa*
    (C) *Staphylococcus aureus*
    (D) *Clostridium difficile*
    (E) herpes simplex

18. Which of the following is (are) employed as antifungal agents?

    I. Natamycin
    II. Clotrimazole
    III. Mafenide

    (A) I only
    (B) III only
    (C) I and II only
    (D) II and III only
    (E) I, II, and III

19. Isotretinoin is used therapeutically

    (A) as a urinary analgesic
    (B) in the treatment of cystic acne
    (C) as an antifungal agent
    (D) in the treatment of resistant tuberculosis
    (E) as an osmotic diuretic

20. An agent that would be most likely to cause drug-induced bronchospasm is

    (A) nedocromil
    (B) enalapril
    (C) isoproterenol
    (D) pindolol
    (E) theophylline

21. Dopamine (Intropin) is a (an)

    I. norepinephrine precursor
    II. $alpha_1$ and $beta_1$ agonist
    III. antihypertensive agent

    (A) I only
    (B) III only
    (C) I and II only
    (D) II and III only
    (E) I, II, and III

22. Which of the following is (are) dopaminergic antiparkinson agents?

    I. Bromocriptine (Parlodel)
    II. Pergolide (Permax)
    III. Selegiline (Eldepryl)

    (A) I only
    (B) III only
    (C) I and II only
    (D) II and III only
    (E) I, II, and III

23. Albuterol (Proventil, Ventolin) is a (an)

    (A) alpha-receptor antagonist
    (B) alpha-receptor agonist
    (C) beta-receptor antagonist
    (D) beta-receptor agonist
    (E) alpha- and beta-receptor agonist

24. Which of the following drugs is (are) histamine antagonists?

    I. Brompheniramine
    II. Pyrilamine
    III. Ranitidine

    (A) I only
    (B) III only
    (C) I and II only
    (D) II and III only
    (E) I, II, and III

25. Agents that are employed as gastric stimulants include

    I. omeprazole
    II. cisapride

III. metoclopramide

(A) I only
(B) III only
(C) I and II only
(D) II and III only
(E) I, II, and III

26. Effects expected as a result of inhaling the smoke of cannabis (marijuana) include

I. vascular congestion of the eye
II. perceptual changes
III. decreased pulse rate

(A) I only
(B) III only
(C) I and II only
(D) II and III only
(E) I, II, and III

27. Of the following glucocorticoids, which one has the greatest anti-inflammatory potency when administered systemically?

(A) Hydrocortisone (Cortef)
(B) Dexamethasone (Decadron)
(C) Triamcinolone (Aristocort)
(D) Prednisone (Meticorten)
(E) Cortisone (Cortone)

28. Benzoyl peroxide is commonly employed in the treatment of

(A) psoriasis
(B) pinworms
(C) acne
(D) trichomonal infections
(E) seborrheic dermatitis

29. Zosyn is a product that contains pipericillin sodium and tazobactam sodium. Tazobactam sodium

(A) is an antifungal agent
(B) prevents the urinary excretion of pipericillin sodium
(C) prevents first-pass metabolism of pipericillin sodium
(D) is a buffer
(E) inhibits beta-lactamase enzymes

30. Which one of the following hormones is released from the posterior pituitary gland?

(A) Oxytocin
(B) Adrenocorticotropic hormone (ACTH)
(C) Thyroid-stimulating hormone (TSH)
(D) Follicle-stimulating hormone (FSH)
(E) Growth hormone

31. During ovulation, peak plasma concentration(s) of which of the following hormone(s) will be reached?

I. Progesterone
II. Follicle-stimulating hormone (FSH)
III. Luteinizing hormone (LH)

(A) I only
(B) III only
(C) I and II only
(D) II and III only
(E) I, II, and III

32. Liotrix is a thyroid preparation that contains

I. liothyronine sodium
II. levothyroxine sodium
III. desiccated thyroid

(A) I only
(B) III only
(C) I and II only
(D) II and III only
(E) I, II, and III

33. Methimazole (Tapazole) is used for the same therapeutic indication as

(A) methoxsalen
(B) danazol
(C) propylthiouracil
(D) omeprazole
(E) azathioprine

34. A phenothiazine derivative commonly used for its antihistaminic effect is

    (A) promethazine
    (B) promazine
    (C) chlorpromazine
    (D) prochlorperazine
    (E) thioridazine

35. Carbamazepine (Tegretol) is indicated for the treatment of

    I. insomnia
    II. epilepsy
    III. trigeminal neuralgia

    (A) I only
    (B) III only
    (C) I and II only
    (D) II and III only
    (E) I, II, and III

36. Of the following anxiolytic agents, the one that possesses the least sedating action is

    (A) diazepam (Valium)
    (B) oxazepam (Serax)
    (C) meprobamate (Miltown, Equanil)
    (D) chlordiazepoxide (Librium)
    (E) buspirone (Buspar)

37. Which of the following is (are) NOT true of theophylline?

    I. Chemically related to caffeine
    II. Increases the contractile force of the heart
    III. Causes CNS depression

    (A) I only
    (B) III only
    (C) I and II only
    (D) II and III only
    (E) I, II, and III

38. Penicillins are believed to exert their antibacterial effect by which one of the following mechanisms?

    (A) Detergent effect on the bacterial cell membrane
    (B) Inhibition of protein synthesis
    (C) Destruction of the bacterial cell nucleus
    (D) Inhibition of bacterial cell wall synthesis
    (E) Steric hindrance of membrane amino acids

39. The antibacterial mechanism of the penicillins is most similar to that of

    (A) lincomycin (Lincocin)
    (B) tetracycline HCl (Achromycin)
    (C) ciprofloxacin (Cipro)
    (D) cefuroxime (Ceftin)
    (E) gentamicin (Garamycin)

40. Which one of the following agents can be administered with ampicillin and other penicillins to achieve higher blood levels of the penicillin?

    (A) Clavulanic acid
    (B) Penicillamine (Cuprimine)
    (C) Sulbactam
    (D) Granisetron (Kytril)
    (E) Probenecid (Benemid)

41. Five hundred milligrams of phenoxymethyl penicillin is equivalent to approximately how many units of penicillin activity?

    (A) 125,000
    (B) 200,000
    (C) 1600
    (D) 250,000
    (E) 800,000

42. Which one of the following agents is most similar in action to nafcillin?

    (A) Amoxicillin (Amoxil)
    (B) Bacampicillin (Spectrobid)
    (C) Penicillin V potassium (Pen Vee K)
    (D) Dicloxacillin (Pathocil)
    (E) Benzyl penicillin

43. Chlorhexidine gluconate is most similar in action to

    (A) quinidine gluconate
    (B) chlorpheniramine

(C) calcium gluconate

(D) hexachlorophene

(E) chloroquine phosphate

44. Penicillamine is a drug used therapeutically for the treatment of

   I. Wilson's disease
   II. rheumatoid arthritis
   III. cysteinuria

   (A) I only
   (B) III only
   (C) I and II only
   (D) II and III only
   (E) I, II, and III

45. Polymyxin B is pharmacologically and microbiologically similar to

   (A) ampicillin (Polycillin)
   (B) colistin (Coly-Mycin S)
   (C) gentamicin (Garamycin)
   (D) penicillin G
   (E) tetracycline (Achromycin)

46. Potentially fatal aplastic anemia is a toxic effect associated with

   (A) ciprofloxacin (Cipro)
   (B) cefadroxil (Duracef)
   (C) disopyramide (Norpace)
   (D) clindamycin (Cleocin)
   (E) chloramphenicol (Chloromycetin)

47. Which one of the following agents is effective against penicillinase-producing staphylococci?

   (A) Piperacillin (Pipracil)
   (B) Penicillin V potassium (V-Cillin K)
   (C) Ticarcillin (Ticar)
   (D) Dicloxacillin (Pathocil)
   (E) Amoxicillin (Amoxil)

48. Sulfonamides exert a bacteriostatic effect by competitively inhibiting the action of

   (A) monoamine oxidase
   (B) xanthine oxidase

(C) pyrimidine

(D) para-aminobenzoic acid

(E) uric acid

49. Sulfones such as dapsone are employed commonly in the treatment of

   (A) urinary tract infections
   (B) psoriasis
   (C) Bright's disease
   (D) Hansen's disease
   (E) Cushing's disease

50. Which one of the following tetracyclines has the longest duration of action?

   (A) Doxycycline (Vibramycin) 15-24°
   (B) Tetracycline (Achromycin) 6-12°
   (C) Demeclocycline (Declomycin) 12-16°
   (D) Minocycline (Minocin) 11-18°
   (E) Oxytetracycline (Terramycin) 8-12°

51. Tricyclic antidepressants are believed to exert their antidepressant action by

   (A) potentiating GABA activity
   (B) increasing the effect of neurotransmitters on postsynaptic receptor sites
   (C) blocking alpha-adrenergic receptors
   (D) increasing the metabolic breakdown of biogenic amines
   (E) blocking beta-adrenergic receptors

52. Agent(s) indicated for the treatment of depression include(s)

   I. bupropion (Wellbutrin)
   II. fluoxetine (Prozac)
   III. phenelzine (Nardil)

   (A) I only
   (B) III only
   (C) I and II only
   (D) II and III only
   (E) I, II, and III

53. A common adverse effect associated with the chronic use of aluminum antacids is

    (A) nausea and vomiting
    (B) gastrointestinal bleeding
    (C) flatulence
    (D) diarrhea
    (E) constipation

54. Enhanced clotting ability of the blood is associated with the administration of

    I. tocopherol
    II. ticlopidine
    III. phytonadione

    (A) I only
    (B) III only
    (C) I and II only
    (D) II and III only
    (E) I, II, and III

55. Carbidopa can best be classified as a drug that

    (A) reverses symptoms of Parkinson's disease
    (B) exerts an anticholinergic action
    (C) is a dopa-decarboxylase inhibitor
    (D) is a neuromuscular blocking agent
    (E) is a skeletal muscle relaxant

56. Methylxanthines such as caffeine and theophylline exert all of the following pharmacologic effects EXCEPT

    (A) cardiac stimulation
    (B) peripheral vasoconstriction
    (C) relaxation of smooth muscle
    (D) diuresis
    (E) CNS stimulation

57. Which one of the following anorexiant drugs is more likely to cause CNS depression than stimulation?

    (A) Diethylpropion HCl (Tepanil)
    (B) Phentermine (Fastin)
    (C) Fenfluramine HCl (Pondimin)
    (D) Phendimetrazine tartrate (Plegine)
    (E) Mazindol (Mazanor)

58. Lactase enzyme is available for the treatment of

    (A) lactose intolerance
    (B) galactokinase deficiency
    (C) cystic fibrosis
    (D) phenylketonuria
    (E) Crohn's disease

59. Isotretinoin (Accutane) is a drug employed in the treatment of severe recalcitrant cystic acne. Which one of the following is NOT an adverse effect associated with its use?

    (A) Hyperglycemia
    (B) Hypertriglyceridemia
    (C) Pseudotumor cerebri
    (D) Conjunctivitis
    (E) Fetal abnormalities

60. Which one of the following is true of isotretinoin (Accutane)?

    (A) Commonly causes cheilitis
    (B) A derivative of vitamin D
    (C) Is applied topically to severe acne lesions
    (D) Contraindicated in patients with diabetes
    (E) May be used safely in pregnant patients after the first trimester

61. Endorphins are

    (A) endogenous opioid peptides
    (B) a new class of topical anti-inflammatory agents
    (C) neuromuscular blocking agents
    (D) biogenic amines believed to cause schizophrenia
    (E) endogenous chelating agents

62. Which of the following statements is (are) true of "crack"?

    I. It is generally injected intravenously.
    II. It is a free-base form of cocaine.
    III. Its use results in CNS stimulation.

    (A) I only
    (B) III only

(C) I and II only

(D) II and III only

(E) I, II, and III

63. A uricosuric drug is one that

(A) decreases flow of urine

(B) increases flow of urine

(C) blocks excretion of uric acid in the urine

(D) aids in the tubular reabsorption of uric acid

(E) promotes excretion of uric acid in the urine

64. Alteplase (Activase) is employed clinically as a (an)

(A) xanthine oxidase inhibitor

(B) tissue plasminogen activator

(C) proton pump inhibitor

(D) ulcer adherent complex

(E) proteolytic enzyme

65. A disadvantage in the use of cimetidine (Tagamet) is its ability to cause

(A) cheilosis

(B) aplastic anemia

(C) gastric hyperparesis

(D) inhibition of hepatic enzyme activity

(E) decreased prolactin secretion

66. A drug that decreases the formation of uric acid is

(A) allopurinol

(B) famotidine

(C) probenecid

(D) phenylbutazone

(E) propylthiouracil

67. Hypoparathyroidism is a disorder that would most logically be treated with

(A) dihydrotachysterol

(B) prednisone

(C) liothyronine

(D) phytonadione

(E) propylthiouracil

68. Drugs employed in reducing elevated serum cholesterol include(s)

    I. simvastatin (Zocor)

    II. quinapril (Accupril)

    III. mexiletine (Mexitil)

(A) I only

(B) III only

(C) I and II only

(D) II and III only

(E) I, II, and III

69. Which one of the following is NOT an anabolic steroid?

(A) Stanozolol

(B) Nandrolone

(C) Oxandrolone

(D) Oxymetholone

(E) Norethindrone

70. Nerves in the human body that transmit their impulses by releasing acetylcholine are known as _____ nerves.

(A) adrenergic

(B) choleretic

(C) sympathetic

(D) cholinergic

(E) neurogenic

71. Pentoxifylline (Trental) can best be classified pharmacologically as a (an)

(A) bronchodilator

(B) antihyperlipidemic agent

(C) histamine H_2 antagonist

(D) hemorheologic agent

(E) antipsychotic

72. Methadone is a (an)

   I. narcotic antagonist
   II. controlled substance
   III. analgesic drug

(A) I only
(B) III only
(C) I and II only
(D) II and III only
(E) I, II, and III

73. An example of a pure narcotic antagonist is

(A) butorphanol (Stadol)
(B) buprenorphine (Buprenex)
(C) nalbuphine HCl (Nubain)
(D) naloxone (Narcan)
(E) sufentanil (Sufenta)

74. Which of the following agents is (are) indicated for the treatment of migraine headaches?

   I. Nabumetone
   II. Sumatriptan succinate
   III. Ergotamine tartrate

(A) I only
(B) III only
(C) I and II only
(D) II and III only
(E) I, II, and III

75. Morphine can be expected to produce which of the following pharmacologic effects?

   I. Constriction of the pupils
   II. Respiratory depression
   III. Constipation

(A) I only
(B) III only
(C) I and II only
(D) II and III only
(E) I, II, and III

76. An active metabolite of the anticonvulsant drug primidone (Mysoline) is

(A) methadone

(B) dopamine
(C) phenytoin
(D) phenobarbital
(E) trimethadione

77. Etidronate disodium (Didronel) is an agent primarily indicated for the treatment of

(A) Crohn's disease
(B) Ménière's syndrome
(C) Paget's disease
(D) Hansen's disease
(E) Parkinson's disease

78. An agent used for the same indication as alendronate sodium (Fosamax) is

(A) dantrolene (Dantrium)
(B) pancuronium bromide (Pavulon)
(C) carmustine (BiCNU)
(D) chenodiol (Chenix)
(E) salmon calcitonin (Miacalcin)

79. Prednisone is an agent that is employed in the treatment of

   I. rheumatic disorders
   II. Crohn's disease
   III. bacterial infections

(A) I only
(B) III only
(C) I and II only
(D) II and III only
(E) I, II, and III

80. Which one of the following agents is indicated for use as an antiemetic agent?

(A) Colestipol (Colestid)
(B) Guanfacine (Tenex)
(C) Ondansetron (Zofran)
(D) Methoxsalen (Oxsoralen)
(E) Difenoxin (Motofen)

81. Amrinone (Inocor) is most similar in action to

(A) digoxin (Lanoxin)
(B) lidocaine (Xylocaine)

(C) hydralazine (Apresoline)

(D) disopyramide (Norpace)

(E) nadolol (Corgard)

82. Which one of the following is a vasodilating drug with marked platelet-suppressing activity?

(A) Nitroglycerin

(B) Dipyridamole (Persantine)

(C) Pentaerythritol tetranitrate (Peritrate)

(D) Acetaminophen

(E) Hydralazine (Apresoline)

83. Lactulose (Cephulac, Chronulac)

   I. is a laxative

   II. increases blood ammonia levels

   III. is an artificial sweetener

(A) I only

(B) III only

(C) I and II only

(D) II and III only

(E) I, II, and III

84. Ricinolate is an active component of

(A) milk of magnesia

(B) cod liver oil

(C) cascara sagrada

(D) citrate of magnesia

(E) castor oil

85. The dose of liothyronine sodium that is approximately equivalent to 60 mg of Thyroid USP in its ability to produce a clinical response is

(A) 120 µg

(B) 0.4 µg

(C) 250 µg

(D) 25 µg

(E) 100 µg

86. Acid rebound is likely to occur with the use of large doses of which of the following antacids?

   I. Aluminum hydroxide

   II. Sodium bicarbonate

   III. Calcium carbonate

(A) I only

(B) III only

(C) I and II only

(D) II and III only

(E) I, II, and III

87. Chronic use of aluminum hydroxide gel may deplete a patient of

(A) ammonia

(B) vitamin B_{12}

(C) medium chain triglycerides

(D) phosphate

(E) potassium

88. Patients who are sensitive to aspirin should avoid the use of

   I. codeine

   II. meperidine

   III. ibuprofen

(A) I only

(B) III only

(C) I and II only

(D) II and III only

(E) I, II, and III

89. Aspirin is believed to inhibit clotting by its action on which of the following endogenous substances?

(A) Endorphin A

(B) Xanthine oxidase

(C) Fibrinogen

(D) Thromboxane

(E) Dopa decarboxylase

90. The primary site of action of triamterene (Dyrenium) and spironolactone (Aldactone) is the

(A) distal tubule

(B) descending loop of Henle

(C) ascending loop of Henle

(D) proximal tubule

(E) glomerulus

91. Which of the following beta-adrenergic blocking agents also exhibit alpha₁-adrenergic blocking action?

    I. Labetalol (Normodyne, Trandate)
    II. Sotalol (Betapace)
    III. Timolol (Blocadren)

    (A) I only
    (B) III only
    (C) I and II only
    (D) II and III only
    (E) I, II, and III

92. Which one of the following drugs is most useful in the relief of acute attacks of gout?

    (A) Alendronate (Fosamax)
    (B) Ergonavine maleate (Ergotrate)
    (C) Buspirone (Buspar)
    (D) Colchicine
    (E) Allopurinol (Zyloprim)

93. Prolonged activity (8–10 hours) is an advantage in the use of which of the following topical decongestants?

    I. Xylometazoline
    II. Oxymetazoline
    III. Phenylephrine

    (A) I only
    (B) III only
    (C) I and II only
    (D) II and III only
    (E) I, II, and III

94. Auranofin (Ridaura) is employed in the treatment of

    (A) ear infections
    (B) psoriasis
    (C) ulcerative colitis
    (D) recalcitrant acne
    (E) rheumatoid arthritis

95. Which of the following agents is NOT likely to reduce blood sugar in a patient with type II diabetes mellitus?

    I. Tolazamide

II. Metformin
III. Glucagon

    (A) I only
    (B) III only
    (C) I and II only
    (D) II and III only
    (E) I, II, and III

96. After oral administration, the greatest amount of iron absorption occurs in the

    (A) ascending portion of the large intestine
    (B) stomach
    (C) sigmoid portion of the large intestine
    (D) transverse portion of the large intestine
    (E) duodenum

97. Iron is required by the body to maintain normal

    (A) digestion
    (B) oxygen transport
    (C) bone growth
    (D) immunologic function
    (E) ascorbic acid absorption

98. Prolonged use of organic nitrates (eg, nitroglycerin) is likely to result in the development of

    (A) hepatotoxicity
    (B) nephrotoxicity
    (C) aplastic anemia
    (D) tolerance
    (E) visual disturbance

99. Which of the following statements is (are) true of regular insulin?

    I. It is a clear product.
    II. It may be administered either SC or IV.
    III. It is a short-acting insulin.

    (A) I only
    (B) III only
    (C) I and II only
    (D) II and III only
    (E) I, II, and III

100. Lovastatin (Mevacor) is contraindicated for use in patients who are

(A) hypersensitive to aspirin
(B) pregnant
(C) chronic asthmatics
(D) more than 25% over ideal body weight
(E) diabetics

101. Which one of the following drugs is available in a transdermal dosage form for use in the prevention of nausea and vomiting associated with motion sickness in adults?

(A) Metoclopramide
(B) Ondansetron
(C) Scopolamine
(D) Clonidine
(E) Granisetron

102. Which one of the following drugs is indicated for the treatment of primary nocturnal enuresis?

(A) Ritodrine (Yutopar)
(B) Amoxapine (Asendin)
(C) Metolazone (Zaroxolyn)
(D) Desmopressin acetate (DDAVP)
(E) Methenamine hippurate (Urex)

103. An example of a benzodiazepine that is not metabolized to active metabolites in the body is

(A) triazolam
(B) chlordiazepoxide
(C) zolpidem
(D) diazepam
(E) halazepam

104. Which one of the following antimicrobial agents would be MOST useful in the treatment of an infection caused by beta-lactamase–producing staphylococci?

(A) Amoxicillin
(B) Cephapirin
(C) Cephalexin
(D) Dicloxacillin
(E) Bacampicillin

105. Gastric intrinsic factor is a glycoprotein that is required for the gastrointestinal absorption of

(A) medium chain triglycerides
(B) folic acid
(C) iron
(D) tocopherols
(E) cyanocobalamin

106. Gingival hyperplasia, hirsutism, and ataxia are adverse effects associated with the use of

(A) minoxidil (Loniten)
(B) chlorpromazine (Thorazine)
(C) ginseng root
(D) phenytoin (Dilantin)
(E) ciprofloxacin (Cipro)

107. Levobunolol (Betagan) is a drug used in the treatment of glaucoma. Which one of the following best describes the action it exerts on the eye?

(A) Miotic
(B) Decreases the production of aqueous humor
(C) Interferes with the enzyme carbonic anhydrase
(D) Acts as an osmotic diuretic
(E) Mydriatic

108. Cardioselectivity is a property of which of the following beta-adrenergic blocking agents?

I. Carteolol (Ocupress)
II. Metipranolol HCl (OptiPranolol)
III. Betaxolol (Betoptic)

(A) I only
(B) III only
(C) I and II only
(D) II and III only
(E) I, II, and III

109. Which of the following is (are) a property or an action of pilocarpine?

   I. Direct-acting miotic
   II. Ingredient in Ocusert ocular therapeutic system
   III. Similar pharmacologic action to dorzolamide (Trusopt)

   (A) I only
   (B) III only
   (C) I and II only
   (D) II and III only
   (E) I, II, and III

110. Which one of the following is NOT an effect of atropine on the human body?

   (A) Cardiac stimulation
   (B) Diminished sweating
   (C) Mydriasis
   (D) Reduction of gastrointestinal tone
   (E) Stimulation of gastic secretion

111. Which one of the following statements best describes the mechanism of action of antihistaminic drugs?

   (A) They interfere with the synthesis of histamine in the body.
   (B) They form inactive complexes with histamine.
   (C) They stimulate the metabolism of endogenous histamine.
   (D) They block the receptor sites on which histamine acts.
   (E) They are alpha-adrenergic blockers.

112. Haloperidol (Haldol) differs from chlorpromazine (Thorazine) in that haloperidol

   (A) is not an antipsychotic agent
   (B) does not produce extrapyramidal effects
   (C) is not a phenothiazine
   (D) does not cause sedation
   (E) cannot be administered parenterally

113. Tamoxifen (Nolvadex) is an agent that can best be described as a (an)

   (A) gonadotropin-releasing hormone analog
   (B) antiestrogen
   (C) estrogen
   (D) progestin
   (E) androgen

114. Which of the following is (are) true of auranofin (Ridaura)?

   I. May cause thrombocytopenia
   II. Orally administered form of gold therapy
   III. Its use may result in renal impairment

   (A) I only
   (B) III only
   (C) I and II only
   (D) II and III only
   (E) I, II, and III

115. Advantages of acetaminophen over aspirin include all of the following EXCEPT

   (A) no alteration of bleeding time
   (B) less gastric irritation
   (C) no occult blood loss
   (D) no appreciable effect on uric acid excretion
   (E) greater anti-inflammatory action

116. The use of clozapine (Clozaril) has been associated with the development of

   (A) thrombocytopenia
   (B) hypercalcemia
   (C) agranulocytosis
   (D) meningitis
   (E) hyperuricemia

117. Which one of the following statements is true of propoxyphene HCl (Darvon)?

   (A) It has about the same analgesic activity as an equivalent dose of codeine.
   (B) It has significant analgesic and antipyretic properties.
   (C) It has analgesic and anti-inflammatory properties but has no antipyretic properties.
   (D) The analgesic property of this drug resides only in the dextrorotatory isomer (d-propoxyphene).

(E) It is administered with meperidine to reduce meperidine's adverse effects.

118. Although classified as antibiotics, dactinomycin (Cosmegen) and plicamycin (Mithracin) are used in cancer chemotherapy because they have a (an)

(A) immunosuppressant effect
(B) antiviral effect
(C) ability to "sterilize" the blood
(D) anabolic effect
(E) cytotoxic effect

119. The anti-inflammatory effect of aspirin is due to

I. resetting of the hypothalamic "setpoint"
II. adrenal stimulation
III. inhibition of prostaglandin synthesis

(A) I only
(B) III only
(C) I and II only
(D) II and III only
(E) I, II, and III

120. The "first-dose" effect is characterized by marked hypotension and syncope on taking the first few doses of medication. This effect is seen with the use of

I. bepridil (Vascor)
II. terazosin (Hytrin)
III. prazosin (Minipress)

(A) I only
(B) III only
(C) I and II only
(D) II and III only
(E) I, II, and III only

121. Carbon monoxide exerts its toxic effects primarily by

(A) reacting with body enzymes to produce acidic substances
(B) decreasing the oxygen-carrying capacity of the blood
(C) reacting with amino acids in the body to form ammonia

(D) inhibiting the gag reflex
(E) paralyzing the muscles of the diaphragm

122. The most serious potential consequence of ingestion of a liquid hydrocarbon such as kerosene or gasoline is

(A) the aspiration of the poison into the respiratory tract
(B) the corrosive action of the poison on the stomach lining
(C) the paralysis of peristaltic motion of the GI tract
(D) dissolution of the mucoid coat of the esophagus
(E) the destruction of body enzymes by the poison

123. Deferoxamine mesylate is considered to be a specific antidote for the treatment of poisoning caused by

(A) anticholinergic agents
(B) opiate narcotics
(C) benzodiazepines
(D) loop diuretics
(E) iron-containing products

124. Which one of the following agents is classified pharmacologically as a carbonic anhydrase inhibitor?

(A) Indapamide (Lozol)
(B) Acetazolamide (Diamox)
(C) Chlorthalidone (Hygroton)
(D) Torsemide (Demadex)
(E) Amiloride (Midamor)

125. The thiazide diuretics decrease the excretion of

(A) uric acid
(B) urea
(C) sodium
(D) bicarbonate
(E) creatinine

126. The renal excretion of amphetamines can be diminished by alkalinization of the urine. Which of the following would tend to diminish the excretion rate of amphetamine sulfate?

    I. Methenamine mandelate
    II. Sodium bicarbonate
    III. Acetazolamide

    (A) I only
    (B) III only
    (C) I and II only
    (D) II and III only
    (E) I, II, and III only

127. An agent employed in relieving signs and symptoms of spasticity resulting from multiple sclerosis is

    (A) buspirone (Buspar)
    (B) dantrolene (Dantrium)
    (C) ursodiol (Actigall)
    (D) mexiletine (Mexitil)
    (E) amiodarone (Cordarone)

128. Which of the following drugs may interfere with ethanol metabolism?

    I. Metronidazole (Flagyl)
    II. Disulfiram (Antabuse)
    III. Chlorpropamide (Diabinese)

    (A) I only
    (B) III only
    (C) I and II only
    (D) II and III only
    (E) I, II, and III only

129. Which of the following is (are) MAO inhibitors?

    I. Pargyline (Eutonyl)
    II. Tranylcypromine (Parnate)
    III. Cyclobenzaprine (Flexeril)

    (A) I only
    (B) III only
    (C) I and II only
    (D) II and III only
    (E) I, II, and III only

130. A drug that is indicated for the treatment of both diarrhea and constipation is

    (A) bisacodyl (Dulcolax)
    (B) lactulose (Cephulac)
    (C) magnesium sulfate
    (D) senna (Senokot)
    (E) polycarbophil (Mitrolan)

131. Which one of the following is a microsomal enzyme inducer?

    (A) Indomethacin
    (B) Rifampin
    (C) Tolbutamide
    (D) Tobramycin
    (E) Ibuprofen

132. The thiazide derivative diazoxide (Hyperstat)

    (A) is a stronger diuretic than hydrochlorothiazide
    (B) is not a diuretic
    (C) produces about the same diuretic response as an equal dose of hydrochlorothiazide
    (D) produces diuresis in normotensive subjects only
    (E) is a pressor agent

133. Which of the following is (are) broad-spectrum antifungal agents?

    I. Griseofulvin
    II. Ketoconazole
    III. Miconazole

    (A) I only
    (B) III only
    (C) I and II only
    (D) II and III only
    (E) I, II, and III

134. Which one of the following barbiturates is used as an intravenous anesthetic?

    (A) Mephobarbital
    (B) Amobarbital
    (C) Methohexital sodium

(D) Pentobarbital sodium

(E) Secobarbital sodium

135. The most useful drug in the treatment of diabetes insipidus is

(A) chlorpropamide (Diabinese)

(B) glucagon

(C) insulin

(D) glyburide (Micronase)

(E) lypressin (Diapid)

136. A pharmacist receives a prescription order for indomethacin (Indocin) capsules. He/She should consult with the physician if the medication record indicates that the patient

(A) has gout

(B) has arthritis

(C) has a peptic ulcer

(D) has insomnia

(E) is hypertensive

137. The sulfonylureas (eg, Diabinese, Glucotrol) are believed to exert their hypoglycemic effect by

(A) decreasing the desire for sugar consumption

(B) inhibiting the breakdown of endogenous insulin

(C) enhancing the effectiveness of the small amounts of insulin that the diabetic can produce

(D) increasing the peripheral utilization of glucose

(E) stimulating the release of insulin from the pancreas

138. Which one of the following oral hypoglycemic drugs has the longest serum half-life?

(A) Acetohexamide (Dymelor)

(B) Tolbutamide (Orinase)

(C) Glyburide (Diabeta, Micronase)

(D) Chlorpropamide (Diabinese)

(E) All of the above have about the same serum half-life

139. Vidarabine (Vira-A) is an antiviral agent indicated for the treatment of

(A) rubella

(B) smallpox

(C) influenza

(D) pneumocystis carinii pneumonia (PCP)

(E) herpes simplex encephalitis

140. Which of the following statements regarding methenamine mandelate is (are) true?

I. After oral ingestion, formaldehyde is formed in acid urine.

II. It should be given with sulfonamides to enhance the effectiveness of therapy.

III. After parenteral ingestion, ammonia forms in the urinary tract.

(A) I only

(B) III only

(C) I and II only

(D) II and III only

(E) I, II, and III

141. Zidovudine (Retrovir) is indicated for the treatment of patients with

I. influenza A virus infection

II. herpes simplex infections

III. human immunodeficiency virus (HIV) infection

(A) I only

(B) III only

(C) I and II only

(D) II and III only

(E) I, II, and III

142. Which one of the following statements is true of alteplase (Activase)?

(A) It is derived from bovine tissue.

(B) It is a thrombolytic agent.

(C) It is derived from porcine tissue.

(D) It is an anticoagulant.

(E) It is administered intramuscularly.

143. Which of the following agents is (are) employed in the treatment of bronchial asthma?

    I. Dyphylline (Lufyllin)
    II. Salmeterol (Serevent)
    III. Nedocromil sodium (Tilade)

(A) I only
(B) III only
(C) I and II only
(D) II and III only
(E) I, II, and III

144. Oxaprozin (Daypro) is most similar in action to

(A) buspirone (Buspar)
(B) diclofenac sodium (Voltaren)
(C) chlorzoxazone (Paraflex)
(D) dicyclomine (Bentyl)
(E) mecamylamine (Inversine)

145. Cromolyn sodium (Intal, Nasalcrom, Opticrom) is a drug that is

(A) effective in acute asthmatic attacks
(B) a synthetic corticosteroid
(C) a histamine antagonist
(D) a theophylline derivative
(E) a mast cell stabilizer

146. Which of the following calcium channel blockers may be employed parenterally in the treatment of cardiac arrhythmias?

    I. Amlodipine (Norvasc)
    II. Isradipine (DynaCirc)
    III. Verapamil (Isoptin, Calan)

(A) I only
(B) III only
(C) I and II only
(D) II and III only
(E) I, II, and III

147. Which one of the following antibiotics is a third-generation cephalosporin?

(A) Cefoxitin (Mefoxin)
(B) Ceftibuten (Cedax)
(C) Cephalexin (Keflex)
(D) Cefonicid (Monocid)
(E) Cefaclor (Ceclor)

148. Reflex tachycardia is an adverse effect most likely to be associated with the use of which of the following drugs?

(A) Moexipril (Univasc)
(B) Losartan (Cozaar)
(C) Minoxidil (Loniten)
(D) Nadolol (Corgard)
(E) Clonidine (Catapres)

149. Which of the following statements is TRUE of buprenorphine (Buprenex)?

    I. It is available only for parenteral use.
    II. It is a nonphenothiazine antipsychotic agent.
    III. It may cause agranulocytosis in some patients.

(A) I only
(B) III only
(C) I and II only
(D) II and III only
(E) I, II, and III

150. Which one of the following is NOT a progestin?

(A) Norethynodrel
(B) Norethindrone
(C) Ethynodiol diacetate
(D) Levonorgestrel
(E) Mestranol

151. Which one of the following beta-adrenergic blocking agents has intrinsic sympathomimetic activity (ISA)?

(A) Esmolol (Brevibloc)
(B) Atenolol (Tenormin)
(C) Pindolol (Visken)
(D) Metoprolol (Lopressor)
(E) Propranolol HCl (Inderal)

152. Danazol (Danocrine) can best be classified as a (an)

(A) anti-inflammatory corticosteroid

(B) androgen

(C) progestin

(D) neuromuscular blocking agent

(E) estrogen

153. Torsemide (Demadex) is most similar in action to

(A) spironolactone (Aldactone)

(B) risperidone (Risperdal)

(C) bumetanide (Bumex)

(D) chlorthalidone (Hygroton)

(E) acetazolamide (Diamox)

154. Potassium supplementation is LEAST likely to be required in a patient using

(A) ethacrynic acid (Edecrin)

(B) chlorthalidone (Hygroton)

(C) furosemide (Lasix)

(D) acetazolamide (Diamox)

(E) triamterene (Dyrenium)

155. Acyclovir (Zovirax) is indicated for the treatment of

(A) shingles

(B) pseudomembranous enterocolitis

(C) HIV infection

(D) measles

(E) influenza caused by influenza A virus strains

156. A drug that is effective in the treatment of alcohol withdrawal syndromes and in the prevention of delirium tremens is

(A) disulfiram (Antabuse)

(B) methadone (Dolophine)

(C) phenytoin (Dilantin)

(D) chlordiazepoxide (Librium)

(E) haloperidol (Haldol)

157. Which of the following statements is TRUE of bacitracin?

I. It is effective in treating *Pseudomonas* infections.

II. It is an aminoglycoside antimicrobial agent.

III. Nephrotoxicity limits its parenteral use.

(A) I only

(B) III only

(C) I and II only

(D) II and III only

(E) I, II, and III

158. Which of the following agents would be effective when administered orally to relieve symptoms of Parkinson's disease?

I. Selegiline (Eldepryl)

II. Procyclidine (Kemadrin)

III. Methysergide maleate (Sansert)

(A) I only

(B) III only

(C) I and II only

(D) II and III only

(E) I, II, and III

159. Olsalazine sodium (Dipentum) is employed in the treatment of

(A) diabetes mellitus

(B) duodenal ulcers

(C) ulcerative colitis

(D) urinary tract infections

(E) diabetes insipidus

160. An advantage of pirbuterol (Maxair) over isoproterenol (Isuprel) in the treatment of bronchial asthma is that pirbuterol

(A) has more beta-agonist activity than isoproterenol

(B) is more selective for beta$_2$-adrenergic receptors

(C) has alpha-adrenergic activity

(D) has no effect on the heart

(E) has a more rapid onset of action

161. Moexipril HCl can best be classified as a (an)

(A) angiotensin-converting enzyme inhibitor
(B) vasodilator
(C) potassium-sparing diuretic
(D) beta-adrenergic blocking agent
(E) alpha-adrenergic blocking agent

162. Which of the following statements is TRUE of beclomethasone dipropionate (Beclovent, Vanceril) aerosol?

(A) It should only be used in the treatment of an acute asthmatic attack.
(B) It should not be used in a patient who is currently using a theophylline product.
(C) Beclomethasone is not absorbed systemically by this route.
(D) The aerosol form is also useful in the treatment of status asthmaticus.
(E) If used in conjunction with a bronchodilator administered by inhalation, the bronchodilator should be used first.

163. Agents useful in the treatment of bronchial asthma usually

(A) block both alpha- and beta-adrenergic receptors
(B) stimulate alpha and/or beta receptors
(C) stimulate beta receptors but block alpha receptors
(D) stimulate alpha receptors but block beta receptors
(E) inhibit acetylcholinesterase activity

164. Which of the following cancer chemotherapeutic agents is (are) classified as an antimetabolite?

I. Fluorouracil (Adrucil)
II. Mercaptopurine (Purinethol)
III. Cytarabine (Cytosar-U)

(A) I only
(B) III only
(C) I and II only
(D) II and III only
(E) I, II, and III

165. Which one of the following antihistamines would be LEAST likely to cause sedation?

(A) Diphenhydramine (Benadryl)
(B) Cetirizine (Zyrtec)
(C) Clemastine (Tavist)
(D) Dimenhydrinate (Dramamine)
(E) Tripelennamine (PBZ)

166. Which one of the following agents is indicated for the treatment of attention deficit disorder?

(A) Methdilazine
(B) Lithium carbonate
(C) Methylphenidate
(D) Haloperidol
(E) Methoxsalen

167. Which of the following agents are macrolides?

I. Tobramycin
II. Polymyxin B
III. Clarithromycin

(A) I only
(B) III only
(C) I and II only
(D) II and III only
(E) I, II, and III

168. Stavudine (Zerit) is an antiviral agent employed in the treatment of

(A) herpes zoster
(B) influenza A virus
(C) *Helicobacter pylori*
(D) HIV infection
(E) herpes simplex

169. Beta carotene is considered to be a precursor for

(A) betaseron
(B) beta interferon
(C) vitamin D
(D) vitamin A
(E) carteolol

170. Simvastatin (Zocor) is an example of a (an)

    (A) HMG-CoA reductase inhibitor
    (B) xanthine oxidase inhibitor
    (C) cholinesterase inhibitor
    (D) bile sequestrant
    (E) alcohol dehydrogenase inhibitor

171. Which of the following statements is (are) true of fentanyl?

    I. It is available as a transdermal system.
    II. It is available as a transmucosal system.
    III. It is a narcotic agonist analgesic.

    (A) I only
    (B) III only
    (C) I and II only
    (D) II and III only
    (E) I, II, and III

172. Which of the following agents is an anabolic steroid?

    I. Metoprolol
    II. Stanozolol
    III. Oxandrolone

    (A) I only
    (B) III only
    (C) I and II only
    (D) II and III only
    (E) I, II, and III

173. Amrinone is a drug that produces

    (A) bronchodilation
    (B) positive inotropism
    (C) antidepressant action
    (D) narcotic antagonism
    (E) benzodiazepine antagonism

174. Which of the following statements is (are) true of potassium?

    I. It is the principal intracellular ion.
    II. It facilitates the utilization of glucose by cells.
    III. It is a component of hemoglobin.

    (A) I only
    (B) III only
    (C) I and II only
    (D) II and III only
    (E) I, II, and III

175. Finasteride can best be described as a (an)

    (A) estrogen
    (B) estrogen inhibitor
    (C) androgen
    (D) androgen inhibitor
    (E) progestin

176. Which of the following agents is considered to be a cortical stimulant?

    I. Caffeine
    II. Pemoline
    III. Methamphetamine

    (A) I only
    (B) III only
    (C) I and II only
    (D) II and III only
    (E) I, II, and III

177. Danazol (Danocrine) can best be described as a (an)

    (A) estrogen
    (B) antimetabolite
    (C) alkylating agent
    (D) progestin
    (E) androgen

178. Simethicone is found in some antacid products. Its primary function is to act as a (an)

    (A) suspending agent
    (B) antiflatulent
    (C) buffer
    (D) adsorbent
    (E) flavoring agent

179. Which of the following statements is (are) true of phenazopyridine (Pyridium)?

    I. Topical urinary analgesic

    II. Discolors urine

    III. Urinary antiseptic action

(A) I only

(B) III only

(C) I and II only

(D) II and III only

(E) I, II, and III

180. Which of the following statements is (are) true of metronidazole?

    I. It is an antifungal agent.

    II. It is indicated for the treatment of herpes zoster.

    III. It has antiprotozoal activity.

(A) I only

(B) III only

(C) I and II only

(D) II and III only

(E) I, II, and III

Answers and Explanations

1. **(E)** Theophylline products tend to cause insomnia, palpitations, nausea, vomiting, and many other adverse effects. *(6:673)*

2. **(A)** Epinephrine is a sympathomimetic agent that produces alpha$_1$- as well as beta$_1$- and beta$_2$-adrenergic agonist activity. It can, therefore, be expected to produce bronchodilation, cardiac stimulation, increased blood pressure, and vasoconstriction. Because it is rapidly destroyed in the GI tract, it is generally administered by IM or SC injection or by inhalation. *(6:205)*

   [handwritten: α, β_1, β_2]

3. **(C)** Finasteride (Proscar) is an agent that is administered orally for the treatment of benign prostatic hyperplasia (BPH). It acts to inhibit the formation of 5α-dihydrotestosterone, a potent androgen. It is classified as a pregnancy category X drug. Women who are or may become pregnant should avoid contact with crushed finasteride tablets and with semen from patients using the drug. *(3:110c)*

4. **(D)** Dipivefrin (Propine) is a prodrug that is much more rapidly (× 17) absorbed into the anterior chamber of the eye than epinephrine. Once absorbed, the drug is converted to epinephrine by enzymatic hydrolysis. It produces the same therapeutic effects as epinephrine with fewer adverse effects. *(3:478d)*

   [handwritten: → Epi]

5. **(B)** Ticlopidine (Ticlid) is an inhibitor of platelet aggregation that is administered orally, with food, in doses of 250 mg twice daily. Patients using this drug must be monitored for the development of neutropenia (decreased number of white blood cells). *(3:85c)*

6. **(C)** Nicardipine HCl (Cardene) is a calcium channel-blocking agent employed in the treatment of angina pectoris and hypertension. Only the sustained release (SR) form of the drug is employed in the treatment of hypertension. *(3:149n)*

   [handwritten: — SR only HTN]

7. **(A)** Alteplase (Activase) is a tissue plasminogen activator prepared by recombinant DNA technology. It is administered intravenously in order to lyse thrombi in patients with acute myocardial infarction. It is also employed to lyse acute pulmonary emboli. *(3:880)*

8. **(B)** Gold compounds such as auranofin (Ridaura), gold sodium thiomalate (Myochrysine), and aurothioglucose (Solganal) are used to suppress or prevent, but not cure, arthritis and synovitis. Auranofin is administered orally, whereas the other compounds are administered by the IM route. All gold compounds may cause serious adverse effects, including dermatitis, renal damage, and blood dyscrasias. *(3:253d)*

9. **(E)** Procainamide and quinidine are both classified as Group IA antiarrhythmic drugs. These are local anesthetics or membrane stabilizers that depress phase 0 and prolong the duration of the action potential. *(3:145–46)*

10. **(D)** Tocainide (Tonocard), mexiletine (Mexitil), and lidocaine (Xylocaine) are classified as Group IB antiarrhythmic agents. They slightly depress phase 0 and may shorten the action potential. *(3:146f)*

11. **(D)** Acetylcysteine (Mucomyst) is primarily employed as a mucolytic in the treatment of respiratory diseases in which mucus is produced. It is also used as an antidote in the treatment of acetaminophen poisoning. *(3:181a)*

12. **(E)** Epinephrine is available in combination with lidocaine (Xylocaine) in a number of different products. It is used to cause local vasoconstriction, thereby reducing the rate of lidocaine removal from the local injection site. *(6:342)*

13. **(C)** Colestipol (Colestid) is an anion exchange resin that binds bile acids in the intestine, causing them to be removed in the feces. This causes further breakdown of cholesterol to bile acids, as well as a decrease in low-density lipoproteins (LDL) and serum cholesterol levels. *(6:888)*

14. **(D)** Pravastatin (Pravachol) is an HMG-CoA reductase inhibitor. It is employed as an adjunct to diet in treating hypercholesterolemia. It is classified in pregnancy category X. *(3:171u)*

15. **(E)** Nicotinamide, unlike nicotinic acid (niacin), does not lower plasma lipoprotein concentrations or cause vasodilation. It does, however, produce the same vitamin actions as nicotinic acid. *(3:172k)*

16. **(C)** Cyproheptadine (Periactin), an antihistamine, is an H_1-receptor antagonist. Cyproheptadine also antagonizes the action of 5-hydroxytryptamine (5-HT, serotonin), which makes it particularly useful as an antipruritic agent. *(6:261)*

17. **(E)** Dendritic keratitis is an ophthalmic viral infection caused by the action of herpes simplex virus. Idoxuridine (Herplex) blocks herpes simplex virus reproduction and thereby helps to control this condition. *(3:498b)*

18. **(C)** Natamycin (Natacyn) is an antifungal agent used to treat ophthalmic fungal disorders. Clotrimazole is a broad-spectrum antifungal agent used topically. *(3:498a)*

19. **(B)** Isotretinoin (Accutane) is a vitamin A derivative that appears to be useful in the treatment of acne because of its ability to reduce the secretion of sebum. It is classified in pregnancy category X. *(3:543a)*

20. **(D)** Pindolol (Visken) is a nonselective beta-adrenergic blocking agent. Such drugs should be avoided in patients with bronchospastic disorders because they may cause bronchoconstriction. *(6:236)*

21. **(C)** Dopamine (Intropin, Dopastat) is an endogenous catecholamine that is a precursor for norepinephrine. It acts directly and indirectly on $alpha_1$- and $beta_1$-adrenergic receptors to produce an inotropic effect, increased cardiac output, and increased systolic pressure. It is commonly employed in the treatment of shock syndrome. *(6:114)*

22. **(E)** Bromocriptine (Parlodel), pergolide (Permax), and selegiline (Eldepryl) are dopaminergic agents that enhance dopamine activity and provide palliative treatment of Parkinson's disease. *(3:290g)*

23. **(D)** Albuterol is an agonist acting on $beta_1$- and $beta_2$-adrenergic receptors to produce bronchodilation and potential cardiac stimulation. Albuterol is considered to be $beta_2$-selective, making it less likely than many other sympathomimetic agents to cause cardiac stimulation. *(3:174a)*

24. **(E)** Brompheniramine and pyrilamine are H_1-receptor antagonists. They antagonize actions of histamine such as vasodilation. Ranitidine is an H_2-receptor antagonist that reduces gastric acid secretion. *(6:279; 590)*

25. **(D)** Cisapride (Propulcid) and metoclopramide (Reglan) are GI stimulants. They appear to act by increasing the activity of acetylcholine in the GI tract. *(3:307; 308b)*

26. **(C)** Inhalation of the smoke of cannabis generally results in increased pulse rate, perceptual changes, vascular congestion of the eye, and anorexia. *(6:572)*

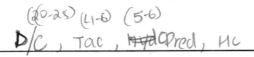

27. **(B)** Dexamethasone is about 25 times as potent as hydrocortisone, 5–6 times as potent as prednisone, 4–6 times as potent as triamcinolone, and 20–25 times as potent as cortisone. *(6:1466)*

28. **(C)** Benzoyl peroxide is an oxidizing agent found in many OTC products that are used in the treatment of acne. It is believed to exert an antibacterial effect, thereby reducing the level of *Propionibacterium acnes* on the skin surface. *(2a:575)*

29. **(E)** Tazobactam sodium is an agent capable of inactivating beta-lactamase enzymes that are often found in microorganisms resistant to penicillin. The addition of tazobactam sodium to pipericillin sodium extends the spectrum of antimicrobial coverage of pipericillin sodium to include beta-lactamase producing organisms. *(6:1098)*

30. **(A)** Oxytocin is an endogenous hormone produced by the posterior pituitary gland. It is a uterine stimulant that promotes uterine contractions, particularly during labor. The other hormones are released by the anterior pituitary gland. *(6:940)*

31. **(D)** During the menstrual cycle, levels of follicle-stimulating hormone (FSH) and luteinizing hormone (LH) vary widely. At the time of ovulation, the concentration of each of these hormones reaches a peak, coinciding with the release of the ovum and the complete development of a mature endometrial wall. *(6:1375)*

32. **(C)** Liotrix consists of a uniform mixture of synthetic levothyroxine sodium (T4) and liothyronine sodium (T3) in a ratio of 4:1 by weight. It is used in products such as Euthroid and Thyrolar as a thyroid hormone supplement. *(6:1395)*

33. **(C)** Methimazole (Tapazole) and propylthiouracil are antithyroid agents that inhibit synthesis of thyroid hormone and thus are useful in the treatment of hyperthyroidism. *(6:1400)*

34. **(A)** Promethazine (Phenergan) is a phenothiazine derivative with antihistaminic as well as antiemetic and sedative properties. The other agents listed are also phenothiazines but do not exert any significant antihistaminic action. *(3:192b)*

35. **(D)** Carbamazepine (Tegretol) is an anticonvulsant drug indicated for the treatment of trigeminal neuralgia as well as a variety of seizure disorders. Patients using this drug must be monitored carefully for the development of aplastic anemia and agranulocytosis. *(6:473)*

36. **(E)** Buspirone (Buspar) is an anxiolytic agent that, unlike the benzodiazepines, barbiturates, and carbamates, does not produce significant sedative, muscle relaxant, or anticonvulsant effects. *(6:425)*

37. **(B)** Theophylline use is associated with bronchodilation, central nervous system and cardiac stimulation, and stimulation of gastric acid secretion. Because theophylline and caffeine are both methylxanthines, they share many common pharmacologic effects. *(6:673)*

38. **(D)** Penicillins and other beta-lactam antimicrobial agents act by being incorporated into an actively growing bacterial cell wall. This causes defects in the cell wall, causing disintegration and destruction of the bacterial cell. Because human cells do not have cell walls, they are not adversely affected by such antimicrobial agents. *(6:1074)*

39. **(D)** The mechanism of action of the penicillins is most similar to cephalosporins such as cefuroxime (Ceftin); both have a beta-lactam ring incorporated into their structure and exhibit a similar mechanism of action. *(6:1074)*

40. **(E)** Probenecid is a uricosuric and renal tubular blocking agent. It is capable of inhibiting the tubular secretion of penicillins and cephalosporins, thereby increasing the plasma levels of these drugs and prolonging their action in the body. *(3:255)*

41. **(E)** Phenoxymethyl penicillin strength is usually measured in milligrams or units. Each milligram of the pure drug is equivalent to 1600 units of activity. Thus, 500 mg of phenoxymethyl penicillin is approximately equivalent to 800,000 units of activity. *(6:1079)*

42. **(D)** Nafcillin and dicloxacillin are both penicillinase-resistant penicillins. They are employed primarily in treating infections caused by penicillinase-producing staphylococci. *(6:1083)*

43. **(D)** Chlorhexidine (Hibiclens) and hexachlorophene (pHisoHex) are antiseptic agents used in surgical scrub and bacteriostatic skin cleanser products. Both provide a residual bacteriostatic effect on the cleansed surface, which helps sustain a lowered bacterial count. Chlorhexidine is also used in antiseptic mouthwash products such as Peridex. *(3:521a; 637)*

44. **(E)** Penicillamine (Cuprimine, Depen) is a chelating agent used in treating Wilson's disease, a disorder characterized by an excessive level of copper in the body. It is also capable of binding with iron, mercury, lead, and arsenic. Penicillamine is also used in the treatment of rheumatoid arthritis and cysteinuria, a condition associated with excess cysteine excretion. *(6:1667)*

45. **(B)** Polymyxin B and colistin (Coly-Mycin S) are closely related chemical compounds that are cationic detergents and act as antimicrobial agents. They have the strongest antimicrobial action against gram-negative organisms. Because of their potential for producing severe nephrotoxicity, they are rarely used systemically. *(6:1143)*

46. **(E)** Chloramphenicol (Chloromycetin) is a broad-spectrum antimicrobial agent. Its use has been associated with the development of serious and sometimes fatal blood dyscrasias, including aplastic anemia. As a result, chloramphenicol is indicated only for the treatment of serious infections that are not responsive to less dangerous drugs. *(6:1132)*

47. **(D)** Dicloxacillin (Dynapen, Pathocil) is one of several antimicrobial drugs resistant to beta-lactamase (penicillinase) enzymes produced by some microorganisms. Other drugs resistant to such enzymes include methicillin, oxacillin, nafcillin, and cloxacillin. *(3:331c)*

48. **(D)** Sulfonamides exert their bacteriostatic action by competitively antagonizing para-aminobenzoic acid (PABA). Sulfonamide resistance may occur if an organism produces excessive amounts of PABA or if PABA-containing products are used concurrently with a sulfonamide drug. *(6:1058)*

49. **(D)** Dapsone is a sulfone that is bactericidal and bacteriostatic against *Mycobacterium leprae*, the organism believed to be the cause of leprosy (Hansen's disease). *(3:412)*

50. **(A)** Doxycycline is the longest acting of the tetracyclines, having a normal serum half-life of 15 to 25 hours. Half-lives for other tetracyclines are tetracycline (6 to 12 hours), demeclocycline (12 to 16 hours), minocycline (11 to 18 hours), and oxytetracycline (6 to 12 hours). *(3:341)*

51. **(B)** Tricyclic antidepressants appear to act by increasing the effect of neurotransmitters on postsynaptic receptor sites. They may also inhibit the reuptake of biogenic amines into adrenergic nerve terminals, induce sedation, and produce peripheral and central anticholinergic actions. *(6:436)*

52. **(E)** Bupropion (Wellbutrin) is an aminoketone antidepressant, whereas fluoxetine (Prozac) is a selective serotonin reuptake inhibitor (SSRI) and phenelzine (Nardil) is an MAO inhibitor. *(3:263l)*

53. **(E)** Aluminum-containing antacids (eg, aluminum hydroxide) may cause constipation because of their astringent effect on the GI tract. They may also bind phosphate, thus potentially lowering serum phosphate levels. *(2a:207)*

54. **(B)** Phytonadione is vitamin K_1, a synthetic analog of vitamin K that promotes the hepatic synthesis of clotting factors. *(3:83)*

55. **(C)** Carbidopa is a dopa-decarboxylase inhibitor that prevents peripheral decarboxylation of levodopa in the body. This reduces the adverse effects associated with peripheral dopa decarboxylation and reduces the dose of levodopa required to control a patient with Parkinson's disease. Carbidopa is available alone (Lodosyn) or in combination with levodopa (Sinemet). *(3:290b)*

56. **(B)** Theophylline and caffeine are methylxanthines. They may act in the body to produce diuresis and bronchodilation, as well as cardiac and central nervous system stimulation. *(6:672–8)*

57. **(C)** Fenfluramine HCl (Pondimin) is an anorexiant which, unlike other anorexiants, depresses rather than stimulates the CNS. The other agents listed are anorexiant drugs that tend to stimulate the CNS. *(3:239b)*

58. **(A)** Lactase enzyme is effective in treating symptoms of lactose intolerance. These symptoms are most evident shortly after consuming a lactose-containing food and may include bloating and diarrhea. Lactase enzyme is available as a liquid (Lactaid), caplets (Lactaid), capsules (Lactrase), or as chewable tablets (Dairy Ease). It is also added to some commercial dairy products. *(3:60k)*

59. **(A)** Hyperglycemia is not a problem commonly associated with the use of isotretinoin (Accutane). Cheilitis (cracked margins of the lips), conjunctivitis, and dry mouth occur in a large proportion of patients receiving this drug. *(6:1600)*

60. **(A)** The use of isotretinoin (Accutane), a vitamin A derivative, is associated with an incidence of cheilitis greater than 90%. The drug is administered orally and must not be used in pregnant women because it carries a high risk of causing fetal deformities. *(3:543a)*

61. **(A)** Endorphins are endogenous (naturally found in the body) opioid peptides that are released in response to stress. *(6:521)*

62. **(D)** Crack is a free-base form of cocaine. It is generally smoked and rapidly absorbed through the respiratory membranes. Within seconds, it reaches the brain and produces central nervous system stimulation and euphoria. Dependence may occur with only a single dose of the drug. *(6:570)*

63. **(E)** A uricosuric drug is one that promotes the excretion of uric acid in the urine. Uricosuric agents such as probenecid (Benemid) and sulfinpyrazone (Anturane) inhibit tubular reabsorption of urate and promote urate excretion. They are used to treat hyperuricemia associated with gout or gouty arthritis. *(6:650)*

64. **(B)** Alteplase (Activase) is a tissue plasminogen activator produced by recombinant DNA technology. It is used in the management of acute myocardial infarction. Once injected into the circulation, alteplase binds to fibrin in a thrombus and converts the entrapped plasminogen to plasmin. This produces local fibrinolysis and assists in reopening a blocked coronary blood vessel. *(3:1352)*

65. **(D)** Cimetidine (Tagamet) is an H_2-histamine receptor antagonist used to decrease gastric acid secretion in patients with peptic ulcer disease. It has been shown to inhibit the hepatic metabolism of drugs metabolized via the cytochrome P-450 pathway, thereby delaying metabolism and increasing serum levels. Cimetidine may affect the metabolism of drugs such as theophylline, some benzodiazepines, phenytoin, and warfarin. *(6:905)*

66. **(A)** Allopurinol (Zyloprim) is a xanthine oxidase inhibitor that does not exert a uricosuric effect but does prevent the conversion of hypoxanthine to uric acid. It is employed in the treatment of gout as well as in the management of patients receiving therapy for leukemia and other malignancies that increase uric acid formation. *(3:256)*

67. (A) Dihydrotachysterol is a synthetic product of tachysterol, a substance similar to vitamin D. It is used in combination with calcium and parathyroid hormone in the treatment of hypoparathyroidism. *(3:4c)*

68. (A) Simvastatin (Zocor) is an HMG-CoA reductase inhibitor that is employed as a cholesterol-lowering agent used to reduce elevated total and LDL cholesterol levels in patients with primary hypercholesterolemia when response to diet and other nondrug approaches have not been successful. Its use is associated with hepatic dysfunction and danger to the developing fetus. *(6:884)*

69. (E) Norethindrone is a progestin. All of the other products are anabolic steroids. *(6:1427)*

70. (D) The autonomic nervous system consists of two major branches: the sympathetic (adrenergic) branch and the parasympathetic (cholinergic) branch. Each branch utilizes different neurotransmitters. For example, the sympathetic branch utilizes norepinephrine, whereas the parasympathetic branch utilizes acetylcholine. *(6:105)*

71. (D) Pentoxifylline (Trental), a methylxanthine derivative, is a hemorheologic agent that enhances blood flow by decreasing blood viscosity and improving erythrocyte flexibility. This is useful in patients with chronic peripheral arterial disease. *(6:676)*

72. (D) Methadone (Dolophine) is a narcotic agonist analgesic with actions similar to those of morphine. It is twice as potent when used parenterally than when used orally. It is employed in the treatment of severe pain and in maintenance treatment of narcotic addiction. *(3:243a)*

73. (D) A pure narcotic antagonist is one that reverses the effects of opioids without producing agonist action of its own. Naloxone (Narcan) is an example of a pure narcotic antagonist. Other drugs listed have agonist and some antagonist activity. *(6:550)*

74. (D) Ergotamine tartrate (Ergostat), an ergot alkaloid, and sumatriptan succinate (Imitrex) a serotonin receptor agonist, are used in treating migraine headaches. *(3:256h, 257d)*

75. (E) Constipation is a common effect because morphine decreases peristaltic activity in the GI tract. Constriction of the pupils, CNS and respiratory depression, and nausea and vomiting are all effects also associated with morphine use. *(6:528)*

76. (D) Primidone (Mysoline) is an anticonvulsant drug used in a variety of convulsive disorders. Primidone and its two active metabolites, phenobarbital and phenylethylmalonamide (PEMA), have anticonvulsant activity. *(6:472)*

77. (C) Etidronate (Didronel) is an agent used in treating Paget's disease of the bone, a condition characterized by abnormal bone resorption and the development of fractures. The use of the drug seems to decrease the dissolution of hydroxyapatite crystals, the building blocks of bone tissue. *(3:555)*

78. (E) Salmon calcitonin (Calcimar, Miacalcin) is a polypeptide hormone derived from salmon. It is similar in action to mammalian calcitonin produced in the thyroid gland. This agent inhibits bone resorption much like etidronate (Didronel) does. *(3:134c)*

79. (C) The naturally occurring adrenal cortical steroids exert both salt-retaining (mineralocorticoid) and anti-inflammatory (glucocorticoid) activity. The synthetic steroids prednisone and prednisolone exert similar actions on the body. The use of these agents is often associated with fluid and sodium retention. *(6:1469)*

80. (C) Ondansetron (Zofran) is a selective serotonin receptor antagonist used for the prevention of nausea and vomiting associated with cancer chemotherapy. It is administered by IV infusion over 15 minutes, beginning 30 minutes before the start of emetogenic chemotherapy. *(3:259l)*

81. **(A)** Amrinone (Inocor), like digoxin, is a drug that produces a positive inotropic effect. In addition, amrinone also produces vasodilation. The drug is used for the short-term management of congestive heart failure in patients who have not responded adequately to digoxin, diuretics, or vasodilators. Use of the drug has been associated with the development of thrombocytopenia, arrhythmias, and GI upset. It is administered by IV bolus or infusion. *(6:833)*

82. **(B)** Dipyridamole (Persantine) inhibits platelet adhesion. It is used as an adjunct to coumarin anticoagulants in the prevention of thromboembolic complications of cardiac valve replacement. It is also used either alone or in combination with aspirin for the prevention of myocardial reinfarction and reduction of mortality after myocardial infarction. (This use is unapproved by the FDA.) *(3:85a)*

83. **(A)** Lactulose (Cephulac, Chronulac), a synthetic disaccharide, is an analog of lactose. Unlike lactose, which is hydrolyzed enzymatically to its monosaccharide components, oral doses of lactulose pass to the colon virtually unchanged. In the colon, bacteria chemically convert the lactulose to low-molecular-weight acids and carbon dioxide. The acids produce an osmotic effect that draws water into the colon and makes the stools more watery. They also permit ammonia in the body to be converted to ammonium ion in the acidic colon and allow it to be eliminated in the stool. *(6:922)*

84. **(E)** Ricinolate, the active agent in castor oil, is formed in the small intestine. It facilitates formation and passage of a fluid stool. *(2a:235)*

85. **(D)** Liothyronine sodium (Cytomel) is a synthetic form of the natural thyroid hormone T3. Approximately 25 μg of liothyronine sodium is equivalent to 60 mg (1 grain) of desiccated thyroid (Thyroid, USP). Liothyronine is useful in patients who are allergic to desiccated thyroid and require thyroid supplementation. *(3:133b)*

86. **(D)** Calcium carbonate and sodium bicarbonate may cause rebound hyperacidity and milk–alkali syndrome, a condition that may appear in an acute or chronic form. These antacids are associated with rebound hyperacidity because they may raise the pH of the stomach to a level high enough (alkaline) to permit release of gastrin, a stimulator of hydrochloric acid release. *(2a:206)*

87. **(D)** Aluminum hydroxide gel may irreversibly bind phosphate in the gut, causing it to be eliminated from the body. This may be used to treat patients with hyperphosphatemia or to prevent the formation of phosphate urinary stones. *(2a:207)*

88. **(B)** Ibuprofen (Motrin) is a nonsteroidal anti-inflammatory agent (NSAID) and should be avoided in patients who are sensitive to aspirin because of possible cross-sensitivity reactions. *(3:251j)*

89. **(D)** Single aspirin doses are known to prolong bleeding time, which is believed to occur by the acetylation of platelet cyclooxygenase by aspirin. This in turn prevents the synthesis of thromboxane, a prostaglandin that is a potent vasoconstrictor and an inducer of platelet aggregation. *(6:1353)*

90. **(A)** Both triamterene (Dyrenium) and spironolactone (Aldactone) inhibit sodium reabsorption in the distal tubule. Spironolactone is an aldosterone antagonist that prevents the formation of a protein important for sodium transport in the distal tubule. Triamterene inhibits sodium reabsorption induced by aldosterone and inhibits basal sodium reabsorption. Triamterene is not an aldosterone antagonist. *(3:138k)*

91. **(A)** Labetalol (Normodyne, Trandate) is a nonselective beta-adrenergic blocking agent primarily used for the management of hypertension. In addition to its beta-blocking action, labetalol is also able to block alpha$_1$-adrenergic receptors. This lowers standing blood pressure and may result in hypotension and syncope. *(3:159d)*

92. **(D)** Colchicine is a substance that may be employed orally or parenterally to relieve the pain of acute gout. It appears to act by reducing the inflammatory response to deposited urate crystals and by diminishing phagocytosis. Although it relieves pain in cases of acute gout, colchicine is not an analgesic or a uricosuric agent. Vomiting, diarrhea, abdominal pain, and nausea have all been reported with the use of colchicine. Bone marrow suppression and thrombocytopenia have also been associated with colchicine use. *(6:648)*

93. **(C)** Oxymetazoline (Afrin, Duration) and xylometazoline (Otrivin), when used as topical nasal decongestants, produce an effect that may persist for 8–12 hours. This is in sharp contrast to other topical nasal decongestant drugs such as phenylephrine, naphazoline, and tetrahydrozoline, which require dosing at 3- to 4-hour intervals. *(2a:142)*

94. **(E)** The use of gold compounds such as auranofin (Ridaura), gold sodium thiomalate (Myochrysine), and aurothioglucose (Solganal) has been associated with a wide variety of adverse effects, including blood dyscrasias, dermatitis, and renal disorders. Patients using such compounds must be monitored constantly for adverse effects. *(6:644)*

95. **(B)** Glucagon is a polypeptide secreted by the pancreas. It acts to enhance gluconeogenesis and glycogenolysis, thereby causing higher levels of glucose in the blood. Glucagon is used to treat severe hypoglycemia. It is generally administered intramuscularly or intravenously. Tolazamide is a sulfonylurea hypoglycemic agent, whereas metformin is a biguanide hypoglycemic agent. *(6:1511)*

96. **(E)** Iron is primarily absorbed in the duodenum and the jejunum by an active transport mechanism. The ferrous salt form is absorbed approximately three times more readily than the ferric form. The presence of food, particularly dairy products, eggs, coffee, and tea, in the GI tract may decrease the absorption of iron significantly, although the concurrent administration of vitamin C maintains iron in the ferrous state, thereby enhancing its absorption from the GI tract. *(6:1320)*

97. **(B)** Iron is an essential component of hemoglobin, myoglobin, and several enzymes. Approximately two-thirds of total body iron is in the circulating red blood cells as part of hemoglobin, the most important carrier of oxygen in the body. *(6:1320)*

98. **(D)** The development of tolerance to the action of nitroglycerin may occur with repeated use. Sensitivity to the action of nitroglycerin is generally restored after several hours of withdrawal from the drug. *(6:764)*

99. **(E)** Regular insulin is secreted by the beta cells of the pancreas. In its unmodified form, regular insulin is clear, has a short (0.5–1 hr) onset of action, and a relatively short (6–8 hr) duration of action. Because it is a clear product, it can be administered either SC or IV. *(3:129f)*

100. **(B)** Lovastatin (Mevacor) is a cholesterol-lowering agent contraindicated for use during pregnancy because of its great potential for causing fetal harm. The drug is in FDA pregnancy category X. *(3:171t)*

101. **(C)** Scopolamine is available in a transdermal patch dosage form (Transderm Scop) for prevention of nausea and vomiting associated with motion sickness in adults. It is applied to the skin behind the ear at least 4 hours before the antiemetic effect is required. The drug is then released from the transdermal product for 3 days. *(3:259e)*

102. **(D)** Desmopressin acetate (DDAVP) is the synthetic analog of naturally occurring human antidiuretic hormone (ADH) produced by the posterior pituitary gland. It is administered intranasally for the treatment of primary nocturnal enuresis. A single dose of the drug will produce an antidiuretic effect lasting from 8 to 20 hours. *(3:117g)*

103. **(A)** Triazolam (Halcion) is a benzodiazepine hypnotic agent that is not metabolized to form active metabolites. Because it has the shortest half-life (1.5–5.5 hr) of any of the benzodiazepine hypnotics, it is often used in elderly patients. The development of anterograde amnesia has been reported in some patients receiving therapeutic doses of triazolam. *(3:272d)*

104. **(D)** Dicloxacillin (Dynapen, Pathocil) is a beta-lactamase–resistant penicillin and would be suitable for treating an infection caused by beta-lactamase–producing staphylococci. Other penicillins that would also be suitable include oxacillin (Prostaphlin, Bactocill), cloxacillin (Cloxapen, Tegopen), nafcillin (Nafcil, Unipen), and methicillin (Staphcillin). All of these products are available for oral use with the exception of methicillin, which is administered either IM or IV. *(3:331c)*

105. **(E)** Cyanocobalamin, or vitamin B_{12}, is essential for proper growth, cell reproduction, formation of blood components, and many other functions. In order for cyanocobalamin to be absorbed properly from the GI tract, it must combine with a glycoprotein called intrinsic factor. In the absence of proper levels of intrinsic factor, cyanocobalamin is administered parenterally. *(3:82)*

106. **(D)** Phenytoin (Dilantin) is an anticonvulsant used in controlling grand mal and psychomotor seizures as well as other convulsive disorders. Adverse effects commonly associated with phenytoin use include nystagmus, gingival hyperplasia, ataxia, and many other neurologic, dermatologic, and hematologic disorders. Because of the high frequency of adverse effects associated with the use of this drug, patients must be monitored closely during therapy. *(3:283)*

107. **(B)** Levobunolol (Betagan) is a noncardioselective beta-adrenergic blocking agent used ophthalmically to reduce intraocular pressure in patients with chronic open-angle glaucoma and other disorders. Although the exact mechanism of action of this and similar ophthalmic beta blockers has not been completely established, it appears to be due to the ability of the drug to reduce the production of aqueous humor. *(6:239)*

108. **(B)** Betaxolol (Betoptic) is a beta-adrenergic blocking agent used ophthalmically to reduce intraocular pressure, particularly in patients with chronic open-angle glaucoma. Unlike other ophthalmic beta blockers, the action of betaxolol is more specific for beta$_1$-adrenergic receptors than for beta$_2$-receptors, making it less likely to affect respiratory function. *(3:478l)*

109. **(C)** Pilocarpine (Isopto Carpine, Pilostat) is a direct-acting miotic agent used to decrease elevated intraocular pressure. By causing miosis (constriction of the pupil), greater outflow of aqueous humor is promoted and intraocular pressure falls. Carbachol (Isopto Carbachol) is another direct-acting miotic used in situations in which pilocarpine is ineffective or causes adverse effects. *(3:480a)*

110. **(E)** Atropine is a belladonna alkaloid capable of causing a wide range of effects in the human body. Cardiac stimulation, diminished sweating, reduction of gastric secretion and tone, and mydriasis (dilation of the pupil of the eye) are commonly associated with its administration. *(6:150)*

111. **(D)** Antihistamines are agents that antagonize histamine competitively at the H$_1$-receptor site but do not bind with histamine to inactivate it. Antihistamines do not block histamine release, antibody production, or antigen–antibody reactions. Many of these agents also produce sedation, anticholinergic, and antipruritic actions. Antihistamines are most commonly used to provide symptomatic relief of symptoms associated with perennial and seasonal allergic rhinitis and the common cold. *(2a:140)*

112. **(C)** Haloperidol (Haldol) is an antipsychotic agent available in oral and parenteral forms. It has pharmacologic actions similar to the phenothiazines (sedation, extrapyramidal effects, etc.). Chemically, haloperidol is a butyrophenone. *(3:267h)*

113. **(B)** Tamoxifen (Nolvadex) is an agent that has potent antiestrogenic effects because of its ability to compete with estrogen for binding sites in target tissues such as the breast. It is used in the treatment of metastatic breast cancer in women. Patients with tumors that are estrogen-receptor–positive appear to respond most favorably to tamoxifen. *(3:668b)*

114. **(E)** Auranofin (Ridaura) is an oral gold product used in the treatment of rheumatoid arthritis. Other gold products, such as gold sodium thiomalate (Myochrysine) and aurothioglucose (Solganal), are administered only by intramuscular injection. Use of gold products has been associated with a wide variety of adverse effects including thrombocytopenia and renal impairment. They do not cure arthritis. *(3:254c)*

115. **(E)** Acetaminophen (Tylenol, APAP) is an agent with analgesic and antipyretic actions similar to aspirin. Unlike aspirin, acetaminophen does not significantly inhibit peripheral prostaglandin synthesis, which may account for its relative lack of anti-inflammatory activity. Acetaminophen does not inhibit platelet function, affect prothrombin time, or produce GI distress. *(6:631)*

116. **(C)** Clozapine (Clozaril) is an antipsychotic agent indicated for use in patients who do not respond to standard antipsychotic therapy (phenothiazines, etc.). Use of clozapine has been associated with the development of agranulocytosis, a potentially life-threatening blood disorder. Patients being treated with clozapine must have a baseline white blood cell (WBC) and differential count performed before initiation of treatment, as well as a WBC count every week during treatment and for 4 weeks after discontinuing clozapine therapy. *(3:267m)*

117. **(D)** Propoxyphene (Darvon, Dolene) is a centrally acting narcotic analgesic with a chemical structure similar to methadone. Its analgesic activity is about one-half to two-thirds that of codeine. The analgesic activity of the drug is only apparent with the use of the dextrorotatory isomer. *(6:545)*

118. **(E)** Dactinomycin (Cosmegen) and plicamycin (Mithracin) are antineoplastic agents classified as antibiotics because they are derived from a microbial source. These agents appear to act in a cytotoxic fashion by interfering with DNA and/or RNA synthesis. Their use is associated with the development of nausea and vomiting as well as with bone marrow depression. *(3:676)*

119. **(B)** The anti-inflammatory and analgesic action of aspirin is believed to result from its inhibition of prostaglandin synthesis. Its antipyretic action probably results from its direct action on the hypothalamus and the production of peripheral vasodilation and sweating. *(6:625)*

120. **(D)** Terazosin (Hytrin) and prazosin (Minipress) are alpha$_1$-adrenergic blocking agents used in the treatment of hypertension. By causing dilation of arterioles and veins, both supine and standing blood pressures are lowered. The first-dose effect is the development of marked hypotension and syncope (fainting) on administration of the first few doses of the drug. It can be minimized by administering low initial doses of the drug at bedtime. Dosage can be increased gradually until the drug is better tolerated. Bepridil (Vascor) is a calcium channel-blocking agent. *(3:163p)*

121. **(B)** Carbon monoxide is a colorless and odorless product of the incomplete combustion of hydrocarbons. When it is inhaled and carried to the blood, it reacts with hemoglobin to form carboxyhemoglobin. This reaction dramatically reduces the oxygen-carrying capacity of the blood and, unless corrected quickly, results in the death of the individual. *(6:1676)*

122. **(A)** Aspiration of a liquid hydrocarbon such as gasoline or kerosene may result in severe inflammation of pulmonary tissues, interference with gas exchange, pneumonitis, and possible death. Emesis or gastric lavage is avoided in such patients to avoid aspiration. Catharsis using magnesium or sodium sulfate may be attempted. Supportive therapy is recommended for such patients unless an-

timicrobial agents are required to treat respiratory infection. *(6:1679)*

123. **(E)** Deferoxamine mesylate (Desferal) is a chelating agent that has a high affinity for ferric iron and a relatively low affinity for calcium. It is usually administered intramuscularly in the treatment of acute iron poisoning. *(6:1668)*

124. **(B)** Acetazolamide (Diamox) is a carbonic anhydrase inhibitor used clinically in the treatment of chronic open-angle glaucoma as well as secondary glaucoma. It is also used for treatment of edema caused by congestive heart failure or drug use, or associated with certain forms of epilepsy. Because acetazolamide increases the excretion of sodium, potassium, bicarbonate, and water, many patients develop an alkaline urine. *(3:139c)*

125. **(A)** Thiazide diuretics such as hydrochlorothiazide (Esidrix, HydroDIURIL) increase the renal excretion of sodium, chloride, and potassium while decreasing the excretion of calcium and uric acid. *(6:701)*

126. **(D)** Acetazolamide is a carbonic anhydrase inhibitor that increases the excretion of sodium, potassium, bicarbonate, and water, thereby alkalinizing the urine. Sodium bicarbonate directly alkalinizes the urine. *(6:691)*

127. **(B)** Dantrolene (Dantrium) is a skeletal muscle relaxant that acts directly by affecting the contractile action of skeletal muscle. It is indicated for the management of spasticity resulting from multiple sclerosis and in some patients with spinal cord injuries. Dantrolene may cause hepatotoxicity. It may also cause drowsiness and phototoxicity. *(3:288l)*

128. **(E)** All of these drugs are aldehyde dehydrogenase inhibitors. They cause an intolerance to alcohol so that consumption of even a small amount may produce a broad array of unpleasant effects. These include flushing, throbbing headaches, nausea, sweating, and palpitations. Disulfiram is used in the management of selected chronic alcoholics. The drug should only be used with the full knowledge and understanding of the patient. *(3:735)*

129. **(C)** Cyclobenzaprine (Flexeril) is a centrally acting skeletal muscle relaxant structurally related to the tricyclic antidepressants, and not related to the MAO inhibitors. It is used as an adjunct to rest and physical therapy for relief of painful muscle spasms. *(3:287n)*

130. **(E)** Polycarbophil (Mitrolan) is a synthetic hydrophilic compound that is capable of absorbing large amounts of water. It is indicated for use as a bulk laxative in the treatment of constipation. It is also employed in the treatment of diarrhea, in which it absorbs excess free fecal water and helps create formed stools. *(3:320)*

131. **(B)** Rifampin is a potent hepatic microsomal enzyme inducer. This action may result in increased metabolism and diminished pharmacologic action of drugs metabolized by these enzymes, such as warfarin, corticosteroids, and oral contraceptives. Patients using rifampin must be monitored carefully for reduced pharmacologic effects and may require dosage adjustment. *(3:386)*

132. **(B)** Diazoxide (Hyperstat) is a nondiuretic antihypertensive agent structurally related to the thiazides. It is used in the emergency reduction of elevated blood pressure. Because diazoxide is rapidly and extensively bound to serum protein, it must be administered by rapid IV injection (bolus). Repeated administration of the drug may cause sodium and water retention and the need for adjuvant diuretic therapy. An oral form of diazoxide (Proglycem) is used in the management of hypoglycemia. *(3:167d)*

133. **(D)** Miconazole (Micatin, Monistat) and ketoconazole (Nizoral) are broad-spectrum antifungal agents effective against yeast infections (*Candida albicans*) as well as dermatophyte infections (tinea cruris, tinea corporis). Griseofulvin (Fulvicin, Grifulvin) is employed primarily in the treatment of tinea infections. *(3:355a)*

134. **(C)** Methohexital sodium (Brevital Sodium) is an ultrashort-acting barbiturate generally administered intravenously and used as a supplement to other anesthetic agents in the induction of anesthesia. Because of its high lipid solubility, methohexital has a very rapid onset of action (30–40 seconds) and a brief duration of action (20–30 minutes), making it a useful agent in brief surgical procedures. *(6:321)*

135. **(E)** Lypressin (Diapid) is a synthetic vasopressin analog possessing antidiuretic activity without producing a pressor or oxytocic effect. It is used clinically in the management of symptoms of diabetes insipidus. Lypressin is administered as a nasal spray. *(3:117b)*

136. *(C)* Indomethacin (Indocin) is a nonsteroidal anti-inflammatory drug (NSAID) used in the treatment of rheumatoid arthritis, ankylosing spondylitis, and other inflammatory conditions such as bursitis. The use of indomethacin and other NSAIDs is associated with serious GI bleeding, ulceration, and gastric distress. Their use should be avoided in patients with a history of peptic ulcer disease. *(3:252a)*

137. **(E)** The sulfonylurea hypoglycemic agents appear to reduce blood glucose levels by stimulating the release of insulin from the beta cells of the pancreas. They are only effective in patients who have some capacity for endogenously producing insulin. *(6:1507)*

138. **(D)** Chlorpropamide (Diabinese) has a serum half-life of about 36 hours. The other sulfonylurea hypoglycemic agents have a serum half-life ranging from 2 to 10 hours. *(3:130j)*

139. **(E)** Vidarabine (Vira-A) is an antiviral agent that possesses activity against herpes simplex virus. It is administered by slow IV infusion for the treatment of herpes simplex encephalitis and is used ophthalmically for the treatment of herpes simplex infections of the eye. *(3:500)*

140. **(A)** Methenamine mandelate (Mandelamine) and methenamine hippurate (Hiprex, Urex) are urinary anti-infectives that are activated in acid urine to produce formaldehyde, which is bactericidal. These agents should not be administered with sulfonamides because of the possible precipitation of the sulfonamide. *(6:1069)*

141. **(B)** Zidovudine (Retrovir) inhibits replication of some retroviruses, including HIV. It is used orally in managing patients with HIV infection who have evidence of impaired immunity. The intravenous form is used for some adult patients with symptomatic HIV infection who have a confirmed presence of pneumocystis carinii pneumonia (PCP). *(6:1205)*

142. **(B)** Alteplase (Activase) is a tissue plasminogen activator produced by recombinant DNA technology. It is used intravenously in the management of acute myocardial infarction (AMI) patients in order to lyse thrombi obstructing coronary arteries. It is administered as soon as possible after the onset of AMI. *(3:88o)*

143. **(E)** Dyphylline is a theophylline derivative, salmeterol is a beta$_2$-adrenergic agonist, and nedocromil sodium is an inhaled anti-inflammatory agent that inhibits mediator release from mast cells. *(3:179e)*

144. **(B)** Oxaprozin (Daypro) and diclofenac sodium (Voltaren) are both nonsteroidal anti-inflammatory drugs (NSAIDs). *(3:252f)*

145. **(E)** Cromolyn sodium (Intal, Nasalcrom, Opticrom) is a drug with antiasthmatic, antiallergy, and mast cell stabilizing activity. It has no bronchodilator or anti-inflammatory activity. Cromolyn appears to inhibit degranulation of sensitized and nonsensitized mast cells that may occur after exposure to certain antigens. Cromolyn products are used prophylactically to treat bronchial asthma, allergic rhinitis, and mastocytosis. Cromolyn should not be used in treating acute asthmatic attacks. *(3:182g; 491c)*

146. **(B)** Verapamil (Calan, Isoptin) is a calcium channel-blocking agent used orally and parenterally in the treatment of cardiac arrhythmias. The other calcium channel-blocking agents listed are used in the treatment of angina pectoris and/or essential hypertension. Oral verapamil is also used for these indications. *(3:150a)*

147. **(B)** Ceftibuten (Cedax) is a third-generation cephalosporin. Third-generation cephalosporins generally have greater gram-negative activity, less gram-positive activity, greater efficacy against resistant organisms, and higher cost than cephalosporins in first- or second-generation groups. *(3:336p)*

148. **(C)** Reflex tachycardia is commonly seen with the use of peripheral vasodilators such as minoxidil (Loniten) and hydralazine (Apresoline). The drop in blood pressure produced by the use of these agents causes increased renin secretion, heart rate, and output as well as sodium and water retention. This may worsen both angina and congestive heart failure. These adverse effects observed with the use of peripheral vasodilators may be managed by the concurrent administration of a beta-adrenergic blocking agent and/or a diuretic. *(3:163r)*

149. **(A)** Buprenorphine (Buprenex) is an opioid analgesic about 30 times as potent as morphine. It is administered intramuscularly or intravenously for the relief of moderate to severe pain. *(3:245h)*

150. **(E)** Mestranol is an estrogen commonly employed in several oral contraceptive products (eg, Norinyl, Ortho-Novum). *(3:108a)*

151. **(C)** Pindolol (Visken) is a nonspecific beta-adrenergic blocking agent that exhibits a high degree of intrinsic sympathomimetic activity (ISA). Drugs with this characteristic tend to reduce resting cardiac output and resting heart rate to a lesser extent than drugs lacking ISA. Other beta-adrenergic blocking agents with this effect are acebutolol (Sectral), carteolol (Cartrol), and penbutolol (Levatol). *(3:157b)*

152. **(B)** Danazol (Danocrine) is a synthetic androgen that suppresses the pituitary–ovarian

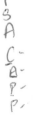

axis by inhibiting the production of pituitary gonadotropins. It is used clinically in the treatment of endometriosis, in which it causes the normal and ectopic endometrial tissue to become inactive and atrophic. Danazol is also employed in the prevention of attacks related to hereditary angioedema. *(3:115u)*

153. **(C)** Torsemide (Demadex) and bumetanide (Bumex) are both loop diuretics. *(3:138c)*

154. **(E)** Triamterene (Dyrenium) is one of three potassium-sparing diuretics currently on the market. The others include spironolactone (Aldactone) and amiloride (Midamor). These drugs are primarily used to enhance the action and counteract the potassium-depleting effect of thiazides and loop diuretics. *(3:138k)*

155. **(A)** Acyclovir (Zovirax) is an antiviral agent used in the treatment of infections caused by herpes simplex virus types 1 and 2 (HSV-1 and HSV-2) and varicella-zoster virus. Shingles is a painful and potentially debilitating disorder caused by varicella-zoster virus. *(3:406u)*

156. **(D)** Chlordiazepoxide (Librium) is a benzodiazepine used in the management of anxiety. It is also indicated in the treatment of symptoms of acute alcohol withdrawal and in the prevention of delirium tremens, a condition developed in chronic alcoholic patients experiencing withdrawal symptoms. *(3:261h)*

157. **(B)** Bacitracin is an antibacterial agent active against a variety of gram-positive and some gram-negative organisms. It is commonly employed in topical antimicrobial products, but is rarely used parenterally because of its ability to cause renal failure due to tubular and glomerular necrosis. When it is used parenterally, renal function of the patient should be assessed both prior to therapy and daily during therapy. If toxicity is evident, the drug should be discontinued. *(6:1147)*

158. **(C)** Selegiline (Eldepryl) is an antiparkinsonian drug that appears to inhibit monoamine oxidase (MAO) type B activity. By inhibiting

MAO, selegiline decreases the breakdown of catecholamines, such as dopamine, norepinephrine, epinephrine, and serotonin, and permits them to accumulate to higher levels in the body. Selegiline is generally used as an adjunct to levodopa/carbidopa therapy in situations in which response is deteriorating. Procyclidine (Kemadrin) is an anticholinergic agent also employed in the treatment of Parkinson's disease. *(3:290h)*

159. **(C)** Olsalazine sodium (Dipentum) is a salicylate compound that is converted to 5-aminosalicylic acid (5-ASA) in the colon. This exerts an anti-inflammatory effect useful in treating ulcerative colitis. *(3:326c)*

160. **(B)** Pirbuterol (Maxair) and isoproterenol (Isuprel) are sympathomimetic bronchodilators that affect predominantly beta$_2$-adrenergic receptors. Pirbuterol is believed, however, to have less beta$_1$-activity than isoproterenol. This would make it less likely to stimulate the heart. *(3:177b)*

161. **(A)** Moexipril HCl (Univasc) is an angiotensin-converting enzyme inhibitor indicated for the treatment of hypertension. When administered orally, antihypertensive action occurs within 1 hour. Peak antihypertensive action is reached within 2 to 6 hours after dosing and persists for 24 hours. This permits single daily dosing. *(3:165l)*

162. **(E)** Beclomethasone dipropionate (Beclovent, Vanceril) is a synthetic corticosteroid used by inhalation to control bronchial asthma. It is generally reserved for patients in whom bronchodilators and other nonsteroidal medications have not been totally successful in controlling asthmatic attacks. When used with a bronchodilator administered by inhalation, the beclomethasone dipropionate should be administered several minutes after the bronchodilator in order to enhance the penetration of the bronchodilator into the bronchial tree. *(3:180b)*

163. **(B)** Sympathomimetic bronchodilators such as albuterol, terbutaline, and isoproterenol are agents that primarily stimulate beta-adrenergic receptors. Some sympathomimetic drugs (eg, ephedrine, epinephrine) also stimulate alpha-adrenergic receptors. Methylated xanthine bronchodilators such as theophylline act by inhibiting the phosphodiesterase enzyme. *(6:664)*

164. **(E)** Antimetabolites are a diverse group of compounds that interfere with normal metabolic processes and thereby disrupt nucleic acid synthesis and normal cell function. *(6:1243)*

165. **(B)** Cetirizine (Zyrtec), loratidine (Claritin), terfenadine (Seldane), and astemizole (Hismanal) are antihistamines that produce a low degree of sedation. The other agents are much more likely to produce sedation as an adverse effect. *(3:188)*

166. **(C)** Methylphenidate (Ritalin) is an amphetamine-like cortical stimulant employed in treating attention deficit disorders as well as narcolepsy. Nervousness and insomnia are common adverse effects associated with methylphenidate use. *(3:268g)*

167. **(B)** Clarithromycin (Biaxin) is a macrolide antimicrobial agent related to erythromycin, azithromycin (Zithromax), and dirithromycin (Dynabac). *(3:242i)*

168. **(D)** Stavudine (Zerit) is an antiviral agent used in treating patients with HIV. Its use has been associated with the development of peripheral neuropathy. *(3:403f)*

169. **(D)** Beta carotene is also known as provitamin A. It is a precursor that is converted to vitamin A in the body. *(3:3)*

170. **(A)** Simvastatin (Zocor) is an HMG-CoA reductase inhibitor. It and similar agents such as fluvastatin, lovastatin, and pravastatin inhibit HMG-CoA reductase, an enzyme that catalyzes an early step in the synthesis of cholesterol in the body. *(3:171m)*

171. **(E)** Fentanyl is a narcotic agonist analgesic that is significantly more potent than morphine. It may be administered parenterally

(IM or IV) for induction or as an adjunct to general anesthesia. It may also be used transdermally (Duragesic) to manage chronic pain for up to 72 hours. It is also available as a transmucosal system (Fentanyl Oralet) for use as a preanesthetic medication or as an adjunct to anesthesia. *(3:242)*

172. **(D)** Anabolic steroids are related to androgens. Their use results in enhanced tissue building. They are used in the treatment of certain types of anemia and in treating metastatic breast cancer in women. *(3:113)*

173. **(B)** Amrinone (Inocor) is an agent that produces a positive inotropic effect as well as vasodilation. It is used to treat congestive heart failure (CHF) in patients who have not responded adequately to digitalis glycosides, diuretics, or vasodilators. *(3:142c)*

174. **(C)** Potassium is the principal intracellular cation of a number of body tissues. It is essential for proper transmission of nerve impulses; contraction of cardiac, skeletal, and smooth muscles; and in the transport of glucose across cell membranes. *(3:15)*

175. **(D)** Finasteride (Proscar) is an androgen hormone inhibitor employed in the treatment of benign prostatic hyperplasia (BPH). Because prostatic development is dependent on androgen activity, finasteride can effectively reduce prostate gland size. *(3:110c)*

176. **(E)** Each of these agents stimulate the central nervous system and increase alertness and a

heightened awareness of surroundings. High doses may produce hyperactivity, autonomic effects on the heart, and muscle tremor. *(3:235; 269a)*

177. **(E)** Danazol (Danocrine) is a synthetic androgen used primarily for the treatment of endometriosis and for the treatment of fibrocystic breast disease. It may cause masculinizing effects in some patients. *(3:115u)*

178. **(B)** Simethicone is a mixture of inert silicon polymers. It is employed as an ingredient in antacid products because of its defoaming action in the GI tract. It acts to reduce the surface tension of gas bubbles, thereby causing them to break and release their entrapped gases. *(2a:216)*

179. **(C)** Phenazopyridine (Pyridium) is a reddish dye that is excreted in the urine. It also produces a topical analgesic effect on the urinary tract mucosa. The drug is employed in reducing urinary burning and discomfort resulting from infection, trauma, or surgery to the urinary tract. *(3:731)*

180. **(B)** Metronidazole (Flagyl) is an agent that is primarily used because of its antiprotozoal activity, particularly in the treatment of trichomoniasis. It is also employed as an antibacterial in treating certain anaerobic bacterial infections. Patients using metronidazole should avoid alcoholic beverages to avoid disulfiram-like effects when the combination is used. *(3:400)*

CHAPTER 2

Pharmaceutical Calculations

As the fraction of prescriptions requiring compounding diminishes, it seems that the importance of pharmaceutical calculations will also decline. However, the continued necessity to compound some prescriptions as well as the increased role of the pharmacist in preparing parenteral admixtures require pharmacists to maintain their calculation skills. In addition, competence in mathematics is essential in order to comprehend the scientific literature.

Most textbooks dealing with pharmaceutical calculations present the reader with many problems to solve. We have attempted to present this topic with a sampling of pharmaceutical calculations that are relevant to current pharmacy practice. Following the lead of the USP/NF, the metric system is the basis for this chapter. Any problems from previous editions that involved the apothecary system have been dropped. Obviously, units that are commonly referred to as "household measures" have been retained.

Questions

DIRECTIONS (Questions 1 through 60): Each of the numbered items or incomplete statements in this section is followed by answers or by completions of the statement. Select the ONE lettered answer or completion that is BEST in each case.

1. Pico, nano, atto, and mega are prefixes associated with which of the following measuring systems?

   I. Avoirdupois
   II. Metric
   III. Systeme International

   (A) I only
   (B) III only
   (C) I and II only
   (D) II and III only
   (E) I, II, and III

2. Five thousand (5000) nanograms equals 5

   (A) centigrams
   (B) grams
   (C) kilograms
   (D) micrograms
   (E) milligrams

3. A patient's serum cholesterol value is reported as 4 mM/L. This concentration expressed in terms of mg/dL will be (mol. wt. cholesterol = 386):

   (A) 0.154 mg/dL
   (B) 1.54 mg/dL
   (C) 154 mg/dL
   (D) 596 mg/dL
   (E) 1540 mg/dL

4. What is the minimum amount of a potent drug that may be weighted on a prescription balance with a sensitivity requirement of 6 mg if at least 98% accuracy is required?

   (A) 6 mg
   (B) 120 mg
   (C) 180 mg
   (D) 200 mg
   (E) 300 mg

5. The upper therapeutic drug concentration for valproic acid is considered to be 100 μg/mL. Express this value in terms of mg/dL.

   (A) 0.1 mg/dL
   (B) 1 mg/dL
   (C) 10 mg/dL
   (D) 100 mg/dL
   (E) 1000 mg/dL

6. Calculate the dose of a drug to be administered to a patient if the dosing regimen is listed as 2 mg/kg/day. The patient weighs 175 lb.

   (A) 78 mg
   (B) 160 mg
   (C) 140 mg
   (D) 350 mg
   (E) 770 mg

7. The adult dose of a drug is 250 mg. What would be the approximate dose for a 6-year-old child weighing 60 lb? (Use Young's Rule.)

   (A) 60 mg
   (B) 85 mg

(C) 100 mg

(D) 125 mg

(E) 180 mg

8. A package insert lists a drug dose for a neonate as being 10 μg/kg/day. The age range for a neonate is considered to be

(A) birth to 1 month *neonates*

(B) 1 month to 6 months

(C) 1 month to 1 year *Infants*

(D) birth to 1 week

(E) 1 year through 5 years *e-childhood*

9. The child's dose of a drug is reported as 1.2 mg/kg body weight. What is the appropriate dose for a child weighing 60 lb?

(A) 6 mg

(B) 9 mg

(C) 32 mg

(D) 72 mg

(E) 126 mg

10. The infusion rate of theophylline established for a neonate is 0.08 mg/kg/hr. How many mg of drug are needed for one daily bottle if the body weight is 16 lb?

(A) 0.58 mg

(B) 14 mg

(C) 30 mg

(D) 150 mg

(E) 8 mg

11. How many mg of codeine phosphate are being consumed daily by a patient taking the following prescription as directed?

```
Rx
   Codeine Phosphate        200 mg
   Dimetapp Elix            q.s. 120 mL

   Sig: ℥ i t.i.d. p.c. & h.s.
```

(A) 6.25 mg

(B) 8.25 mg

(C) 19 mg

(D) 25 mg

(E) 33 mg

12. How many mg of codeine base is in each dose of the cough product used in Question 11? (Mol. wts: codeine = 299; codeine phosphate = 406.)

(A) 6 mg

(B) 8 mg

(C) 11 mg

(D) 16 mg

(E) 24 mg

13. The directions intended for the patient on a prescription read "1 tbsp ac and hs for 10 days." What is the minimum volume the pharmacist should dispense?

(A) 160 mL

(B) 200 mL

(C) 400 mL

(D) 600 mL

(E) 800 mL

14. The USP contains nomograms for estimating body surface area (BSA) for both children and adults. Which of the following measurements must be known in order to use this nomogram?

(A) Age and height

(B) Age and weight

(C) Height and creatinine clearance

(D) Height and weight

(E) Weight and sex

15. The adult dose of a drug is 100 mg. What is an appropriate dose for a child whose BSA is calculated to be 0.75 m²?

(A) 25 mg

(B) 40 mg

(C) 50 mg

(D) 75 mg

(E) 80 mg

16. Blood pressure measurements were made for 1 week on five patients with the following averages:

Patient	1	2	3	4	5
B.P.	140/70	160/84	180/88	190/90	150/70

What is the median systole pressure?

(A) 80
(B) 83
(C) 84
(D) 160
(E) 164

17. After 1 month of therapy, all of the patients listed in Question 16 had a systolic blood pressure reduction of 10 mm with a standard deviation (SD) of 5 mm. What percentage of patients had a reduction between 5 and 15 mm?

(A) 20%
(B) 40%
(C) 50%
(D) 70%
(E) 90%

18. The concentration of sodium fluoride (NaF) in a community's drinking water is 0.6 ppm. Express this concentration as a percentage.

(A) 0.00006%
(B) 0.0006%
(C) 0.006%
(D) 0.06%
(E) 0.6%

19. Lanoxin Pediatric Elixir contains 0.05 mg of digoxin per mL. How many micrograms (μg) are there in 3 mL of the elixir?

(A) 0.15 μg
(B) 0.015 μg
(C) 1.5 μg
(D) 0.0015 μg
(E) None of the above

20. A pharmacist adds 1 pint of Alcohol USP to 1 L of a mouthwash formula. What is the new percentage of alcohol present if the original mouthwash was labeled as 12% V/V ethanol?

(A) 30%
(B) 38%
(C) 45%
(D) 57%
(E) 59%

21. A prescription calls for the dispensing of a 4% Pilocar solution with the directions of "gtt i OU TID." How many mg of pilocarpine hydrochloride is being used per day? Assume that the dropper is calibrated to deliver 20 drops to the mL.

(A) 4 mg
(B) 6 mg
(C) 12 mg
(D) 24 mg
(E) 60 mg

22. The adult intravenous (IV) dose of zidovudine is 2 mg/kg q 4 h six times daily. How many mg will a 180-lb patient receive daily?

(A) 12 mg
(B) 164 mg
(C) 650 mg
(D) 980 mg
(E) 2160 mg

23. A pharmacist dilutes 100 mL of Clorox with 1 quart of water. Express the concentration of sodium hypochlorite in the final dilution as a W/V ratio. Commercial Clorox contains 5.25% W/V sodium hypochlorite.

(A) 1/9
(B) 1/10
(C) 1/100
(D) 1/180
(E) 1/200

Questions 24 and 25

Questions 24 and 25 relate to the following hospital formula for T-A-C Solution.

Cocaine HCl	4%
Tetracaine HCl 2%	0.5 mL
Epinephrine HCl solution	1/2000
Sodium Chloride injection	qs 4 mL

24. How many mg of cocaine HCl is in the final solution?

    (A) 400 mg
    (B) 4 mg
    (C) 20 mg
    (D) 8 mg
    (E) 160 mg

25. How many mL of Adrenalin Chloride Solution (0.1%) may be used to prepare the solution?

    (A) 0.002 mL
    (B) 0.04 mL
    (C) 1 mL
    (D) 2 mL
    (E) 5 mL

Questions 26 and 27

Questions 26 and 27 relate to the following hospital order.

Parenteral Admixture Order
For: Alex Sanders   Room: M 704
Cefazolin sodium   400 mg in 100 mL N/S
Infuse over 20 minute q 6 hr ATC for 3 days

Available in the pharmacy are cefazolin sodium 1-gram vials with reconsititution directions of 2.5 mL SWFI will give 3.0 mL of solution.

26. How many mL of the reconstituted solution are required for each day of therapy?

    (A) 1.2 mL
    (B) 4.8 mL
    (C) 3 mL
    (D) 6 mL
    (E) 12 mL

27. What infusion rate in mL/min should the nurse establish for each bottle?

    (A) 0.15 mL/min
    (B) 0.28 mL/min
    (C) 1.1 mL/min
    (D) 2 mL/min
    (E) 5 mL/min

28. A vial of a lyophilized drug is labeled "10,000 units: to reconstitute, add 17 mL of Sterile Water for Injection to obtain 500 units per mL." How many mL of SWFI must a pharmacist add if a 1000 U/mL concentration is needed by the nurse?

    (A) 7 mL
    (B) 8.5 mL
    (C) 10 mL
    (D) 17 mL
    (E) 20 mL

29. An administration set delivers 60 drops to the mL. How many drops per minute are needed to obtain 20 units of heparin per minute if the IV admixture contains 15,000 units per 250 mL of normal saline?

    (A) 20
    (B) 40
    (C) 60
    (D) 80
    (E) 120

30. Dopamine (Intropin) 200 mg in 500 mL of normal saline at 5 μg/kg/min is ordered for a 155-lb patient. What is the final concentration of solution in μ/mL?

    (A) 0.4 μg/mL
    (B) 2.5 μg/mL
    (C) 40 μg/mL
    (D) 400 μg/mL
    (E) 25 μg/mL

31. Referring to Question 30, at what rate (mL/min) should the solution be infused to deliver the desired dose of 5 μg/kg/min?

    (A) 0.35 mL/min
    (B) 0.40 mL/min
    (C) 0.88 mL/min
    (D) 2.0 mL/min
    (E) 5.0 mL/min

32. A 250-mL infusion bottle contains 5.86 g of potassium chloride (KCl). How many milliequivalents (mEq) of KCl are present? (Mol. wt. KCl = 74.6.)

    (A) 12.7 mEq
    (B) 20 mEq
    (C) 78.5 mEq
    (D) 150 mEq
    (E) None of the above

33. A solution contains 1.5 mEq of calcium per 100 mL. Express the solution's strength of calcium in terms of mg/L. (The atomic weight of calcium is 40.)

    (A) 30 mg/L
    (B) 60 mg/L
    (C) 150 mg/L
    (D) 300 mg/L
    (E) 600 mg/L

34. Calcium chloride ($CaCl_2 \cdot 2H_2O$) has a formula weight of 147. What weight of the chemical is needed to obtain 40 mEq of calcium? (Ca = 40.1; Cl = 35.5; H_2O = 18.)

    (A) 0.80 g
    (B) 2.22 g
    (C) 1.47 g
    (D) 2.94 g
    (E) 5.88 g

35. Polymyxin B Sulfate is available in 10 mL parenteral vials labeled as containing 500,000 units. Which of the following statements are accurate if the pharmacist wants to prepare 30 g of ointment (15,000 U/g)?

    I. The pharmacist will use 9 mL of the Polymyxin B Sulfate solution.

    II. It will be best to incorporate the solution into an absorption base.
    III. The solution should be incorporated into 30 g of ointment base.

    (A) I only
    (B) III only
    (C) I and II only
    (D) II and III only
    (E) I, II, and III

36. A floor nurse requests a 50 mL minibottle to contain heparin injection 100 units/mL. The number of mL of heparin injection 10,000 units/mL needed for this order will be:

    (A) 0.1 mL
    (B) 0.5 mL
    (C) 1 mL
    (D) 2.5 mL
    (E) 5 mL

37. The estimated creatinine clearance rate for a 120-lb patient is 40 mL/min. What maintenance dose should be administered if the normal maintenance dose is 2 mg/lb of body weight?

    (A) 60 mg
    (B) 100 mg
    (C) 120 mg
    (D) 160 mg
    (E) 240 mg

    (handwritten: #7 CrCL = 100 - 120 ml/min)

38. A total parental nutrition (TPN) order requires 500 mL of $D_{30}W$. How many mL of $D_{40}W$ should be used if the $D_{30}W$ is not available?

    (A) 125 mL
    (B) 300 mL
    (C) 375 mL
    (D) 400 mL
    (E) 667 mL

39. A physician requests 1 lb of bacitracin ointment containing 200 U of bacitracin per gram. How many grams of bacitracin ointment (500 U/g) must be used to make this ointment?

(A) 182 g
(B) 200 g
(C) 227 g
(D) 362 g
(E) None of the above

Questions 40 through 43

Questions 40 through 43 relate to the following formula for a psoriasis lotion.

Coal tar solution	5 mL
Salicylic acid	
Urea	aa 5%
Triamcinolone acetonide	0.25 g
Alcohol USP	20 mL
Propylene glycol	qs 120 mL

40. What weight of salicylic acid is needed to prepare 1 pt of the formula listed?

(A) 11.8 g
(B) 12 g
(C) 23.7 g
(D) 24 g
(E) 25 g

41. What percent V/V concentration of alcohol would be listed on the label?

(A) 8%
(B) 15.8%
(C) 16.7%
(D) 19%
(E) 20%

42. How many mL of triamcinolone acetonide aqueous injection (40 mg/mL) will be needed to prepare 240 mL of the formula?

(A) 6.3 mL
(B) 12.5 mL
(C) 1.2 mL
(D) 10 mL
(E) 15 mL

43. Propylene glycol was purchased at a cost of $12.00 per pound. What is the cost of 100 mL

of the liquid? (Specific gravity = 1.04.)

(A) $2.60
(B) $2.64
(C) $2.75
(D) $12.50
(E) $13.00

44. A pharmacist repackages 10 lb of an ointment into jars to be labeled 2 oz (avoir.). How many jars can be filled?

(A) 73
(B) 80
(C) 83
(D) 88
(E) 100

45. How many mL of glycerin would be needed to prepare 1 lb of an ointment containing 5% W/W glycerin? (The density of glycerin is 1.25 g/mL.)

(A) 1.2 mL
(B) 18.2 mL
(C) 22.7 mL
(D) 24 mL
(E) 28.4 mL

46. A hospital clinic requests 2 lb of 2% hydrocortisone ointment. How many grams of 5% hydrocortisone ointment could be diluted with white petrolatum to prepare this order?

(A) 18.2 g
(B) 27.5 g
(C) 45.4 g
(D) 363 g
(E) 545 g

47. How many mL of 2% iodine solution must be mixed with a 7% iodine solution to obtain 1 L of 5% strength?

(A) 200 mL
(B) 300 mL
(C) 400 mL
(D) 500 mL
(E) 600 mL

48. How many grams of pure hydrocortisone powder must be mixed with 60 g of 0.5% hydrocortisone cream if one wishes to prepare a 2.0% W/W preparation?

    (A) 0.90 g
    (B) 0.92 g
    (C) 0.30 g
    (D) 1.2 g
    (E) 1.53 g

49. A ready-to-use enteral nutritional solution has an osmolarity of 470 mOsm/L. How many mL of purified water are needed to adjust 8 fluid ounces of the enteral solution to an osmolarity (280 mOsm/L)?

    (A) 120 mL
    (B) 160 mL
    (C) 240 mL
    (D) 300 mL
    (E) 400 mL

50. How much sodium chloride is needed to adjust the following prescription to isotonicity? (E value for sodium thiosulfate is 0.31.)

Rx	
Sodium thiosulfate	1.2%
Sodium chloride	qs
Purified water	qs 100 mL

    (A) 0.37 g
    (B) 0.45 g
    (C) 0.53 g
    (D) 0.31 g
    (E) 0.90 g

51. How much additional sodium chloride should be added to the following prescription to maintain isotonicity? Zincfrin is an isotonic solution.

Rx	
Zincfrin	15 mL
Sodium chloride	q.s.
Sterile Water for Injection	60 mL

    (A) 0.135 g
    (B) 0.4 g
    (C) 0.54 g
    (D) 0.9 g
    (E) None (because Sterile Water for Injection is already isotonic)

52. Estimate the milliosmolarity (mOsm/L) for normal saline. (Na = 23; Cl = 35.5)

    (A) 150 mOsm/L
    (B) 300 mOsm/L
    (C) 350 mOsm/L
    (D) 400 mOsm/L
    (E) 600 mOsm/L

53. How many milliosmoles are present in a solution prepared by dissolving 1000 mg of sodium chloride in 100 mL D5W? (Na = 23; Cl = 35.5; hydrous dextrose = 198.)

    (A) 30
    (B) 60
    (C) 150
    (D) 300
    (E) 600

54. How many mL of Hydrochloric Acid USP are needed to prepare 4 L of Diluted Hydrochloric Acid USP? The label on the available hydrochloric acid bottle shows that the concentration of the acid is 36.8% W/W and the solution specific gravity is 1.19. The diluted acid is 10% W/V according to the official monograph.

    (A) 147 mL
    (B) 400 mL
    (C) 913 mL
    (D) 1087 mL
    (E) 1294 mL

55. How many grams of glacial acetic acid (99.9% W/W) must be added to 1 gal purified water to prepare an irrigation solution containing 0.25% W/V acetic acid?

    (A) 1.2 g
    (B) 9.5 g
    (C) 12 g

(D) 20 g

(E) 95 g

56. How much elemental iron is present in every 300 mg of ferrous sulfate ($FeSO_4 \cdot 7H_2O$)? (Atomic weights: iron = 55.9; S = 32; O = 16; H = 1. Iron has valences of +2 and +3.)

(A) 30 mg

(B) 60 mg

(C) 110 mg

(D) 120 mg

(E) 164 mg

57. The USP states that 1 g of a chemical is soluble in 10 mL of alcohol. What is the percentage strength of a saturated solution of this chemical if alcohol has a sp. gr. of 0.80?

(A) 10.0% W/V

(B) 10.0% W/W

(C) 11.1% W/V

(D) 11.1% W/W

(E) 12.5% W/V

58. What is the decay constant (k) of the radioisotope ^{32}P if its half-life is 14.3 days? Assume that radiopharmaceuticals follow first-order kinetics.

(A) 0.048/day

(B) 0.07/day

(C) 0.097/day

(D) 0.1/day

(E) 0.15/day

59. A radiopharmacist prepares a solution of ^{99m}Tc (40 mCi/mL) at 6:00 AM. If the solution is intended for administration at 12:00 PM at a dose of 20 mCi, how many mL of the original solution are needed? The half-life of the radioisotope is 6 h.

(A) 0.5 mL

(B) 1.0 mL

(C) 1.5 mL

(D) 2.0 mL

(E) 5.0 mL

60. What concentration of the original ^{99m}Tc solution described in Question 59 will remain 24 h after its original preparation?

(A) 15 mCi

(B) 10 mCi

(C) 7.5 mCi

(D) 5.0 mCi

(E) 2.5 mCi

Answers and Explanations

1. **(D)** The metric system is used exclusively in most nations in the world except the United States. The prefixes in the metric system are based on increasing or decreasing magnitudes of 10, 100, or 1000. Converting from one set of quantities to another simply requires the movement of decimal points. For example, converting 1 kg to g requires moving the decimal point three places to the right. The metric system has been expanded into the Systeme International (SI) measuring system that encompasses all types of measures. The major prefixes in the order of magnitude include:

Prefix	Magnitude	Example
mega	1,000,000 ×	megagram
kilo	1000 ×	kilogram
—	1 ×	gram
centi	0.01 ×	centigram
milli	0.001 ×	milligram
micro	$1 \times 10^{-6} \times$	microgram
nano	$1 \times 10^{-9} \times$	nanogram
pico	$1 \times 10^{-12} \times$	picogram
femto	$1 \times 10^{-15} \times$	femtogram
atto	$1 \times 10^{-18} \times$	attogram

(1:66; 23:46)

2. **(D)** In this example, consider a nano quantity as 0.001 the magnitude of a micro. Therefore, 5000 nanograms equals 5 micrograms. *(1:66; 23:46)*

3. **(C)** An increasing number of laboratory test values and drug doses are being reported in terms of millimoles (mM). Weight quantities expressed in molar amounts allow a more realistic evaluation of the actual number of drug molecules present, for example, when comparing salts of a drug. In this problem,

the mM/L concentration is converted by realizing that 1 mole of cholesterol weighs 386 g and 4 mmoles equals 0.004 moles.

$$\frac{1 \text{ mole}}{386 \text{ g}} = \frac{0.004 \text{ mole}}{x \text{ g}}$$

$x = 1.54$ g in 1 L or 1540 mg in 1 L and 154 mg in 1 dL (100 mL)

(23:108)

4. **(E)** The minimum weight that can be measured on any balance can be determined if the balance's sensitivity requirement (SR) and the acceptable percentage of error has been established. The equation is:

SR = (minimum weighable amount) × (acceptable error)

In this problem, the SR was given as 6 mg and an accuracy of at least 98% or an error of not more than 2% is permissible.

$$6 \text{ mg} = (x \text{ mg}) (2\%)$$

$$6 \text{ mg} = (x \text{ mg}) (0.02)$$

$$x = 300 \text{ mg}$$

(23:35)

5. **(C)** Because 1000 µg = 1 mg and 100 mL = 1 dL, 100 µg/mL = 0.1 mg/mL = 10 mg/dL

Or, by dimensional analysis,

$$\frac{100 \text{ µg}}{1 \text{ mL}} \times \frac{1 \text{ mg}}{1000 \text{ µg}} \times \frac{100 \text{ mL}}{1 \text{ dL}} = 10 \text{ mg/dL}$$

Note that when dimensional analysis is used, all of the units cancel except those appropriate for the final answer. *(23:47–48; 13)*

6. **(B)** Because 1 kg = 2.2 lb

$$175 \text{ lb} \times \frac{1 \text{ kg}}{2.2 \text{ lb}} \times 2 \text{ mg} = 160 \text{ mg}$$

7. **(B)** Young's Rule relates a child's dose to the child's age.

$$\text{Child's dose} = \frac{\text{Age (yr)}}{(\text{Age [yr]} + 12)} \times \text{Adult dose}$$

$$\text{Dose} = \frac{6}{(6 + 12)} \times 250 \text{ mg}$$

$$\text{Dose} = 83.3 \text{ or } 85 \text{ mg}$$

Although well intended, rules like Young's (child's age), Cowling's (age at next birthday divided by 24), Clark's (weight divided by average weight of an adult [150 lb]) are only rough estimates. Pharmacists should check the literature for individual drug dosing for children. In some instances, the child's dose will be similar to that for the adult. *(1:82; 23:65–66)*

8. **(A)** Neonates have an age span from birth to 1 month of age. Infants are 1 month to 1 year, early childhood is 1 through 5 years, late childhood is 6 through 12 years. *(23:65)*

9. **(C)**
$$60 \text{ lb} \times \frac{1 \text{ kg}}{2.2 \text{ lb}} \times \frac{1.2 \text{ mg}}{\text{kg}} = 32 \text{ mg}$$

(23:82)

10. **(B)** The body weight will be

$$16 \text{ lb} \times \frac{1 \text{ kg}}{2.2 \text{ lb}} = 7.27 \text{ kg}$$

$$\frac{0.08 \text{ mg}}{\text{kg}} \times 7.27 \text{ kg}$$
$$= 0.58 \text{ mg per hour or } 14 \text{ mg daily}$$

The low dosing of theophylline is correct because the metabolism pathway in young babies has yet to develop sufficiently. *(19:19–17; 23:67)*

11. **(E)** In today's health practice, the symbol "℥ i" is used to represent a 1 teaspoon dose. The symbol's original meaning as a drachm (weight) or fluidrachm (volume) quantities is archaic and should not be used. Because a standard teaspoon is considered to be 5 mL,

the patient in this prescription is receiving four daily doses for a total of 20 mL.

$$\frac{200 \text{ mg codeine}}{120 \text{ mL of Rx}} = \frac{x \text{ mg codeine}}{20 \text{ mL of Rx}}$$

(23:61–64; 225)

12. **(A)** The weight of codeine phosphate present in each dose is

$$\frac{200 \text{ mg}}{120 \text{ mL}} = \frac{x \text{ mg}}{5 \text{ mL}}$$

$$x = 8.3 \text{ mg per teaspoon}$$

The relationship between codeine and codeine phosphate is easily seen when viewed as a chemical reaction.

$$\begin{array}{ccc} & & \text{(wt. of codeine} \\ \text{(wt. of codeine)} & & \text{phosphate)} \end{array}$$

codeine + phosphoric acid = codeine phophate
(mol. wt. = 299)   (mol. wt. = 406)

$$\frac{x \text{ mg}}{299} = \frac{8.3 \text{ mg}}{406}$$

$$x = 6 \text{ mg of codeine}$$

(1:1199; 23:305)

13. **(D)** One tablespoonful (tbsp) delivers 15 mL of liquid. In this prescription, the patient is receiving four doses per day for 10 days. Therefore,

$$15 \text{ mL} \times 4 \times 10 \text{ days} = 600 \text{ mL total}$$

(23:61–64)

14. **(D)** The nomogram in the USP consists of three parallel vertical lines. The left line is calibrated with height measurements in both centimeters and inches, whereas the right line lists weights in kilograms and pounds. Using data based on the patient's measurements, a line is drawn between the two outside parallel lines. The intercept on the middle line, which is calibrated in square meters of body surface area, allows the estimation of the patient's BSA. *(23:68–71)*

15. **(B)** The average adult BSA is estimated to be 1.73 m². A child's dose can be estimated by:

$$\frac{\text{BSA (child)}}{\text{BSA (adult)}} \times \text{Adult dose} = \text{Child's dose}$$

In this question,

$$\frac{0.75 \text{ m}^2}{1.73 \text{ m}^2} \times 100 \text{ mg} = 43 \text{ mg}$$

(1:82; 23:68)

16. **(D)** The median value in a series of numbers is that value in the middle (ie, the number of values lower than the median value is equal to the number of values higher than the median value). The median may not be the same as the average value, which is obtained by adding all of the values together and dividing by the number of values. *(23:260)*

17. **(D)** A standard deviation is calculated mathematically for experimental data. It shows the dispersion of numbers around the mean (average value). One SD will include approximately 67% to 70% of all values, whereas 2 SDs will include approximately 97% to 98%. *(1:97; 23:261)*

18. **(A)** Sodium fluoride is a solid chemical. The 0.6 ppm concentration indicates 0.6 g of sodium fluoride per 1,000,000 mL of solution. Therefore, the grams present in 100 mL will be:

$$\frac{0.6 \text{ g NaF}}{1,000,000 \text{ mL}} = \frac{x \text{ g NaF}}{100 \text{ mL}}$$

$$x = 0.00006 \text{ g or } 0.00006\% \text{ W/V}$$

(23:109)

19. **(E)** 1 mg = 1000 μg. Therefore, 0.15 mg of digoxin contained in 3 mL of the elixir would be equivalent to 150 μg of drug. *(23:49)*

20. **(B)** Alcohol USP contains 95% V/V ethanol. Therefore,

$$473 \text{ mL} \times 95\% = 449 \text{ mL of ethanol}$$
$$1000 \text{ mL} \times 12\% = \underline{120 \text{ mL}}$$
$$\text{total} = \overline{569 \text{ mL}} \text{ of ethanol}$$

$$\frac{569 \text{ mL}}{1473 \text{ mL}} = 38\% \text{ V/V}$$

(23:129)

21. **(C)** The patient is placing 1 drop in each eye three times a day, thus a total of 6 drops. This equates to 0.3 mL since the dropper calibration was 20 drops to a mL.

$$\frac{20 \text{ drops}}{1 \text{ mL}} = \frac{6 \text{ drops}}{x \text{ mL}}$$

$$x = 0.3 \text{ mL}$$

A 4% Pilocar solution contains 4000 mg of drug per 100 mL.

$$\frac{4000 \text{ mg}}{100 \text{ mL}} = \frac{x \text{ mg}}{0.3 \text{ mL}}$$

$$x = 12 \text{ mg}$$

(23:62)

22. **(D)** First, convert the weight in pounds to kilograms.

$$180 \text{ lb} \times \frac{1 \text{ kg}}{2.2 \text{ lb}} = 82 \text{ kg}$$

Second, determine the total daily dose.

$$82 \text{ kg} \times 2 \text{ mg} \times 6 \text{ doses} = 980 \text{ mg}$$

(23:67)

23. **(E)** One hundred mL of Clorox will contain 5.25 g of sodium hypochlorite. The final dilution will be 100 mL + 946 mL of water for a total of 1046 mL. The ratio strength will be:

$$\frac{5.25 \text{ g}}{1046 \text{ mL}} = \frac{1}{x}$$

$$x = 200, \text{ or } 1:200 \text{ W/V of sodium hypochlorite}$$

In actual practice, Clorox is recommended as a disinfectant for HIV-contaminated equipment when used in a 1:10 dilution. However, this designation refers to 1 mL of *Clorox* in every 10 mL of final dilution. *(23:106)*

24. **(E)** Four milliliters of a 4% cocaine HCl solution will contain .16 g, or 160 mg, of cocaine HCl (4 mL × 4%), or, by proportions:

$$\frac{4000 \text{ mg}}{100 \text{ mL}} = \frac{x \text{ mg}}{4 \text{ mL}}$$

$$x = 160 \text{ mg}$$

(23:98)

25. **(D)** Use the equation of

$$(Q_1)(C_1) = (Q_2)(C_2)$$

$$(4 \text{ mL})\left(\frac{1}{2000}\right) = (x \text{ mL})\left(\frac{1}{1000}\right)$$

$$\frac{4}{2000} = \frac{x}{1000}$$

$$x = 2 \text{ mL}$$

(20:246; 23:120)

26. **(B)** The dosing regimen for this patient consists of 400 mg of cefazolin every 6 hours. When the pharmacist reconstitutes the 1000-mg vials, the strength will be 1000 mg/3 mL of solution.

$$\frac{1000 \text{ mg}}{3 \text{ mL}} = \frac{1600 \text{ mg}}{x \text{ mL}}$$

$$x = 4.8 \text{ mL}$$

(23:172)

27. **(E)** The original order requested that the solution be infused over a 20-minute time span. Therefore, 100 mL divided by 20 minutes equals 5 mL/minute. *(23:180)*

28. **(A)** When some drug powders, especially bulky antibiotics, are reconstituted, the volume occupied by the bulk powder once it has dissolved must be considered. In this example, the final volume of solution is:

$$\frac{500 \text{ U}}{1 \text{ mL}} = \frac{10,000 \text{ U}}{x \text{ mL}}$$

$$x = 20 \text{ mL}$$

The previously listed volume means that the volume occupied by the bulk powder must have been 20 − 17 mL = 3 mL. When a concentration of 1000 U/mL is desired, the total volume of solution that must be prepared will be:

$$\frac{1000 \text{ U}}{1 \text{ mL}} = \frac{10,000 \text{ U}}{x \text{ mL}}$$

$$x = 10 \text{ mL}$$

Therefore, the pharmacist must add 7 mL of SWFI to the vial. When the powder has dis-

solved, the resulting volume will be 10 mL. *(23:168–73)*

29. **(A)** Step 1: Determine the drug concentration present in every milliliter.

$$\frac{15,000 \text{ U}}{250 \text{ mL}} = \frac{x \text{ U}}{1 \text{ mL}}$$

$$x = 60 \text{ U/mL}$$

Step 2: Determine the mL needed to obtain the concentration requested.

$$\frac{60 \text{ U}}{1 \text{ mL}} = \frac{20 \text{ U}}{x \text{ mL}}$$

$$x = 0.33 \text{ mL}$$

Step 3: Calculate the number of drops needed, based on the administration set being used, to obtain the required volume.

$$\frac{60 \text{ drops}}{1 \text{ mL}} = \frac{x \text{ drops}}{0.33 \text{ mL}}$$

$$x = 19.8 \text{ or } 20 \text{ drops}$$

(23:82)

30. **(D)** 200 mg dopamine in 500 mL = 0.4 mg/mL. Because 1 mg = 1000 μg, 0.4 mg = 400 mcg; therefore, the final concentration of dopamine will be 400 μg/mL. *(23:174)*

31. **(C)**

$$155 \text{ lb} \times \frac{1 \text{ kg}}{2.2 \text{ lb}} \times \frac{5 \text{ μg}}{\text{kg} \times 1 \text{ min}} = 352 \text{ μg/min}$$

Because the solution concentration is 400 μg/mL, divide the dosage rate by the concentration:

$$\frac{352 \text{ μg/min}}{400 \text{ μg/mL}} = 0.88 \text{ mL/min}$$

(23:180)

32. **(C)** 1 equivalent weight of KCl = 74.6 g
1 milliequivalent (mEq)   = 74.6 mg

$$\frac{1 \text{ mEq}}{74.6 \text{ mg}} = \frac{x \text{ mEq}}{5860 \text{ mg}}$$

$$x = 78.5 \text{ mEq}$$

Or the problem may be solved by using the equation:

$$\text{mg of chemical} = \frac{(\text{mEq}) \, (\text{mol. wt.})}{(\text{valence})}$$

$$5860 \, \text{mg} = \frac{(x) \, (74.6)}{(1)}$$

$$x = 78.5 \, \text{mg}$$

(23:159)

33. **(D)** Because the valence of calcium is +2, 1 mEq equals 40 mg divided by 2 = 20 mg. Therefore, 1.5 mEq = 30 mg. If there are 30 mg/dL of solution, there will be 300 mg/L.

Or, by using the equation:

$$\text{mg of chemical} = \frac{(\text{mEq}) \, (\text{mol. wt.})}{(\text{valence})}$$

$$x \, \text{mg} = \frac{(1.5 \, \text{mEq}) \, (40)}{(2)}$$

$$x = 30 \, \text{mg/dL}$$
or 300 mg/L

(23:158–59)

34. **(D)** One equivalent of calcium chloride = 147 (mol. wt.) divided by 2 (valence of calcium) = 73.5 g and 1 mEq = 73.5 mg. Therefore, 40 mEq = 40 × 73.5 mg = 2940 mg, which is 2.94 g.

Or, the problem can be solved by the equation:

$$\text{mg of chemical} = \frac{(\text{mEq}) \, (\text{mol. wt.})}{(\text{valence})}$$

$$x \, \text{mg} = \frac{(40 \, \text{mEq}) \, (147)}{(2)}$$

$$x = 2940 \, \text{mg, or } 2.94 \, \text{g}$$

It must be remembered that 40 mEq of calcium combines with 40 mEq of chloride to form 40 mEq of calcium chloride. *(1:91; 23:157)*

(A–incorrect) This answer is obtained if one multiplies the 40 mEq desired by the atomic weight of calcium and then divides by the +2 valence. The use of the atomic weight of calcium is incorrect because the official hydrated calcium chloride is being weighed to obtain the correct amount of calcium. The

right answer can be obtained by adding this step:

$$\frac{0.80 \, \text{g (Ca)}}{40 \, (\text{atomic wt. Ca})} = \frac{x \, \text{g (hydrated calcium chloride)}}{147 \, (\text{formula wt. hydrated salt})}$$

$$x = 2.94 \, \text{g hydrated calcium chloride}$$

(B–incorrect) The answer of 2.22 g is incorrect because it assumes that anhydrous calcium chloride (molecular weight of 111) was used. However, the problem specified that the official form, which contains two waters of hydration, was available.

(E–incorrect) The answer of 5.88 g is obtained if one ignores the +2 valence of calcium.

35. **(C)**

$$\frac{500,000 \, \text{U}}{10 \, \text{mL}} = \frac{(15,000 \, \text{U} \times 30 \, \text{g})}{x \, \text{mL}}$$

$$x = 9 \, \text{mL}$$

To incorporate 9 mL of an aqueous solution into an ointment, water absorption bases such as Aquaphor or hydrophilic petrolatum are suitable. The pharmacist would not incorporate 9 mL of antibiotic solution directly into 30 g of ointment base because the incorrect concentration of drug would result. Instead, 9 mL should be mixed with a total of 21 g of base.

36. **(B)**

$$50 \, \text{mL} \times 100 \, \text{U/mL} = 5000 \, \text{U total}$$

$$\frac{10,000 \, \text{U}}{1 \, \text{mL}} = \frac{5,000 \, \text{U}}{x \, \text{mL}}$$

$$x = 0.5 \, \text{mL}$$

(23:192)

37. **(B)** The normal maintenance dose would be:

$$120 \, \text{lb} \times 2 \, \text{mg/lb} = 240 \, \text{mg}$$

Because the normal creatinine clearance rate is 100 to 120 mL per minute:

$$\frac{40 \, \text{mL/min}}{100 \, \text{mL/min}} \times 240 \, \text{mg} = 96, \text{ or } 100 \, \text{mg}$$

(23:208)

38. (C) 500 mL of $D_{30}W$ will contain 150 g of dextrose. $D_{40}W$ contains 40 g of dextrose per 100 mL.

$$\frac{40 \text{ g dextrose}}{100 \text{ mL of solution}} = \frac{150 \text{ g dextrose}}{x \text{ mL of solution}}$$

$$x = 375 \text{ mL}$$

Or, this problem may be solved by using the equation:

$$(Q_1)(C_1) = (Q_2)(C_2)$$

$$(x \text{ mL})(40\%) = (500 \text{ mL})(30\%)$$

$$x = 375 \text{ mL}$$

(23:133)

39. (A) One avoirdupois pound contains 454 g. The total number of bacitracin units required is $454 \text{ g} \times 200 \text{ U/g} = 90{,}800 \text{ U}$.

$$\frac{500 \text{ U}}{1 \text{ g}} = \frac{90{,}800 \text{ U}}{x \text{ g}}$$

$$x = 182 \text{ g}$$

(23:188–90)

40. (C)

$$\frac{5 \text{ g salicylic acid}}{100 \text{ mL of lotion}} = \frac{x \text{ g}}{473 \text{ mL of lotion}}$$

$$x = 23.7 \text{ g}$$

(23:101)

41. (B) When concentrations of alcohol are listed on labels, the percent V/V is based on absolute alcohol (100% ethanol), although this form of alcohol is seldom used during manufacturing or compounding. Alcohol USP was specified for the formula. Its strength is 95% V/V.

$$20 \text{ mL} \times 95\% = 19 \text{ mL}$$

$$\frac{19 \text{ mL}}{120 \text{ mL}} = 15.8\% \text{ V/V}$$

(23:277)

42. (B)

$$\frac{0.25 \text{ g}}{120 \text{ mL}} = \frac{x \text{ g}}{240 \text{ mL}}$$

$$x = 500 \text{ mg pure triamcinolone}$$

$$\frac{40 \text{ mg}}{1 \text{ mL}} = \frac{500 \text{ mg}}{x \text{ mL}}$$

$$x = 12.5 \text{ mL of the injection solution}$$

(23:120)

43. (C) The mL in 1 lb of propylene glycol can be calculated as

$$SG = \frac{W}{V}$$

$$1.04 = \frac{454 \text{ g}}{x \text{ mL}}$$

$$x = 436 \text{ mL of propylene glycol in 1 lb}$$

$$\frac{\$12.00}{436 \text{ mL}} = \frac{\$x}{100 \text{ mL}}$$

$$x = \$2.75$$

(1:74; 23:88)

44. (B) Ten pounds contain $454 \text{ g} \times 10 = 4540 \text{ g}$. Two ounces (avoir.) consist of 28.4 g/oz, or 56.8 g. Thus, 4540 g divided by 56.8 g = 80 jars. *(23:232)*

45. (B) A density or SG of 1.25 indicates that 1 mL of the liquid weighs 1.25 g.

Because 1 lb of the ointment contains 5% W/W glycerin,

$$454 \text{ g} \times 5\% \text{ W/W} = 22.7 \text{ g of glycerin}$$

$$\text{Density} = \frac{W}{V}$$

$$1.25 = \frac{22.7 \text{ g}}{x \text{ mL}}$$

$$x = 18.2 \text{ mL}$$

(1:74; 23:88)

46. (D) Two pounds would contain $454 \times 2 = 908$ g of ointment. The final preparation would contain 908 g $\times$ 2% = 18.18 g of pure hydrocortisone. Because the available hydrocortisone ointment is 5% strength, one would need:

$$\frac{5\,g}{100\,g} = \frac{18.6\,g}{x\,g}$$

$$x = 363.2\,g \text{ of the 5\% ointment}$$

Or, using the equation: $(Q_1)\,(C_1) = (Q_2)\,(C_2)$

$$(908\,g)\,(2\%\ W/W) = (x\,g)\,(5\%\ W/W)$$

$$x = 363.2\,g$$

(23:131)

47. (C) This problem can be solved by the alligation alternate or simple parts method

```
7%  |        | 3 parts
    |   5%   |
2%  |        | 2 parts
```

Thus, the final solution will contain 2 parts of 2% iodine for every 3 parts of 7% iodine.

$$\frac{2\ parts}{x} = \frac{5\ parts\ total}{1000\ ml\ total}$$
$$= 400\ mL \text{ of 2\% iodine solution}$$

(23:130–34)

48. (B) Because the amount of 0.5% hydrocortisone creams is exactly 60 g, the final weight of the cream will be greater when hydrocortisone powder is added. Therefore, the problem may be solved by the alligation alternate method or by simple algebra.

```
100% HC  |        | 1.5 parts
         |   2%   |
0.5%     |        | 98 parts
```

$$\frac{60\,g\ of\ 0.5\%}{98\ parts} = \frac{x\,g\ of\ 100\%}{1.5\ parts}$$

$$x = 0.92 \text{ grams}$$

Or, by algebra, let x = weight of 100% HC powder

$$(x\,g)\,(100\%) + (60\,g)\,(0.5\%) = (60\,g + x\,g)\,(2\%)$$

$$x + 0.3 = 1.2 + .02\,x$$

$$x = 0.92\,g$$

(23:130)

49. (B) One of the most convenient methods of solving this problem is using the equation:

$$(Q_1)\,(C_1) = (Q_2)\,(C_2)$$

$$(240\ mL)\,(470\ mOsm/L) = (x\ mL)\,(280\ mOsm/L)$$

$$280\,x = 112{,}800$$

$$x = 403\ mL \text{ of final product}$$

Therefore, the amount of water diluent = $403 - 240 = 163$ mL.

(1:615; 23:162)

50. (C) Step 1. Determine amount of sodium thiosulfate in the Rx.

$$100\ mL \times 1.2\% = 1.2\,g, \text{ or } 1200\ mg$$

Step 2. Multiply the amount of chemical by its "E" value

$$1200\ mg \times 0.31 = 372\ mg$$
$$\text{(equivalent amount of NaCl)}$$

Step 3. Determine amount of NaCl needed as if no other chemical was present.

$$100\ mL \times 0.9\% = 900\ mg$$

Step 4. Subtract contribution by chemical (Step 2) from the amount of NaCl (Step 3)

$$900\ mg - 372\ mg = 528\ mg,$$
(the amount of NaCl needed to render the solution isotonic)

(1:620–21)

51. (B) Only 45 mL of the prescription must be adjusted to isotonicity because the 15 mL of Zincfrin is already isotonic. An isotonic solution of sodium chloride contains 0.9% sodium chloride:

$$45 \text{ mL} \times 0.009 = 0.4 \text{ g}$$

(1:620–21)

52. **(B)** One liter of normal saline contains 0.9% NaCl, or 9 g. To calculate the milliosmolarity of the solution:

Step 1. Determine the moles present.

$$\frac{\text{Wt. of chemical}}{\text{Mol. wt.}} = \frac{0.9 \text{ g}}{58.5}$$

$$= 0.154 \text{ moles, or } 154 \text{ millimoles}$$

Step 2. Multiply the millimoles by the "i" value. The "i" value is the theoretical number of ions or particles formed by one molecule of chemical assuming complete ionization.

$$154 \text{ millimoles} \times 2 = 308 \text{ milliosmoles/L}$$

(1:615; 23:162)

53. **(B)** Unlike the previous problem, this question asks for mOsm/100 mL and there are two chemicals present. It is best to calculate the mOsm of each separately, then add the amounts.

$$\text{NaCl: } \frac{1000 \text{ mg}}{58.5} = 17.1 \text{ mM} \times 2 = 34.2 \text{ mOsm}$$

$$\text{Dextrose: } \frac{5000 \text{ mg}}{198} = 25.3 \text{ mM} \times 1$$

$$= 25.3 \text{ mOsm}$$

$$34.2 \text{ mOsm} + 25.3 \text{ mOsm} = 59.5 \text{ mOsm total}$$

(1:615; 23:162)

54. **(C)** Step 1: How many grams of pure HCl are needed?

$$4000 \text{ mL} \times 10\% \text{ W/V} = 400 \text{ g}$$

Step 2: How much of the available 36.8% W/W HCl acid will provide 400 g of pure HCl?

$$\frac{36.8 \text{ g pure HCl}}{100 \text{ g of solution}} = \frac{400 \text{ g pure HCl}}{x \text{ g of solution}}$$

$$x = 1087 \text{ g of acid}$$

Step 3: What volume of concentrated HCl acid is equivalent to 1087 g if its specific gravity is 1.19?

$$SG = \frac{\text{Wt.}}{\text{Vol.}}$$

$$1.19 = \frac{1087 \text{ g}}{x \text{ mL}}$$

$$x = 913 \text{ mL}$$

Thus, 4 L of diluted HCl is prepared by measuring 913 mL of Hydrochloric Acid USP and diluting it with sufficient purified water to measure 4000 mL. *(23:126)*

55. **(B)** One gallon contains 3785 mL.

$$3785 \text{ mL} \times 0.25\% = 9.46 \text{ or } 9.5 \text{ g}$$

Because the volume contributed by the acetic acid is insignificant when compared to 3785 mL, it does not enter into the calculation of the final volume. *(23:101)*

56. **(B)** The formula weight of ferrous sulfate is 278. The amount of iron present in 300 mg of the chemical will be:

$$\frac{\text{Atomic wt. Fe}}{\text{Form. wt. salt}} = \frac{55.9}{278} = \frac{x \text{ mg}}{300 \text{ mg}}$$

$$x = 60.4 \text{ mg}$$

Choices A or D would be obtained if the correct answer was either doubled or halved to reflect the +2 valence of iron. The valence of iron has no significance in this type of problem because only one atom of iron is present in each molecule of ferrous sulfate.

Choice C assumes that the ferrous sulfate is anhydrous with a molecular weight of 152. This is incorrect, because the 300-mg weight is based on a chemical formula containing 7 waters of hydration.

Choice E is the amount of anhydrous ferrous sulfate present in each 300 mg. The question asks for iron (Fe) only. *(23:306)*

57. **(D)** A saturated solution of the chemical consists of 1 g of chemical plus 10 mL of alcohol. The exact volume of this soluton is unknown because the volume occupied by 1 g of the chemical when dissolved cannot be deter-

mined. Therefore, the concentration of the saturated solution must be calculated as a percent W/W, not a percent W/V. The weight of alcohol present will be 8 g, because its specific gravity is 0.80.

$$\frac{\text{solute}}{\text{solute} + \text{solvent}} = \frac{1\,\text{g}}{1\,\text{g} + 8\,\text{g}} = \frac{1\,\text{g}}{9\,\text{g}}$$
$$= 11.1\%\ \text{W/W}$$

(23:101)

58. **(A)** First-order half-lives relate to kinetic constant rate values by the equation:

$$t_{0.5} = \frac{0.693}{k}$$

$$14.3\ \text{days} = \frac{0.693}{k}$$

$$k = 0.048/\text{day, or } 4.8\% \text{ per day}$$

(23:218)

59. **(B)** Because the time interval between preparation and administration is 6 h, and the half-life of the radiopharmaceutical is 6 h, approximately one-half of the original strength has decayed. Therefore, 1 mL of the solution now assaying at 20 mCi/mL is needed. *(23:219)*

60. **(E)** The loss in first-order kinetics is a constant fraction of the immediate past concentration. In this example, the half-life of 6 h allows a quick comparison of the amount of radioactivity remaining.

Original Activity	40 mCi/mL
After 6 h	20 mCi/mL
After 12 h	10 mCi/mL
After 18 h	5 mCi/mL
After 24 h	2.5 mCi/mL

(13:308; 23:218–19)

CHAPTER 3

Pharmacy

Definitions of pharmacy differ from one dictionary to another. Some contain the simple, traditional statement, "the art of preparing and dispensing drugs." Others expand on the definition by including "the art or practice of preparing, preserving, compounding, and dispensing drugs plus administering drugs and discovering new drugs through research."

Today, pharmacy encompasses all aspects of drug preparation and dispensing, as well as evaluation of therapeutic effects in patients. The term "pharmaceutical care" is being used to stress the duty of the pharmacist to ensure that drug therapy produces maximum beneficial outcomes. This chapter includes basic material with which the practicing pharmacist should be familiar in order to dispense drug products successfully and to serve as the resource person to other health professionals and the general public. This includes knowledge of the manufacture and characteristics of the dosage form, trade names and generic names, drug strengths and commercial dosage forms, packaging, dispensing advice, recognition of significant drug interactions, and the selection of over-the-counter products. Actually, this chapter is intended to include topics and information not specifically designated in the other book chapters. Subsequent chapters stress the pharmacokinetics and therapeutic actions of drugs in the body, the selection of specific drugs to treat various diseases, and the evaluation of therapeutic outcomes.

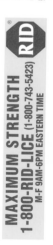

Questions

DIRECTIONS (Questions 1 through 197): Each of the numbered items or incomplete statements in this section is followed by answers or by completions of the statement. Select the ONE lettered answer or completion that is BEST in each case.

1. Official standards for individual drugs and chemicals formulated into dosage forms are published in

   (A) *USP/NF*
   (B) *USP DI* Volume I
   (C) *USP DI* Volume II
   (D) *USP DI* Volume III
   (E) *PDR*

2. Which one of the following chemicals is NOT suitable as a drug excipient?

   (A) Butyl paraben
   (B) Lactose
   (C) Glycerin
   (D) Benzocaine
   (E) Gelatin

3. According to the USP, the instruction "protect from light" in a monograph indicates storage in a

   (A) dark place
   (B) amber glass bottle
   (C) light-resistant container
   (D) hermetic container
   (E) tight glass container

4. According to the National Bureau of Standards (NBS), the initial calibration mark on a 100-mL graduate should be

   (A) 5 mL
   (B) 10 mL
   (C) 15 mL
   (D) 20 mL
   (E) 30 mL

5. The USP describes several tests for evaluating prescription balances. These tests include all of the following EXCEPT

   (A) arm ratio
   (B) rest point
   (C) rider and graduated beam
   (D) sensitivity requirement
   (E) shift

6. According to USP standards, a refrigerator can be used to store pharmaceuticals that specify storage in a

   I. freezer
   II. cool place
   III. cold place

   (A) I only
   (B) III only
   (C) I and II only
   (D) II and III only
   (E) I, II, and III

7. Which of the following alkaloids exhibits good water solubility?

I. Morphine HCl
II. Cocaine
III. Atropine

(A) I only
(B) III only
(C) I and II only
(D) II and III only
(E) I, II, and III

8. All of the following physicochemical constants may be useful when predicting the solubility of a chemical EXCEPT

(A) dielectric constants
(B) pH of solution
(C) pKa of the chemical
(D) solubility parameters
(E) valence of the chemical

9. Descriptions of the Federal Controlled Substances Act, Approved Drug Products with Therapeutic Equivalence Evaluations, and USP/NF dispensing requirements may be found in the

(A) *USP DI* Volume I
(B) *USP DI* Volume II
(C) *USP DI* Volume III
(D) *Facts and Comparisons*
(E) *PDR*

10. Prescription drug descriptions expressed in layperson's terms and useful as handouts for patients may be photocopied from the

(A) *USP DI* Volume I — HCP info
(B) *USP DI* Volume II — Pt info
(C) *USP DI* Volume III bioequivalency OB info
(D) *Facts and Comparisons*
(E) *Remington's Pharmaceutical Sciences*

11. Solubility of a substance may be expressed in several ways. When a quantitative statement of solubility is given in the USP, it is generally expressed as

(A) g of solute soluble in 1 mL of solvent
(B) g of solute soluble in 100 mL of solvent
(C) mL of solvent required to dissolve 1 g of solute
(D) mL of solvent required to dissolve 100 g of solute
(E) mL of solvent required to prepare 100 mL of saturated solution

12. If a bottle of tablets has an expiration date of "Dec 1999," the pharmacist may continue to dispense the product

(A) up to 1 year after the expiration date
(B) only through January 31, 2000
(C) only through December 15, 1999
(D) only through December 31, 1999
(E) if the pharmacist informs the patient to discard unused tablets in 6 months

13. The expiration date on a pharmaceutical container states "Expires July 2000." This statement means that by that expiration date, the product may have lost

(A) up to 5% of its activity
(B) up to 10% of its activity
(C) up to 20% of its activity
(D) up to 50% of its activity
(E) sufficient activity to be outside USP monograph requirements

14. Which one of the following practices would NOT be classified as "alternative medicine" in the United States?

(A) Allopathy
(B) Chiropractic
(C) Naturopathy
(D) Nutraceutical
(E) Reflexology

15. An alternative medical practice that stresses the use of extremely small doses of drugs is known as

(A) folk medicine
(B) holistic medicine
(C) homeopathic medicine
(D) orthomolecular medicine
(E) faith healing

16. Which of the following chemicals may be included in a drug solution as a chelating agent?

    (A) Ascorbic acid
    (B) Hydroquinone
    (C) Edetate
    (D) Sodium bisulfite
    (E) Fluorescein sodium

17. Which of the following ions may be effectively chelated?

    I. Sodium
    II. Lithium
    III. Lead

    (A) I only
    (B) III only
    (C) I and II only
    (D) II and III only
    (E) I, II, and III

18. Which of the following forms of the basic drug haloperidol will have good water solubility?

    I. Hydrochloride
    II. Lactate
    III. Decanoate

    (A) I only
    (B) III only
    (C) I and II only
    (D) II and III only
    (E) I, II, and III

19. An early sign of a decomposing epinephrine solution is the presence of a

    (A) brown precipitate
    (B) pink color
    (C) white precipitate
    (D) crystal
    (E) red color

20. On exposure to air, aminophylline solutions may develop

    (A) crystals of theophylline
    (B) a gas

    (C) a precipitate of aminophylline
    (D) a precipitate of ethylenediamine
    (E) a straw color

21. The process of grinding a substance to a very fine powder is termed

    (A) levigation
    (B) sublimation
    (C) trituration
    (D) pulverization by intervention
    (E) maceration

22. The term "impalpable" refers to a substance that is

    (A) bad tasting
    (B) not perceptible to the touch
    (C) greasy
    (D) nongreasy
    (E) tasteless

23. Dosage forms of cafergot include

    I. oral tablets
    II. rectal suppositories
    III. parenteral solution

    (A) I only
    (B) III only
    (C) I and II only
    (D) II and III only
    (E) I, II, and III

24. The term "chiral" is related to a drug's

    (A) chelating ability
    (B) eutectic properties
    (C) stereoisomerism
    (D) partition coefficient
    (E) water solubility

25. Different crystalline forms (polymorphs) of the same drug exhibit different

    I. metabolism rates
    II. melting points
    III. solubilities

    (A) I only
    (B) III only

(C) I and II only

(D) II and III only

(E) I, II, and III

26. Benzalkonium chloride is a germicidal surfactant that is rendered inactive in the presence of

(A) organic acids

(B) gram-negative organisms

(C) cationic surfactants

(D) soaps

(E) inorganic salts

27. The shrinkage that occurs when alcohol and purified water are mixed is primarily due to

(A) attractive van der Waals forces

(B) covalent bonding

(C) hydrogen bonding

(D) ionic bonding

(E) temperature changes

28. Although most drugs in pharmaceutical dosage forms are expected to decompose following first-order kinetics, an exception is drugs formulated in

(A) capsules

(B) oral solutions

(C) oral suspensions

(D) tablets

(E) suppositories

29. According to the Poiseuille equation, the factor that has the relatively greatest influence on the rate of flow of liquid through a capillary tube is the

(A) length of the tube

(B) viscosity of the liquid

(C) pressure differential on the tube

(D) radius of the tube

(E) temperature of the liquid

30. Patients following low-sodium diets may resort to the use of sodium-free salt substitutes such as NoSalt. The major ingredient in these products is

(A) ammonium chloride

(B) calcium chloride

(C) potassium chloride

(D) potassium iodide

(E) none of these

31. Potassium supplements are administered in all of the following manners EXCEPT

(A) IV infusion

(B) IV bolus

(C) elixirs, po

(D) effervescent tablets

(E) slow-release tablets, po

32. Which of the following statements concerning fluorouracil is NOT true?

(A) Its chemical structure is a modified pyrimidine similar to uracil and idoxuridine.

(B) It is effective only when administered by injection.

(C) Anorexia and nausea and vomiting are very common side effects.

(D) The drug interferes with the synthesis of ribonucleic acid.

(E) Leukopenia is a major clinical toxic effect.

33. The agency in the United States responsible for selecting appropriate nonproprietary names for drugs is the

(A) AMA

(B) APhA

(C) FDA

(D) USAN

(E) USP

34. The product inserts for many drug products contain cautionary statements. Which one of the following sequences lists the three types of cautions in the order of least serious to most serious?

(A) contraindication, precaution, warning

(B) precaution, warning, contraindication

(C) warning, contraindication, precaution

(D) warning, precaution, contraindication

(E) contraindication, warning, precaution

35. A comparison of individual amino acids present in commercial amino acids injection solutions may be found in

    I. *Facts and Comparisons*
    II. *Trissel's Handbook on Injectable Drugs*
    III. *Remington's Pharmaceutical Sciences*

(A) I only
(B) III only
(C) I and II only
(D) II and III only
(E) I, II, and III

36. "Winged" needles are most closely associated with which type of injections?

(A) Intradermal
(B) Intramuscular
(C) Intrathecal
(D) Intravenous
(E) Subcutaneous

37. Hypodermic needle sizes are expressed by gauge numbers. The gauge number refers to the

(A) bevel size
(B) external diameter of the cannula
(C) internal diameter of the cannula
(D) length of the needle
(E) size of the lumen opening

38. Insulin preparations are usually administered by

(A) intradermal injection
(B) intramuscular injection
(C) intravenous bolus
(D) intravenous infusion
(E) subcutaneous injection

39. Which one of the following needles is most suited for the administration of insulin solutions?

(A) 16G ⁵/₈″
(B) 21G ¹/₂″
(C) 21G ⁵/₈″
(D) 25G ⁵/₈″
(E) 25G 1″

40. Which of the following are used to prepare "targeted drug delivery systems"?

    I. Liposomes
    II. Nanoparticles
    III. Transdermal patches

(A) I only
(B) III only
(C) I and II only
(D) II and III only
(E) I, II, and III

41. The quantities of all ingredients present in parenteral solutions must be specified on the label EXCEPT for

    I. antimicrobial preservatives
    II. isotonicity adjustors
    III. pH adjustors

(A) I only
(B) III only
(C) I and II only
(D) II and III only
(E) I, II, and III

42. Which one of the following commonly available large-volume dextrose solutions for intravenous use is isotonic?

(A) 2.5%
(B) 5.0%
(C) 10%
(D) 20%
(E) 50%

43. The term "venoclysis" is most closely associated with

(A) intravenous injections
(B) intrathecal injections
(C) intravenous infusions
(D) intrapleural withdrawals
(E) peritoneal dialysis

44. The designation "minibottles" refers to

(A) partially filled parenteral bottles with 50- to 150-mL volumes

(B) any parenteral bottle with a capacity of less than 1 L

(C) 10- to 30-mL glass vials

(D) prescription bottles with capacities of 4 oz or less

(E) vials with a capacity of less than 10 mL

45. The term "piggyback" is most commonly associated with

(A) intermittent therapy

(B) intrathecal injections

(C) intravenous bolus

(D) slow intravenous infusions

(E) total parenteral nutrition

46. What is the approximate maximum volume of fluid that should be administered daily by intravenous infusion to a stabilized patient?

(A) 1 L

(B) 4 L

(C) 8 L

(D) 12 L

(E) 16 L

47. Which one of the following injectable solutions may result in a precipitate when added to D5W or NS?

(A) Diazepam (Valium)

(B) Folic acid (Folvite)

(C) Furosemide (Lasix)

(D) Gentamicin sulfate (Garamycin)

(E) Succinylcholine chloride (Anectine)

48. Official forms of water include

I. Water for Injection

II. Bacteriostatic Water for Injection

III. Sterile Water for Inhalation

(A) I only

(B) III only

(C) I and II only

(D) II and III only

(E) I, II, and III

49. The method of preparation must be indicated on labels for

(A) Bacteriostatic Water for Injection USP

(B) Milk of Magnesia USP

(C) Purified Water USP

(D) Sterile Water for Injection USP

(E) Water for Injection USP

50. The Norplant implant system is

I. inserted under the skin

II. effective for only 1 year   → specific organ No, No!!!

III. classified as a targeted delivery system

(A) I only

(B) III only

(C) I and II only

(D) II and III only

(E) I, II, and III

51. The usual expiration dating that should be placed on a parenteral admixture prepared in a hospital pharmacy is

(A) 1 hour

(B) 24 hours

(C) 48 hours

(D) 72 hours

(E) 1 week

52. Which one of the following designations is most appropriate for a medical order requiring an intravenous bolus injection?

(A) per IV

(B) IVP

(C) IVPB

(D) po

(E) KVO

53. Although isotonicity is desirable for almost all parenterals, it is particularly critical for which injections?

(A) Intra-articular

(B) Intradermal

(C) Intramuscular

(D) Intravenous

(E) Subcutaneous ✓

54. The osmotic pressure of a 0.1 molar dextrose solution will be approximately how many times that of a 0.1 molar sodium chloride solution?

   (A) 0.5
   (B) 1
   (C) 2
   (D) 3
   (E) 4

55. Parenteral solutions that are isotonic with human red blood cells have an osmolality of approximately how many mOsm/L?

   (A) 20
   (B) 40
   (C) 50
   (D) 150
   (E) 300

56. Which of the following injectables is (are) isotonic with human red blood cells?

   I. D5W
   II. D5W/NS
   III. D5W/.45NS

   (A) I only
   (B) III only
   (C) I and III
   (D) II and III
   (E) I, II, and III

57. A suspension is NOT a suitable dosage form for what type of injection?

   (A) Intra-articular
   (B) Intradermal
   (C) Intramuscular
   (D) Intravenous
   (E) Subcutaneous

58. Which one of the following parenteral solutions is considered to most closely approximate the extracellular fluid of the human body?

   (A) Dextrose 2½% and sodium chloride 0.45% injection
   (B) Lactated Ringer's injection
   (C) Ringer's injection
   (D) Sodium chloride injection
   (E) Sodium lactate injection

59. Even distribution of a drug into the blood after an IV bolus injection can be expected

   (A) instantaneously
   (B) within 4 minutes
   (C) in 5 to 10 minutes
   (D) within 30 minutes
   (E) only after a few hours

60. Which one of the following routes of administration is NOT considered suitable for Heparin Sodium Injection USP?

   (A) Continuous IV infusion
   (B) Intermittent IV infusion
   (C) Intramuscular
   (D) Subcutaneous
   (E) All are suitable

61. The IV fluid systems that use glass bottles may be divided into two types according to the

   (A) presence or absence of a vacuum in the bottle
   (B) presence or absence of an airway tube in the bottle
   (C) use of amber versus clear glass
   (D) size (volume) of the available solutions
   (E) presence or absence of pressure in the bottle

62. Which of the following facts concerning insulin is (are) true?

   I. Degradation occurs only in the liver
   II. Product is available without a prescription
   III. Drug has a short plasma half-life

   (A) I only
   (B) III only
   (C) I and III
   (D) II and III
   (E) I, II, and III

63. Simethicone is most likely to be included in what type of OTC product?

   (A) Antacid
   (B) Cough product
   (C) Decongestant
   (D) Laxative
   (E) Weight control

64. Which one of the following parenteral antibiotics is the most stable in an aqueous solution?

   (A) Gentamicin sulfate
   (B) Methicillin sodium
   (C) Oxacillin sodium
   (D) Tetracycline hydrochloride
   (E) Vancomycin hydrochloride

65. Which of the following vitamins possesses antioxidant properties?

   I. Ascorbic acid
   II. Ergocalciferol
   III. Pantothenic acid

   (A) I only
   (B) III only
   (C) I and III
   (D) II and III
   (E) I, II, and III

66. Naturally occurring vitamin K_1 is also called

   (A) menadione
   (B) phytonadione
   (C) tocopherol
   (D) pantothenic acid
   (E) biotin

67. Which of the following is likely to have the greatest water solubility?

   (A) Butane
   (B) Tertiary butanol
   (C) Tertiary pentanol
   (D) n-Butanol
   (E) n-Pentanol

68. Methylparaben is an ester of

   (A) benzoic acid
   (B) p-hydroxybenzoic acid
   (C) para-aminosalicylic acid
   (D) propionic acid
   (E) benzyl alcohol

69. Biologicals can be used to obtain either active or passive immunity. Which one of the following pairs is NOT correct?

   (A) Antiserum, passive immunity
   (B) Antitoxin, passive immunity
   (C) Human immune serum, active immunity
   (D) Toxoid, active immunity
   (E) Vaccine, active immunity

70. Which one of the following is a vaccine used for active immunization against measles (rubeola)?

   (A) Attenuvax
   (B) Fluogen
   (C) Recombivax HB
   (D) Havrix
   (E) Sabin

71. All of the following biologicals are used for active immunization EXCEPT

   (A) antiserums
   (B) bacterial vaccines
   (C) bacterial antigens
   (D) multiple antigen preparations
   (E) toxoids

72. Immune serum globulin (gamma globulin) is usually administered by what type of injection?

   (A) Intradermal
   (B) Intramuscular
   (C) Intravenous
   (D) Subcutaneous
   (E) Any of the usual methods of injection

73. Tuberculin syringes are

    I. only suitable for administration of TB vaccine
    II. prefilled syringes
    III. 1 mL units with 0.05 mL accuracy

    (A) I only
    (B) III only
    (C) I and III
    (D) II and III
    (E) I, II, and III

74. The intermediate tuberculin skin test (intermediate strength PPD) contains

    (A) 2 tuberculin units
    (B) 5 tuberculin units
    (C) 25 tuberculin units
    (D) 250 tuberculin units
    (E) 500 tuberculin units

75. All of the following are used for the prophylaxis or treatment of diseases EXCEPT

    (A) antitoxins
    (B) antivenins
    (C) globulins
    (D) serums
    (E) serum albumin

76. The usual storage condition specified for biologicals is

    (A) below 2° C
    (B) 2–8° C
    (C) a cool place
    (D) 8–15° C
    (E) room temperature

77. All of the following statements concerning toxoids are true EXCEPT

    (A) toxoids are detoxified toxins
    (B) toxoids are antigens
    (C) toxoids produce permanent immunity
    (D) toxoids are often available in a precipitated or adsorbed form
    (E) toxoids produce artificial active immunity

78. The DTP series of injections is intended for administration to

    (A) infants
    (B) children
    (C) children 6 years and older
    (D) children and adults
    (E) only after puberty

79. All of the following are viral infections EXCEPT

    (A) influenza
    (B) measles
    (C) mumps
    (D) hepatitis
    (E) typhoid fever

80. All of the following are bacterial infections EXCEPT

    (A) cholera
    (B) plague
    (C) rabies
    (D) pertussis
    (E) tuberculosis

81. Which of the following preparations will induce passive rather than active immunity?

    (A) Tetanus toxoid
    (B) Botulism antitoxin
    (C) Typhoid vaccine
    (D) Mumps virus vaccine, attenuated
    (E) Cholera vaccine

82. For which one of the following categories of chemicals is denaturation a major stability problem?

    (A) Amino acids
    (B) Benzodiazepines
    (C) Catecholamines
    (D) Cephalosporins
    (E) Proteins

83. Which of the following is considered effective in the treatment of accidental drug poisoning?

I. Activated charcoal

II. Ipecac syrup

III. "Universal antidote"

(A) I only

(B) III only

(C) I and II only

(D) II and III only

(E) I, II, and III

84. Which one of the following compounds is NOT adsorbed by activated charcoal?

(A) Acetaminophen

(B) Cyanide

(C) Phenothiazines

(D) Salicylates

(E) Tricyclic antidepressants

85. A cough syrup is labeled as containing 20% alcohol by volume. Which of the following statements is (are) true?

I. Each 100 mL of syrup contains exactly 20 mL Alcohol USP.

II. There is the equivalent of 20 mL of absolute alcohol present in every 100 mL of syrup.

III. The strength of this product may be expressed as 40 proof.

(A) I only

(B) III only

(C) I and II only

(D) II and III only

(E) I, II, and III

86. Which of the following chemicals is (are) included in topical formulas as sunscreens?

I. Benzophenones

II. Cinnamates

III. Methyl salicylate

(A) I only

(B) III only

(C) I and II only

(D) II and III only

(E) I, II, and III

87. A fair-skinned client claims that he normally begins to sunburn in approximately 30 minutes when exposed to the midday sun. What maximum length of protection could he expect using a sun lotion with a SPF of 12?

(A) 1 hour

(B) 2 to 3 hours

(C) 4 to 6 hours

(D) 10 to 12 hours

(E) 24 hours

88. Colostomy pouches are classified by

I. an open vs closed design

II. size of stoma

III. whether for a male or female

(A) I only

(B) III only

(C) I and II only

(D) II and III only

(E) I, II, and III

89. The most hygroscopic of the following liquids is

(A) acetone

(B) alcohol USP

(C) glycerin

(D) mineral oil

(E) PEG 400

90. Which of the following statements concerning medicinal oxygen therapy is (are) true?

I. Medical oxygen has a prescription-only status.

II. The usual flow rate for the relief of hypoxemia is 2 liters/minute.

III. Compressed oxygen in tanks is the only form available for home use.

(A) I only

(B) III only

(C) I and II only

(D) II and III only

(E) I, II, and III

91. The containers used to package drugs may consist of several components and/or be composed of several materials. The release of an ingredient from packaging components into the actual product is best described by the term

    (A) adsorption
    (B) diffusion
    (C) leaching
    (D) permeation
    (E) porosity

92. Techniques used in the development of "biotechnological drugs" include

    I. gene splicing
    II. preparation of monoclonal antibodies
    III. lyophilization

    (A) I only
    (B) III only
    (C) I and II only
    (D) II and III only
    (E) I, II, and III

93. Most of the recently developed biotechnological drugs are formulated into which dosage form?

    (A) Inhalation solutions
    (B) Parenteral
    (C) Capsules
    (D) Tablets
    (E) Topicals

94. Which one of the following drugs is NOT prepared by recombinant DNA technology?

    (A) Epoetin
    (B) Erythropoietin
    (C) Humulin
    (D) Interferon
    (E) Urokinase

95. Which of the following home diagnostic tests incorporates monoclonal antibodies into the testing procedure?

    I. Fecal occult blood
    II. Ovulation prediction
    III. Pregnancy determination

    (A) I only
    (B) III only
    (C) I and II only
    (D) II and III only
    (E) I, II, and III

96. Uses for surfactants in pharmaceutical products include

    I. percutaneous absorption enhancers
    II. cleansing agents
    III. therapeutic activity

    (A) I only
    (B) III only
    (C) I and II only
    (D) II and III only
    (E) I, II, and III

97. The HLB system is most applicable for the classification of which surfactants?

    (A) Anionic
    (B) Ampholytic
    (C) Cationic
    (D) Nonionic
    (E) Either anionic or cationic

98. An example of a nonionic surfactant would be

    (A) ammonium laurate
    (B) cetylpyridinium chloride
    (C) dioctyl sodium sulfosuccinate
    (D) sorbitan monopalmitate
    (E) triethanolamine stearate

99. Vehicles for nasal medications should possess all of the following properties EXCEPT

    (A) an acid pH
    (B) isotonicity
    (C) high buffer capacity
    (D) ability to resist growth of microorganisms
    (E) all of the above are important properties; no exceptions

100. Which one of the following statements concerning bisacodyl is NOT true?

(A) Laxative action occurs within 6 hours after oral administration.
(B) Action of suppositories occurs within 1 hour of insertion.
(C) Suppositories may cause rectal irritation with continued administration.
(D) Tablets should be swallowed whole.
(E) Tablets should be administered with milk to avoid gastric irritation.

101. Most iron salts are administered orally. A commercially available parenteral product is

(A) Chel-Iron
(B) Feosol
(C) Simron
(D) InFeD
(E) Troph-Iron

102. Which one of the following chemicals is an effective and safe drug in the treatment of either diarrhea or constipation?

(A) Activated charcoal
(B) Bismuth salts
(C) Kaolin
(D) Attapulgite
(E) Polycarbophil

103. All of the following OTC laxative products contain phenolphthalein EXCEPT

(A) Agoral (Warner Wellcome Consumer) (mineral oil)
(B) Alophen (Warner Wellcome Consumer)
(C) Perdiem (Ciba Self-Medication)
(D) Correctol (Phillips Bayer Consumer)
(E) Modane (Savage Labs)

104. Insoluble bismuth salts are used as adsorbents and also possess useful astringent and protective properties. A commercial product containing a bismuth compound is

(A) Bisacodyl
(B) Donnagel
(C) Kaopectate
(D) Pepto-Bismol
(E) Rheaban

105. Which of the following antidiarrheal products contains the adsorbent clay attapulgite?

I. Donnagel
II. Kaopectate suspension
III. Parepectolin

(A) I only
(B) III only
(C) I and II only
(D) II and III only
(E) I, II, and III

106. A sympathomimetic often present in OTC appetite suppressants is

(A) caffeine
(B) ephedrine
(C) phenylephrine
(D) phenylpropanolamine
(E) pseudoephedrine

107. Which of the following internal analgesic products contain ketoprofen?

(A) Actron
(B) Advil
(C) Haltran
(D) Nuprin
(E) Valprin

108. Which of the following drugs have label warnings against their use during pregnancy especially during the last trimester?

I. Acetaminophen
II. Aspirin
III. Ibuprofen

(A) I only
(B) III only
(C) I and II only
(D) II and III only
(E) I, II, and III

109. All of the following products contain buffered aspirin EXCEPT

    (A) Ascriptin
    (B) Cope
    (C) Arthritis Strength Bufferin
    (D) Excedrin
    (E) Vanquish

110. Which one of the following OTC internal analgesics contains magnesium salicylate?

    (A) Bromo-Seltzer
    (B) Doan's Original
    (C) Ecotrin
    (D) Pamprin
    (E) Sinarest

111. Advantages of dextromethorphan as a cough suppressant include all of the following EXCEPT

    (A) as effective as codeine on a weight/weight basis
    (B) does not cause respiratory depression
    (C) is nonaddicting
    (D) doses of 10 to 15 mg suppress coughing for at least 4 hours
    (E) maximum daily adult dose is 30 mg

112. When dispensing Emetrol, which of the following consultations is (are) appropriate?

    I. Indicated for both nausea and vomiting due to an upset stomach
    II. Take 15 to 30 mL every 15 minutes for not more than five doses
    III. If desired, dilute with water to ease administration

    (A) I only
    (B) III only
    (C) I and II only
    (D) II and III only
    (E) I, II, and III

113. Disadvantages of calcium carbonate as an antacid include all of the following EXCEPT

    (A) some patients may develop hypercalcemia

    (B) capacity for acid neutralization is poor
    (C) may cause constipation
    (D) may induce gastric hypersecretion
    (E) prolonged use may induce renal calculi and decreased renal function

114. Which of the following products contain calcium carbonate as the active ingredient?

    I. Basaljel capsules
    II. Rolaids chewable tablets
    III. Titralac chewable tablets

    (A) I only
    (B) III only
    (C) I and II only
    (D) II and III only
    (E) I, II, and III

115. Which one of the following antacid products is a chemical combination of aluminum and magnesium hydroxides?

    (A) Gelusil
    (B) Maalox
    (C) Mylanta
    (D) Riopan
    (E) Tums

116. The prime purpose for which of the following types of coating may be to mask the bitter taste of an orally administered drug?

    I. Enteric
    II. Film
    III. Sugar

    (A) I only
    (B) III only
    (C) I and II only
    (D) II and III only
    (E) I, II, and III

117. Advantages to the manufacturer for tablet film coating when compared to sugar coating include

    I. shorter production times
    II. less gross weight
    III. lower incidence in coat chipping

(A) I only
(B) III only
(C) I and II only
(D) II and III only
(E) I, II, and III

118. Tablet friability most closely relates to a tablet's

(A) dissolution
(B) disintegration
(C) cohesiveness
(D) heat resistance
(E) weight

119. Which of the following is NOT used primarily as a diluent in tablet formulations?

(A) Magnesium stearate
(B) Dicalcium phosphate
(C) Lactose
(D) Mannitol
(E) Starch

120. Which of the following is NOT a function of the lubricant in a tablet formulation?

(A) Improving flow properties of granules
(B) Reducing powder adhesion onto the dies and punches
(C) Improving tablet wetting in the stomach
(D) Reducing punch and die wear
(E) Facilitating tablet ejection from the die

121. Aspartame may be included in a drug product as a (an)

(A) buffer
(B) source of calories
(C) solubilizer
(D) sweetener
(E) stimulant

122. Characteristics of drugs intended for formulation into sustained release dosage forms include:

I. possess short half-lives (<2 hr)
II. be intended for treatment of chronic conditions
III. have a high therapeutic index

(A) I only
(B) III only
(C) I and II only
(D) II and III only
(E) I, II, and III

123. An antihypertensive drug product that is based on circadian rhythm is

(A) Catapres (clonidine)
(B) Covera-HS (verapamil)
(C) Aldomet (methyldopa)
(D) Monopril (fosinopril)
(E) Vasotec (enalapril)

124. Which of the following trademarked dosage forms is enteric coated?

(A) Enduret
(B) Enseal
(C) Extentab
(D) Filmtab
(E) Spansule

125. A sweetener that is widely employed in chewable tablet formulas is

(A) aspartame
(B) glucose
(C) lactose
(D) mannitol
(E) sucrose

126. Mannitol may be included in lyophilized products as a

(A) buffer
(B) bulking agent
(C) preservative
(D) sweetener
(E) tonicity adjuster

127. Benzyl alcohol is present in some parenteral solutions as a (an)

    (A) antimicrobial preservative
    (B) antioxidant
    (C) chelating agent
    (D) buffering agent
    (E) tonicity adjuster

128. Which of the following properties is desirable in a pharmaceutic suspension?

    I. Caking
    II. Pseudoplastic flow
    III. Thixotropy

    (A) I only
    (B) III only
    (C) I and II only
    (D) II and III only
    (E) I, II, and III

129. Characteristics of inhalation aerosol dosage forms include

    I. avoid first-pass effect
    II. rapid onset of action
    III. can administer large amounts of drug to intended site

    (A) I only
    (B) III only
    (C) I and II only
    (D) II and III only
    (E) I, II, and III

130. Which of the following ingredients is (are) available in OTC aerosol asthmatic products?

    I. Epinephrine
    II. Ephedrine
    III. Metaproterenol

    (A) I only
    (B) III only
    (C) I and II only
    (D) II and III only
    (E) I, II, and III

131. An ileostomy differs from a colostomy in which of the following characteristics?

    I. The discharge from an ileostomy is more viscous.
    II. The stoma is significantly larger.
    III. The discharge is more irritating to the skin.

    (A) I only
    (B) III only
    (C) I and II only
    (D) II and III only
    (E) I, II, and III

132. Which one of the following narcotics may NOT be used for medicinal purposes in this country?

    (A) Diacetylmorphine
    (B) Ethylmorphine
    (C) Dihydrocodeinone
    (D) Methylmorphine
    (E) All are permitted

133. Burns are classified according to relative severity. Characteristics of a first-degree burn are

    (A) erythema, pain, no blistering
    (B) erythema, pain, blistering
    (C) blisters, pain, skin will regenerate
    (D) no blisters, leathery appearance of skin, skin grafting necessary
    (E) blackened skin, danger of deep infection

134. Effective local anesthetics present in OTC burn remedies include

    I. benzocaine
    II. lidocaine
    III. phenol

    (A) I only
    (B) III only
    (C) I and II only
    (D) II and III only
    (E) I, II, and III

135. Which one of the following statements concerning dextranomer (Debrisan by Johnson & Johnson) is NOT correct?

(A) Aids in the removal of wound exudates

(B) Can be used to treat decubitus ulcers

(C) Consists of spherical hydrophilic beads

(D) Is effective in the healing of both secreting and nonsecreting wounds

(E) Must be physically removed after treatment

136. For effectiveness as a local anesthetic, the level of benzocaine in a topical preparation should be AT LEAST

(A) 0.1%

(B) 1.0%

(C) 2.0%

(D) 5.0%

(E) 25%

137. Rectal clinical thermometers differ from oral thermometers in

(A) bulb shape

(B) stem length

(C) distance between graduation marks on the stem

(D) standards for accuracy

(E) stem shape

138. A basal thermometer is

(A) a rectal thermometer

(B) used to estimate time of ovulation

(C) used to determine basal metabolic rate

(D) graduated only in Celsius degrees

(E) used vaginally

139. The scale most commonly used in this country for denoting urinary catheter sizes is the

(A) American

(B) English

(C) French

(D) Stubbs

(E) Foley

140. Which one of the following statements concerning allergic reactions to insect bites and stings is NOT true?

(A) Cross-sensitization to bites of different insects (ants, wasps, bees, etc.) can be expected.

(B) Death may occur due to anaphylactic reaction.

(C) The initial systemic reaction will usually occur within 20 minutes of the time of the bite.

(D) The toxicity of the venom is the prime cause of the severe reaction or death.

(E) Subsequent sting episodes usually cause more severe reactions than the earlier stings.

141. Emergency insect sting and bite kits usually contain all of the following except

(A) antiseptic pads

(B) antihistamines

(C) epinephrine HCl injection

(D) tourniquet

(E) tweezers

142. Which one of the following is most appropriate as a primary covering over a small (2 × 2 inch) second-degree burn?

(A) Butter

(B) Cotton gauze

(C) Absorbent pad

(D) Petrolatum gauze

(E) White vaseline

143. Ingredients in Debrox drops include

I. alcohol

II. carbamide peroxide

III. glycerin

(A) I only

(B) III only

(C) I and II only

(D) II and III only

(E) I, II, and III

144. Which one of the following procedures would NOT improve the absorption of a drug into the skin?

    (A) Applying the ointment and covering the area with an occlusive bandage or Saran wrap
    (B) Incorporating an oil-soluble drug in polyethylene glycol ointment rather than white ointment
    (C) Applying the medicated ointment on the back of the hand rather than on the palms
    (D) Increasing the concentration of the active drug in the ointment bases
    (E) Using an ointment base in which the active drug has excellent solubility

145. Aqueous solutions can be directly incorporated into all of the following ointment bases EXCEPT

    (A) Aquaphor
    (B) lanolin
    (C) Polysorb
    (D) Unibase
    (E) white ointment

146. Melatonin is available is some products as a (an)

    (A) amino acid supplement
    (B) sleep aid
    (C) digestant
    (D) noncaloric sweetener
    (E) coloring agent

147. Alphosyl cream contains allantoin, which is present as a (an)

    (A) antibacterial agent
    (B) antifungal agent
    (C) antipruritic
    (D) emollient
    (E) vulnerary (healing agent)

148. Which of the following drugs is NOT available in a suppository dosage form?

    (A) Acetaminophen
    (B) Ergotamine

    (C) Phenazopyridine
    (D) Prochlorperazine
    (E) Promethazine

149. Characteristics of rectal drug administration include all of the following EXCEPT

    (A) neutral pH of colon fluids lessens possible drug inactivation by stomach acidity
    (B) drugs may avoid first-pass hepatic inactivation
    (C) drugs intended for systemic activity can be administered
    (D) the release and absorption of drugs is predictable
    (E) irritating drugs have less effect on the rectum than on the stomach

150. Most commercial vaginal suppositories use a base of

    (A) beeswax
    (B) cocoa butter
    (C) glycerin
    (D) glycerinated gelatin
    (E) polyethylene glycols

151. An excellent choice of diluent for a compressed vaginal tablet formulation would be

    (A) lactose
    (B) starch
    (C) sucrose
    (D) talc
    (E) all are equally effective

152. Which of the following vaginal suppository products have contraceptive properties?

    I. Norforms
    II. Terazol
    III. Semicid

    (A) I only
    (B) III only
    (C) I and II only
    (D) II and III only
    (E) I, II, and III

153. Starch may be included in tablet formulations as a

    I. binder
    II. disintegrant
    III. lubricant

    (A) I only
    (B) III only
    (C) I and II only
    (D) II and III only
    (E) I, II, and III

154. Carbomers may be included in a topical product as

    (A) antimicrobial preservatives
    (B) buffers
    (C) penetration enhancers
    (D) sweeteners
    (E) thickening agents

155. How many minutes is the usual time allowed for the disintegration of most uncoated tablets?

    (A) 30
    (B) 60
    (C) 90
    (D) 120
    (E) 180

156. Which one of the following statements concerning tablet dissolution is NOT true?

    (A) Disintegration precedes dissolution.
    (B) In vivo disintegration is usually a good predictor of dissolution.
    (C) Changing a drug's crystalline state may change dissolution rates.
    (D) Increasing tablet compression will increase dissolution rates.
    (E) Micronization of drug powder will decrease dissolution times.

157. The colligative properties of a solution are related to the

    (A) total number of solute particles
    (B) pH
    (C) number of ions

    (D) number of unionized molecules
    (E) the ratio of the number of ions to the number of molecules

158. Colligative properties are useful in determining

    (A) tonicity
    (B) pH
    (C) solubility
    (D) sterility
    (E) stability

159. For a solution to be isotonic with blood, it should have the same

    (A) salt content
    (B) pH
    (C) fluid pressure
    (D) osmotic pressure
    (E) specific gravity

160. Mixing a hypertonic solution with red blood cells may cause _____ of the red blood cells.

    (A) bursting
    (B) chelating
    (C) crenation
    (D) hemolysis
    (E) hydrolysis

161. Sodium chloride equivalents are used to estimate the amount of sodium chloride needed to render a solution isotonic. The sodium chloride equivalent or "E" value may be defined as the

    (A) amount of sodium chloride that is theoretically equivalent to 1 gram of a specified chemical
    (B) amount of a specified chemical theoretically equivalent to 1 gram of sodium chloride
    (C) milliequivalents of sodium chloride needed to render a solution isotonic
    (D) weight of a specified chemical that will render a solution isotonic
    (E) percent sodium chloride needed to make a solution isotonic

162. A second method for adjusting solution to isotonicity is based on

    (A) boiling point elevation
    (B) blood coagulation time
    (C) freezing point depression
    (D) milliequivalent calculation
    (E) refractive index

163. All aqueous solutions that freeze at −0.52° C are isotonic with red blood cells. They are also isosmotic with each other. Which of the following apply?

    (A) Both statements are true.
    (B) Both statements are false.
    (C) The first statement is true but the second is false.
    (D) The second statement is true but the first is false.
    (E) There is no correlation between freezing points and osmotic pressures of solutions.

164. One disadvantage in calculating isotonicity adjustments using either the sodium chloride equivalent or freezing point depression method is

    (A) D values are not accurate
    (B) E values are not accurate
    (C) it is difficult to locate the values in the literature
    (D) only sodium chloride can be used for tonicity adjustments
    (E) the adjusted solution will be isosmotic but may not be isotonic

165. The main reason why methylcellulose and similar agents are included in ophthalmic solutions is to

    (A) increase drop size
    (B) increase ocular contact time
    (C) reduce inflammation of the eye
    (D) reduce tearing during instillation of the drops
    (E) reduce drop size

166. The presence of *Pseudomonas aeruginosa* would be of particular danger in an ophthalmic solution of

    (A) atropine sulfate
    (B) fluorescein sodium
    (C) pilocarpine hydrochloride
    (D) silver nitrate
    (E) zinc sulfate

167. A second microorganism that has resulted in ophthalmic infections in patients using contact lens solutions is

    (A) *Acanthamoeba*
    (B) *Aspergillus*
    (C) *Escherichia*
    (D) *Heliobacter*
    (E) *Trichophyton*

168. The combination of preservatives that appears to be most effective for ophthalmic use consists of

    (A) benzalkonium chloride and edetate
    (B) benzalkonium chloride and chlorobutanol
    (C) chlorobutanol and EDTA
    (D) methyl and propyl paraben
    (E) phenylmercuric nitrate and phenylethyl alcohol

169. Which of the following ophthalmic solutions do NOT require storage in the refrigerator?

    I. Chloroptic
    II. Eppy
    III. Sodium Sulamyd

    (A) I only
    (B) III only
    (C) I and II only
    (D) II and III only
    (E) I, II, and III

170. All of the following have been included in ophthalmic solutions as viscosity builders EXCEPT

    (A) hydroxypropylmethylcellulose

(B) polyvinyl alcohol
(C) polyvinylpyrrolidone
(D) methylcellulose
(E) veegum

171. The function of papain in a soft contact lens product is to

(A) remove oil films
(B) disinfect
(C) keep the lens soft
(D) remove proteinaceous residues
(E) prevent dehydration of the lens

172. The presence of sodium bisulfite in a drug solution implies that the drug

(A) has poor water solubility
(B) is heat labile
(C) is susceptible to oxidation
(D) requires an alkaline media
(E) will sustain growth of microorganisms

173. Which one of the following side effects occur in some individuals who are sensitive to bisulfites?

(A) difficulty in breathing
(B) a dry cough
(C) diarrhea
(D) dizziness
(E) upset stomach

174. Which one of the following would be most irritating if instilled into the eye?

(A) Purified water
(B) 0.7% sodium chloride solution
(C) 0.9% sodium chloride solution
(D) 1.2% sodium chloride solution
(E) Either 0.7% or 1.2% sodium chloride solution

175. Which of the following descriptions is (are) correct concerning the sterilization by membrane filtration of an extemporaneously prepared solution?

I. Suitable for heat labile drug solutions
II. Convenient for sterilizing small volumes

III. Greater assurance of sterility than using autoclaving

(A) I only
(B) III only
(C) I and II only
(D) II and III only
(E) I, II, and III

176. The capacity of the human eye for instilled ophthalmic drops is approximately

(A) 0.01 to 0.05 mL
(B) 0.1 mL
(C) 0.5 mL
(D) 1.0 mL
(E) 2.0 mL

177. pH is mathematically

(A) the log of the hydroxyl ion concentration
(B) the negative log of the hydroxyl ion concentration
(C) the log of the hydronium ion concentration
(D) the negative log of the hydronium ion concentration
(E) none of the above

178. Data required to determine the pH of a buffer system include

I. molar concentration of the weak acid present
II. the pKa of the weak acid
III. the volume of solution present

(A) I only
(B) III only
(C) I and II only
(D) II and III only
(E) I, II, and III

179. pH is equal to pKa at

(A) pH 1
(B) pH 7
(C) the neutralization point
(D) the end point
(E) the half-neutralization point

180. Units for expressing radioisotope decay include the

    I. rad
    II. curie
    III. becquerel

    (A) I only
    (B) III only
    (C) I and II only
    (D) II and III only
    (E) I, II, and III

181. The decay of radioactive atoms occurs

    (A) at a constant rate
    (B) as a first-order reaction
    (C) as a zero-order reaction
    (D) as a second-order reaction
    (E) at constantly increasing rates

182. A radioisotope generator is a (an)

    (A) pharmaceutic product labeled with a radioactive substance
    (B) ion-exchange column on which a nuclide has been adsorbed
    (C) ionization chamber
    (D) high-energy–yielding radioactive isotope that produces one or more isotopes emitting low-energy radiation
    (E) apparatus in which radioactive isotopes are incorporated into biologic molecules

183. Which of the following widely used radioisotopes is considered to be an almost ideal isotope for medical applications and is commercially available as a radioisotope generator?

    (A) ^{131}I (iodine)
    (B) ^{99m}Tc (technetium)
    (C) ^{32}P (phosphorus)
    (D) ^{59}Fe (iron)
    (E) ^{198}Au (gold)

184. Isotopes are atomic species having the same number of

    (A) protons and neutrons
    (B) protons and electrons
    (C) protons but a different number of electrons
    (D) neutrons but a different number of protons
    (E) protons but a different number of neutrons

185. Which one of the following forms of radiation has the greatest penetrating power?

    (A) Alpha radiation
    (B) Beta radiation
    (C) Gamma radiation
    (D) X-rays
    (E) Ultraviolet radiation

186. Which one of the following general characteristics is NOT true for alkaloids?

    (A) Contain nitrogen in the molecule
    (B) Have good alcohol solubility
    (C) Have pKa's less than 7
    (D) Often exhibit stereoisomerism
    (E) Have poor water solubility

187. Which of the following is (are) true of the ergot alkaloids?

    I. Natural source is a fungus
    II. Their salts would be compatible with acids
    III. Used as oxytocic or antimigraine drugs

    (A) I only
    (B) III only
    (C) I and II only
    (D) II and III only
    (E) I, II, and III

188. The degree of dissociation of acids is often expressed in terms of pKa. A pKa for an acid is

    (A) directly measured by titration of the acid with sodium hydroxide to pH of 7
    (B) calculated by determining the acid's buffer capacity
    (C) directly determined by conductivity measurements
    (D) the natural log of the acid's dissociation constant

(E) the reciprocal log of the dissociation constant

Questions 189 through 191

Answer questions 193 through 195 by referring to the following table as necessary.

TABLE OF pKa VALUES FOR ACIDS

Acid	pKa
Acetic	4.76
Acetylsalicylic	3.49
Boric	9.24
Lactic	3.86
Salicylic	2.97

189. Which one of the following acids would have the greatest degree of ionization in water?

(A) Acetic
(B) Boric
(C) Hydrochloric
(D) Lactic
(E) Salicylic

190. Which one of the following acids would be considered the weakest (with the least amount of ionization) in water?

(A) Acetic
(B) Acetylsalicylic
(C) Boric
(D) Lactic
(E) Salicylic

191. To prepare a buffer system with the greatest buffer capacity at a pH of 4.0, one would use which one of the following acids?

(A) Acetic
(B) Acetylsalicylic
(C) Boric
(D) Lactic
(E) Salicylic

192. Ibuprofen has a pKa of 5.5. If the pH of a patient's urine is 7.5, what would be the ratio of dissociated to undissociated drug?

(A) 2:1
(B) 100:1
(C) 20:1

(D) 1:2
(E) 1:100

193. Drugs with which of the following half-lives are the best candidates for oral sustained release dosage formulations?

(A) <1 hour
(B) 1–2 hours
(C) 2–8 hours
(D) 8–12 hours
(E) 12 hours

194. Valium (diazepam) is available in which of the following dosage forms?

 I. Elixir
 II. Injection solution
 III. Tablet

(A) I only
(B) III only
(C) I and II only
(D) II and III only
(E) I, II, and III

195. All of the following OTC products contain benzoyl peroxide EXCEPT

(A) Pernox
(B) Benoxyl
(C) Clearasil Maximum Strength
(D) Fostex BPO
(E) Pan Oxyl

196. Topical products for acne may contain salicylic acid as a (an)

(A) antimicrobial preservative
(B) bactericide
(C) emollient
(D) keratolytic
(E) local anesthetic

197. Which of the following trademarked sustained-release systems are based on encapsulated drug particles that will dissolve at various rates?

 I. Sequels
 II. Spansules
 III. Extentabs

(A) I only
(B) III only
(C) I and II only
(D) II and III only
(E) I, II, and III

198. Drugs that are available as sustained-release dosage forms utilizing ion-exchange resins include

 I. Ionamin
 II. Contact
 III. Fero-Gradumet

(A) I only
(B) III only
(C) I and II only
(D) II and III only
(E) I, II, and III

199. Drug products that utilize the osmotic pressure–controlled drug delivery system include

 I. Efidac/24
 II. Acutrim
 III. Contac

(A) I only
(B) III only
(C) I and II only
(D) II and III only
(E) I, II, and III

DIRECTIONS (Questions 200 through 203): For each of the following drug tradenames, select the dosage strength(s) that is (are) commercially available for oral administration. Use the response key of

(A) I only
(B) III only

(C) I and II only
(D) II and III only
(E) I, II, and III

200. Inderal

 I. 10 mg
 II. 20 mg
 III. 40 mg

201. Coumadin

 I. 5 mg
 II. 10 mg
 III. 20 mg

202. Prozac

 I. 5 mg
 II. 10 mg
 III. 20 mg

203. Zolof

 I. 50 mg
 II. 100 mg
 III. 250 mg

Questions 204 through 207

MATCH the lettered term concerning hypodermic needles with the associated numbered description.

(A) Bevel
(B) Cannula
(C) Hub
(D) Heel of bevel
(E) Lumen

204. Extension of needle that fits onto the syringe.

205. Portion of needle that is ground for sharpness.

206. Shaft portion of the needle.

207. The hole in the needle.

DIRECTIONS (Questions 208 through 212): SELECT the brandname product(s) that may be substituted for the numbered brandname product when filling a hospital medication order. Assume that a formulary system that allows same drug substitution is in effect. Use the response key of

(A) I only
(B) III only
(C) I and II only
(D) II and III only
(E) I, II, and III

208. Trimox

I. Amoxil
II. Polymox
III. Wymox

209. Proventil

I. Atrovent
II. Vanceril
III. Ventolin

210. V-Cillin K

I. Betapen-VK
II. Veetids
III. Principen

211. Coumadin

I. Hytrin
II. Sofarin
III. Panwarfin

212. Tylox

I. Percocet-5
II. Elocon
III. Vicodin

DIRECTIONS (Questions 213 through 303): Each group of items in this section consists of lettered answers followed by numbered questions. Select the letter answer that is most closely associated with each question. A lettered answer may be selected once, more than once, or not at all.

Questions 213 through 224

MATCH the lettered manufacturer with the associated numbered trademarked dosage form.

(A) Robins
(B) Abbott
(C) Lilly
(D) Schering
(E) Sandoz

213. Filmtab

214. Pulvule

215. Enseal

216. Spacetab

MATCH the following lettered manufacturer with the associated numbered trademarked dosage form.

(A) Mead-Johnson
(B) Robins
(C) Schering
(D) Lakeside
(E) Abbott

217. Gradumet

218. Dividose

219. Repetab

220. Oros

MATCH the following lettered manufacturer with the associated numbered trademarked dosage form.

(A) Smith Kline & French
(B) Schering-Plough
(C) Ciba
(D) Parke-Davis
(E) Bayer

221. Filmseal

222. Chronotabs

223. Spansule

224. Transderm

Questions 225 through 227

MATCH the lettered brand name of anesthetic with the numbered nonproprietary name most closely related to it.

  (A) Marcaine
  (B) Carbocaine
  (C) Novocaine
  (D) Xylocaine
  (E) Tronothane

225. Lidocaine

226. Bupivacaine

227. Procaine

Questions 228 through 237

MATCH the lettered dosage strength with its most closely corresponding numbered drug brand name.

  (A) 10 mg
  (B) 20 mg
  (C) 50 mg
  (D) 100 mg
  (E) 250 mg

228. Glucotrol

229. Ultram

230. Sporanox

231. Lopid

232. Toradol

233. Paxil

234. Azithromycin

MATCH the lettered dosage strength with its most closely corresponding numbered drug brand name.

  (A) 1 mg
  (B) 10 mg
  (C) 50 mg
  (D) 60 mg
  (E) 80 mg

235. Hygroton

236. Tenex

237. Sudafed

Questions 238 through 245

MATCH the lettered generic name most closely corresponding to the numbered drug brand name.

  (A) Nizatidine
  (B) Etodolac
  (C) Paroxetine
  (D) Oxaprozin
  (E) Triamterene

238. Daypro

239. Axid

240. Dyazide

241. Lodine

242. Paxil

MATCH the lettered generic name most closely corresponding to the numbered drug brand name.

  (A) Sertraline
  (B) Pentoxifylline
  (C) Methyldopa
  (D) Simvastatin
  (E) Benztropine

243. Zocor

244. Zoloft

245. Trental

246. Cogentin

MATCH the lettered trade name most closely corresponding to the numbered generic name.

   (A) Inderal
   (B) Serevent
   (C) Tramadol
   (D) Tenormin
   (E) Toprol

247. Atenolol

248. Metoprolol

249. Propranolol

250. Salmeterol

MATCH the lettered generic name most closely corresponding to the numbered trade name.

   (A) Nifedipine
   (B) Enalapril
   (C) Diflunisal
   (D) Ramipril
   (E) Misoprostol

251. Dolobid

252. Procardia

253. Cytotec

254. Altace

255. Vasotec

Questions 256 through 259

MATCH the lettered drug brand name having the same active therapeutic ingredient as the numbered drug brand name.

   (A) Procan SR
   (B) Calan
   (C) Esidrix
   (D) Sorbitrate
   (E) Ventolin

256. Pronestyl

257. Isordil

258. Proventil

259. Isoptin

Questions 260 through 263

   (A) ERYC
   (B) Nilstat
   (C) Larobec
   (D) Erythrocin
   (E) Lithane

260. Pediamycin

261. Eskalith

262. E-Mycin

263. Mycostatin

Questions 264 through 268

MATCH the lettered trade name of each of the following topical decongestant products with the related numbered nonproprietary name.

   (A) Benzedrex
   (B) Duration
   (C) Privine
   (D) Neo-Synephrine Extra
   (E) Otrivin

264. Phenylephrine

265. Propylhexedrine

266. Oxymetazoline

267. Naphazoline

268. Xylometazoline

Questions 269 through 273

MATCH the lettered antacid ingredients with the corresponding numbered commercial antacid product.

(A) Aluminum hydroxide
(B) Mixture of aluminum and magnesium hydroxides
(C) Mixture of aluminum hydroxide, magnesium trisilicate, and sodium bicarbonate
(D) Calcium carbonate
(E) Sodium bicarbonate

269. Amphojel suspension

270. Gaviscon tablets

271. Mylanta suspension

272. Titralac tablets

273. Maalox suspension

Questions 274 through 277

MATCH the lettered manufacturer with the associated numbered parenteral syringe system.

(A) Lyphomed
(B) Pfizer
(C) Roche
(D) Squibb
(E) Wyeth

274. Bristoject

275. Isoject

276. Tubex

277. Unimatic

Questions 278 through 280

MATCH the lettered manufacturer with the associated numbered parenteral container system.

(A) Abbott
(B) Baxter

(C) Lilly
(D) McGaw
(E) Wyeth

278. Excell

279. Lifecare

280. Viaflex

Questions 281 through 284

MATCH the lettered nonproprietary name with the associated numbered vitamin B.

(A) Cyanocobalamin
(B) Pyridoxine
(C) Thiamine
(D) Riboflavin
(E) Pantothenic acid

281. B_1

282. B_2

283. B_6

284. B_{12}

Questions 285 through 287

Alcohol has many pharmaceutical uses and is available in several concentrations. MATCH the lettered concentration (% V/V) with the associated numbered official product.

(A) 49%
(B) 70%
(C) 92%
(D) 95%
(E) 100%

285. Alcohol

286. Diluted Alcohol

287. Rubbing Alcohol

Questions 288 through 291

As a pharmacist you may be asked for advice in selecting a suitable product for a skin condition. MATCH the lettered OTC ointment with the most appropriate numbered request.

    (A) Calamine
    (B) Hydrogen peroxide
    (C) Coal tar
    (D) Ichthammol
    (E) Sulfur

288. To treat inflammation and boils

289. An astringent/protective

290. To treat a mild case of scabies

291. To treat a mild eczematic condition

DIRECTIONS (Questions 292 through 295): It is often desirable to formulate a dosage form so that its pH approximates that of the area to which it is administered. MATCH the lettered pH value that is nearest to the pH usually found in the numbered body areas. Answers may be used once, more than once, or not at all.

    (A) 4.0–4.5
    (B) 5.5
    (C) 6.4
    (D) 7.0
    (E) 7.4

292. Blood

293. Eye

294. Skin

295. Vagina

Questions 296 through 299

MATCH the lettered formulation design that best describes the mechanism of release for each of the following sustained-release drug delivery systems.

    (A) Encapsulated dissolution
    (B) Ion-exchange
    (C) Matrix diffusion
    (D) Matrix dissolution
    (E) Osmotic pump

296. Drug is bound to a resin and released due to changes in pH

297. Drug is compressed into tablets with a slowly soluble polymer

298. Drug is compressed into tablets with an insoluble polymer

299. Drug particles are microencapsulated and a mixture of the particles is placed into the dosage form.

Questions 300 through 303

MATCH the numbered delayed-release or sustained-action principle with the corresponding lettered drug product.

    (A) Ornade
    (B) Tussionex
    (C) Rynatan
    (D) Demazin Repetab
    (E) Procan SR

300. Ion-exchange resin

301. Matrix diffusion

302. Tablet with inner core

303. Complexation with tannic acid

Answers and Explanations

1. **(A)** Official standards in the form of drug monographs are presented in the United States Pharmacopeia/National Formulary (USP/NF). These monographs may describe therapeutically active drugs or other ingredients, known as excipients, that are essential for formulating a stable drug product. *(24:116)*

2. **(D)** Pharmaceutical excipients are selected for specific characteristics that will improve the drug formulation. This includes solvents (glycerin), ointment bases (petrolatum), tablet diluents (lactose), antioxidants (sodium bisulfite), and antimicrobial preservatives (the parabens). Because they must be relatively inert therapeutically, the local anesthetic benzocaine would not be suitable. *(24:111)*

3. **(C)** A container that reduces light transmission in the range between 290 and 450 nanometers to the level specified in the USP may be considered light resistant and suitable protection from light. The container may be constructed of glass or plastic. Although amber units are most common, other colored or opaque containers may meet the official requirements. *(18c:VI–5)*

4. **(D)** The NBS specifications state that a graduate shall have an initial interval of not less than one-fifth nor more than one-fourth of the capacity of the graduate. Therefore, a 100-mL graduate would probably have either a 20- or 25-mL calibration mark as the initial calibration. This regulation is intended to discourage small-volume measurements in large graduates when a smaller graduate should be used. For some measurements, the conical graduate is less accurate than the cylindrical graduate. NBS specifications state that graduates holding 10 mL or less must be cylindrical. Whatever the shape and size of the graduate, one should not attempt to measure volumes less than one-fourth to one-fifth of the total capacity. *(1:73)*

5. **(B)** The rest point is the position at which the indicator pointer on a balance rests when the weights on the pans are in equilibrium. In current practice, it is more convenient and faster to simply observe the swinging of the pointer. When it swings equal distance in both directions, the weights are in equilibrium. All of the other choices are important tests to evaluate the accuracy of a prescription balance. *(1:70)*

6. **(B)** A cold place indicates a temperature not exceeding 8° C (46° F). A refrigerator is a cold place in which the temperature is maintained between 2 and 8° C (36–46° F).

    A cool place refers to areas maintained between 8 and 15°. A freezer is defined as a storage area held between −10 and −20°. *(18c:VI–6; 24:146)*

7. **(A)** Naturally occurring alkaloids which are weak organic bases have relatively poor water solubility but are soluble in alcohol. Most pharmaceutical products use the alkaloid salts such as morphine HCl, cocaine HCl, and atropine sulfate to increase the drugs' water solubility. *(1:398)*

8. **(E)** Valences of atoms do not accurately reflect the solubility characteristics of chemicals. *(12:215)*

(A and D–both incorrect) Dielectric constants and solubility parameters of solutes and solvents reflect relative polarities. The closer the solute and solvent values, the greater the potential solubility. *(12:219,224)*

(B and C–both incorrect) The pKa of a weak acid or base and the pH of the final solution will determine the species of chemical that will be present and the corresponding degree or extent of solubility. *(12:234)*

9. **(C)** Federal drug laws and regulations are described in the *USP Dispensing Information (DI)*, Volume III, which also contains listings of therapeutic equivalent drugs and drugs that are biologically inequivalent. The latter information is from the FDA's "Orange Book." *(18c:VI–52)*

10. **(B)** Volume II of the *USP DI* contains drug monographs written for the layperson. Pharmacists have permission to photocopy individual drug descriptions for distribution to the patient when dispensing the drug. Volume I of the *USP DI* contains drug information for health professionals. It includes more detailed and more scientific information than Volume II. *(18b; 18c)*

11. **(C)** For example, boric acid solubility in water is expressed as 1:18. This indicates that 1 gram of boric acid added to exactly 18 mL of purified water will result in a saturated solution. When compounding, it is advisable to use excess solvent because saturated solutions are difficult to prepare and may precipitate if there are changes in temperature. *(1:194)*

12. **(D)** When expiration dates are expressed only in terms of month and year, the intended expiration date is the end of the last day of the stated month. *(1:639)*

13. **(E)** The expiration date for a pharmaceutical is based on the length of time during which the product continues to meet the specified monograph requirements. Requirements are stated in terms of amount of active ingredient that is present as determined by suitable assay. Most drug products are considered us-

able until approximately 10% of the drug or drug activity has been lost. However, some monographs specify other ranges. For example, digoxin tablets must assay between 92% and 108% of label claim. *(1:639)*

14. **(A)** Allopathy is the treating of disease by using remedies that produce effects on the body that differ from those produced by the disease. This new set of conditions is incompatible with or antagonistic to the original symptoms of the disease. The term is now used when referring to standard or orthodox medical practice. *(1:840; 27:47)*

(C–incorrect) Naturopathy indicates healing by the exclusive use of natural remedies (heat, light, vegetables, fruits, etc.) but no surgery or drugs.

(D) Nutraceutical practice is one in which foods are used to promote healing and health.

15. **(C)** Homeopathy involves the use of substances that produce symptoms similar to the symptoms of the disease (the law of similar). The drugs used, mainly herbals, are administered as very high dilutions, that is, in extremely low doses. *(27:721)*

(B–incorrect) Holistic medicine refers to therapies that treat the whole person—both mind and body. *(1:840)*

16. **(C)** A chelating agent is a compound formed by the combination of an electron donor with a metal ion to form a ring structure. The molecule that forms the ring structure is called a ligand or chelating agent. The metals that may be chelated must have valences of two or more. A major pharmaceutical use for chelating agents is to bind trace metals such as iron and copper that would otherwise catalyze oxidation of active drugs. Edetate (ethylenediamine tetra-acetic acid) is commonly used in parenteral solutions. *(24:118)*

17. **(B)** Edetate calcium disodium (Versenate) is usually administered by intramuscular parenteral injection to reduce blood levels and depot stores of lead in acute and chronic lead poisoning and lead encephalopathy. The chelate formed with lead is stable, water-

soluble, and readily excreted by the kidneys. The other choices, lithium and sodium, are monovalent ions and will not complex with EDTA. *(1:935)*

18. **(C)** Haloperidol is a butyrophenone derivative and the base form has very poor water solubility (1 g in more than 10,000 mL). The hydrochloride salt is water soluble, as is the lactate salt, which is utilized in preparing the aqueous injection of haloperidol. Haloperidol decanoate is the ester form that is dissolved in an oil vehicle. This injection product is injected intramuscularly and has a half-life of approximately 3 weeks. *(1:1184)*

19. **(B)** Epinephrine, a catecholamine, is very sensitive to oxidation, which results in biologically inactive products. The first indication of oxidation is the development of a pink color that darkens to form a brown precipitate. *(1:989)*

20. **(A)** Aminophylline consists of theophylline, which has been reacted with ethylenediamine to improve its water solubility. On exposure to air, carbon dioxide is absorbed and free theophylline forms. Addition of small amounts of ethylenediamine redissolves these crystals. A note in the monograph for Aminophylline Injection USP states: Do not use the injection if crystals have separated. *(1:972)*

21. **(C)** The term trituration usually refers to reducing the particle size of powders often in a mortar and pestle. However, trituration has also been used to describe the simple mixing of two or more powders in the mortar. *(1:1612)*

    (A–incorrect) Levigation is the process of reducing the particle size of solids by adding a small amount of a liquid or an ointment base to make a paste, which is then rubbed with a spatula on an ointment tile. *(1:1612)*

    (B-incorrect) Sublimation is the conversion of a solid to a vapor without passing through a liquid phase. *(1:1612)*

    (D–incorrect) Pulverization by intervention is a process for reducing particle size by using a second agent that can then be readily

removed. For example, camphor is reduced by the intervention of alcohol. *(1:1612)*

    (E–incorrect) Maceration is an extraction process in which the ground drug is soaked in a solvent until the cellular structure is penetrated and the soluble constituents have been dissolved. *(1:1521)*

22. **(B)** Powders that are either directly applied to the skin or are incorporated into topical products should be extremely fine or impalpable. Trituration is often needed to reduce particles to an extremely fine size so that the patient will not discern individual particles when the product is rubbed on the skin. Usually a particle size of 50 microns or smaller is desired.

23. **(C)** Cafergot is available as tablets (1 mg ergotamine tartrate + 100 mg caffeine) and suppositories (2 mg ergotamine tartrate + 100 mg caffeine). Other ergot-containing products include Ergomar and Wigraine. Ergot is classified as an antimigraine agent. *(3; 10)*

24. **(C)** Chiral relates to the optical activity of a molecule. Stereoisomers of a specific drug may exhibit distinctly different degrees of therapeutic activity. For some drugs the activity or major side effects may be due to only one of the isomers present. *(1:155)*

25. **(D)** Polymorphs differ in their melting points, x-ray diffractions, infrared spectra, and dissolution rates. For example, riboflavin has three polymorphs, each with significantly different solubilities. Theobroma oil (cocoa butter) can exist in four forms, each differing in melting points. Gentle heating of cocoa butter will favor the formation of the stable beta polymorph. This crystalline form is desired because it melts at 34.5° C, which is close to but lower than body temperature. Metabolic rates of a drug's polymorphs will not vary because once the drug has dissolved, the polymorphs no longer exist. *(1:168)*

26. **(D)** Benzalkonium chloride is a cationic surface active agent. In the presence of anionic agents such as soaps, benzalkonium chloride

and similar cationic agents are inactivated because the combination of large cations with large anions of soaps form inactive products. *(1:1264)*

27. **(C)** Hydrogen bonding is an attractive force between hydrogen atoms and electronegative atoms such as oxygen, fluorine, and nitrogen. Although weak, hydrogen bonds can bring about the miscibility of certain solvents or the solubility of certain chemicals. Hydrogen bonding is also responsible for the shrinkage phenomenon that occurs when mixing certain liquids. For example, when equal volumes of Alcohol USP and purified water are mixed, there is approximately 3% shrinkage from the theoretical volume. If one wishes to prepare 100 mL of Diluted Alcohol USP, a solution that contains 49% V/V ethanol plus purified water, equal volumes of each are used. However, one must also remember to use an excess of at least 3% of each ingredient to assure obtaining the required volume. *(12:23,213)*

28. **(C)** Drugs in suspensions are likely to follow zero-order kinetics because the limiting factor is the amount of drug actually in solution. The classic example is aspirin suspension. *(12:286)*

29. **(D)** The equation may be expressed as:

$$V = \frac{r^4 \times t \times \Delta P}{8 \times 1 \times \eta}$$

The volume of liquid (V) passing during a unit of time (t) is directly proportional to the radius of the tube (r) and the pressure differential (ΔP) at each end of the tube and inversely proportional to the length of the tube (l) and the viscosity of the liquid (η). Because the radius is raised to the fourth power, doubling the radius would cause a 16-fold change in the flow provided all other factors remained constant. The capillary can be envisioned as a simple glass tube or a human blood vessel. *(1:295; 12:462)*

30. **(C)** Potassium chloride is an obvious substitute for sodium chloride because it has a similar salty taste, is crystalline, and is an electrolyte already present in the body. However, the use of these salt substitutes is contraindicated in patients with severe kidney disease or oliguria. Symptoms such as weakness, nausea, and muscle cramps indicate excessive sodium depletion. Increased sodium intake is warranted. *(10)*

31. **(B)** IV injection of high concentrations of potassium may cause cardiac arrest. Intravenous administration must be by slow infusion to allow dilution of the potassium to occur. When plasma potassium levels are above 2.5 mEq/L, rates up to 10 mEq/h (total of 100 to 200 mEq/day) may be set. In more serious conditions, with plasma levels below 2 mEq/L, rates of 40 mEq/h (total of 400 mEq/day) have been employed. Available injection forms contain 10–80 mEq per vial. IV admixtures are prepared by diluting these solutions to 250–1000 mL. Oral dosage forms include Kay Ciel elixir, Kaon tablets, K-Lor, and K-Lyte packets. Slow-K tablets have a wax matrix from which the KCl slowly dissolves in the GI tract. *(1:930)*

32. **(B)** Topical dosage forms are used. For example, both creams and solutions are available under the tradenames of Efudex and Fluoroplex. In fact, however, fluorouracil is usually administered by IV injection. It is not given orally because of irregular absorption from the GI tract. *(3:2881; 6:1249)*

33. **(D)** The United States Adopted Names (USAN) Council establishes nonproprietary drug names. The Council is jointly sponsored by the AMA, United States Pharmacopoeial Convention, and the APhA. Because the USAN is not an official government agency, the chosen names are not formally recognized until they are published in the *Federal Register*. *(24:30)*

34. **(B)** A "precaution" is intended to advise the physician of possible problems that may occur with the use of a drug. For example, the use of tetracycline may result in overgrowth of nonsusceptible microorganisms. A "warning" signifies a more serious problem with

greater potential for harm to a patient. For example, renal impairment may require reduction in the drug dose. A "contraindication" is the most restrictive limitation because it refers to an absolute prohibition against the use of a drug under certain conditions. For example, the use of penicillin derivatives is prohibited in patients known to be sensitive to penicillin. (24:51)

35. **(C)** Both *Facts and Comparisons* and the *Handbook on Injectable Drugs* present tables comparing the commercial amino acid injections. (21:26–27; 10)

36. **(D)** The winged (scalp–vein, scalp, or butterfly) needle consists of a stainless steel needle with two flexible plastic winglike projections. The wings serve two purposes: They ease manipulation of the needle during insertion into the vein and then allow the needle to be anchored with tape to the skin. (13:326)

37. **(B)** Hypodermic needle sizes are expressed by a gauge system based on the external diameter of the cannula: the larger the number, the smaller the diameter of the needle. For example, the 21-gauge needle is smaller in diameter than the 19-gauge needle. Generally, the length of the cannula is also specified. This measurement, expressed in inches, represents the distance from the needle tip to the junction with the hub. (13:325)

38. **(E)** Insulin is usually administered by subcutaneous injection into the arm or thigh. Absorption of the insulin is good, and this route is both convenient and safe for self-administration of the drug. Some studies indicate that the absorption rate from the arm is 50% faster than from the thigh. (13:110)

39. **(D)** Insulin solutions have low viscosities, and only small volumes are injected. Therefore, small-bore needles (25G up to 30G) may be used. Short ($^3/_8$″ to $^5/_8$″) needles are adequate for the usual subcutaneous route of insulin administration. (13:327)

40. **(C)** Liposomes consist of phospholipids that when dispersed in water form multilamellar

vesicles. These liposomes can be utilized as drug carriers delivering drugs to specific body sites. Nanoparticles refer to dispersed drug consisting of colloidal size particles with diameters between 200 and 500 nm. After IV injection, the nanoparticles will be taken up by the reticuloendothelial system and localize in the liver. Transdermal delivery systems allow diffusion of drug through the skin into the general circulation. They do not "target" specific sites for drug delivery. (1:598,1673–4; 24:220)

41. **(D)** The pH of solutions is often adjusted during the manufacturing procedure by the addition of either acid (hydrochloric acid) or alkali (sodium hydroxide). The amount needed may vary from batch to batch. Therefore, the label cannot specify an exact quantity. Also, isotonicity adjusters may be listed by name only with a statement as to their purpose. (18c:VI–8)

42. **(B)** Either 5% or 5.5% dextrose in water is isotonic, depending on whether the anhydrous or hydrous form of dextrose is used. (1:916)

43. **(C)** The term "venoclysis" is synonymous with intravenous infusion. (13:115)

44. **(A)** Partially filled glass containers (minibottles) usually consist of 250-mL bottles containing 50, 100, or 150 mL of either D5W or NS. To these bottles one can easily add drug solutions, taking advantage of the vacuum present in the minibottle. Plastic bags are also employed for preparing parenteral admixtures. The plastic units do not have a vacuum but are flexible enough to accommodate additional liquids. (1:1551,1553)

45. **(A)** Intermittent therapy refers to administration of parenteral drugs at spaced intervals. One of the most convenient methods for administration is for the pharmacist to prepare a minibottle containing active drug solution such as an antibiotic added to a diluent. This unit is attached to the tubing of a large-volume parenteral (LVP) bottle already hanging on the patient. This "piggyback"

concept saves the patient from multiple injections and assures high blood levels of the additive drug because the minibottle solution is infused in a short period of time. *(1:1551–53; 13:145)*

46. **(B)** Although the maximum volume will vary depending on the condition of the patient, the normal daily water requirement is approximately 25 to 40 mL/kg of body weight. Daily volumes greater than 3 to 4 L in normal (nondehydrated) patients may cause a fluid overload. A dehydrated patient will require larger quantities. Water replacement therapy (hydration therapy) in an adult may be 70 mL/kg. Thus, a 50kg patient will need 3500 mL (replacement) plus 2400 mL (maintenance). *(24:324)*

47. **(A)** The pH of diazepam solution is slightly acidic (pH of 6.2–6.9). To solubilize diazepam, a mixed solvent system of 40% propylene glycol, 10% alcohol and water was necessary. When diazepam solution is added to an aqueous solution, a portion of the diazepam may precipitate. *(21:333)*

48. **(E)** All three forms, as well as Purified Water, Sterile Water for Injection, and Sterile Water for Irrigation, are official. Water for Injection (WFI) is a solvent, free from pyrogens, that is used mainly by manufacturers. Bacteriostatic Water for Injection is used in reconstitution of powders in small vials. Sterile Water for Inhalation is labeled for inhalation use only. It is sterile and free of bacterial endotoxins. It does not contain an antimicrobial agent except when intended for use in a humidifier. *(18c:III–499)*

49. **(C)** Purified Water USP may be prepared by distillation, ion-exchange treatment, reverse osmosis, or other suitable processes, provided that assay requirements are met. Labels must indicate the method of preparation. One possible disadvantage of ion exchange is the high microbial count which may occur in deionized water if the resin beds become contaminated with organic matter. *(18c:III–499)*

50. **(A)** Wyeth-Ayerst Norplant system consists of levonorgestrel in a silastic polymer. The rods are inserted under the skin of the upper arm and slowly release drug for up to 5 years. It is considered a reversible contraceptive system. However, it is not classified as a targeted delivery system, which would imply the delivery of drug only to a specific organ or area. *(1:1671)*

51. **(B)** Although many of the parenteral admixtures are chemically stable for long periods of time, potential contamination of the products during preparation by the pharmacist is of prime concern. Usually no significant microbial growth will occur until after 24 hours. Therefore, an expiration date of 24 hours is safest unless the solution is known to be less stable chemically. Refrigeration also helps to retard microbial growth. *(13:247)*

52. **(B)** The abbreviation of IVP represents intravenous push (bolus) administration indicating fast injection (usually <1 minute) of the parenteral solution. IVPB requests a minibottle or minibag setup known as the piggyback arrangement. These bottles are usually infused over a time span of 20 minutes to 1 hour. KVO means to "keep the vein open" by setting up a large volume parenteral (LVP) of 5% dextrose or 0.9% sodium chloride injection for very slow infusion. The intent is to allow the quick hookup of additional drug solutions without having to enter the vein several times. *(13:92,145)*

53. **(E)** A subcutaneous injection will come into contact with a large number of nerve endings and may remain at the injection site for a long period of time. Pain will be experienced if the solution is not isotonic. The potential effects of hypotonic or hypertonic intravenous solutions are offset by their dilution in the large volume of blood into which they are injected, provided the volume injected is not excessive and the rate of injection is slow. *(1:61;24:290)*

54. **(A)** The osmotic pressure of the dextrose solution will be approximately one-half that of an equimolar sodium chloride solution. The

osmotic pressure of a substance in solution is an example of a colligative property. Equimolar concentrations of nonelectrolytes will have similar osmotic pressures. However, electrolytes ionize to form particles that quantitatively increase the magnitude of the colligative property. Because sodium chloride ionizes into two particles, a 0.1 molar solution has twice the osmotic pressure of a 0.1 molar solution of a nonelectrolyte such as dextrose. Deviations from this simple theory arise from interionic attractions, solvation, and other factors. (1:164)

55. (E) Osmolarity, expressed as mOsm/L, is included on the labels of large-volume parenteral (LVPs). Those injections with a value of approximately 300 mOsm/L will be isoosmotic and presumably isotonic with the blood. For example, 5% dextrose injection has a value of 280 mOsm/L, whereas 0.9% sodium chloride injection has a value of 308 mOsm/L. One calculates the osmolarity of a solution by first determining the millimoles of chemical present, then multiplying by the number of ions formed from one molecule. One liter of 0.9% sodium chloride solution contains 9 g of sodium chloride (MW = 58.4). The millimole concentration will be:

$$\frac{9\,g}{58.4} = 0.154 \text{ mol or } 154 \text{ mM}$$

The milliosmole (mOsm) concentration will be:

$$154\,mM \times 2 \text{ (ions present in NaCl)} = 308 \text{ mOsm}$$

(1:1615)

56. (A) Dextrose 5% solution has an osmolarity of approximately 300 mOsm/L, as does 0.9% sodium chloride solution. If one mixes in the same liter both 50 grams of dextrose and 9 grams of sodium chloride, the resulting osmolarity will be approximately 600 mOsm/L (D5W = 278 mOsm + N/S = 308 mOsm). Although both D5W/NS and D5W/.45NS solutions are hypertonic, they are safe for IV infusion because the hypertonic solution is rapidly diluted by the blood. (1:515; 23:163)

57. (D) There is the potential danger of suspension particles blocking blood vessels. Also, relatively insoluble suspension particles may dissolve faster than desired if injected into the relatively large volume of systemic blood. Only insulin solution is injected intravenously. (24:317)

58. (B) Except for the lactate concentration and the absence of sodium bicarbonate, lactated Ringer's (Hartmann's) solution closely approximates the extracellular fluid. Although the injection has a pH of 6 to 7.5, it has an alkalinizing effect because the lactate is metabolized to bicarbonate. (1:915)

59. (B) Factors affecting the distribution of a drug in the blood after an IV bolus include the blood volume, heart rate, and injection rate. Assuming that even distribution occurs within 4 minutes, drug sampling may be initiated after that time. (1:616)

60. (C) Not only will an intramuscular injection be painful, but it may cause a localized hematoma. (1:923)

61. (B) The Baxter and McGaw systems use a plastic airway tube that extends from the rubber stopper to above the fluid surface when the bottle is inverted for administration. The Abbott system uses a filtered airway that is an integral part of the administration set. (1:1551)

62. (D) There are two main sites of degradation for insulin—the liver and the kidneys. Insulin is filtered through the glomeruli and reabsorbed by the tubules, where some degradation occurs. When injected by the IV route, the half-life is estimated to be 5 to 6 minutes. Approximately 50% of the insulin that reaches the liver through the portal vein is destroyed. U100 insulin is available over-the-counter. (10)

63. (A) Simethicone is a mixture of inert silicon polymers that may be used as a defoaming agent to relieve GI tract gas. This antiflatulent ingredient is present in Mylicon drops and Phazyme tablets. Simethicone

is included in a number of combination antacid products (Mylanta, Riopan, and Gelusil). A newer antiflatulent agent is alpha-Galactosidase, an enzyme that breaks down oligosaccharides before they form intestinal gas. A commercial product is Beano. *(2a:216; 2b:130–31)*

64. **(A)** Gentamicin sulfate (Garamycin) is stable for 2 years at room temperature. Of the five antibiotics listed, it is the only one marketed as an aqueous solution, ready for injection. The others are packaged as powders for reconstitution. *(21:502)*

65. **(A)** Although vitamin C's main attribute is in the prevention and cure of scurvy, it has been advocated for the prevention and alleviation of symptoms of the "common cold," to facilitate absorption of iron by maintaining iron in the ferrous state, and as an antioxidant in both pharmaceuticals and foods. The fat-soluble vitamin E also possesses antioxidant properties, especially within the body. *(1:1115–16)*

    Vitamin D_2 prevents or treats rickets and is used in the management of hypoparathyroidism and hypocalcemia. *(1:1114)*

    Pantothenic acid is biologically important as a component in coenzyme A (CoA). *(1:1120)*

66. **(B)** Vitamin K occurs naturally in two forms, vitamin K_1 and K_4. Phytonadione (Mephyton) is a naturally occurring vitamin K_1. Menadione (K_4) is an inactive synthetic derivative that is transformed by the liver into active vitamin K_1. *(1:1113)*

67. **(B)** Water solubility decreases with an increase in the number of carbons in an alkane chain. Therefore, the butanols will be more soluble than the pentanols. Because side chains tend to improve water solubility, tertiary butanol would be more soluble than n-butanol. *(1:206)*

    (A–incorrect) The absence of hydroxyl groups in butane would indicate poor water solubility.

68. **(B)** Esters of p-hydroxybenzoic acid are used as preservatives to protect against mold and yeast growth in pharmaceuticals. Toxicity, preservative effect, and lipid solubility all increase as the molecular weight increases. Of the four esters—methyl, ethyl, propyl, and butyl—the latter two are more suitable for oils and fats. They are often used in combination with each other, but these chemicals are slow acting and are now unacceptable as ophthalmic antimicrobial preservatives *(1:1573)*

69. **(C)** Human immune serum is obtained from human blood. It contains specific antibodies reflecting the diseases contracted by the donor. The immunity is passive because the recipient's body does not actively develop either antibodies or sensitized lymphocytes in response to a foreign antigen. Passive immunity does not last long; usually not more than 2 or 3 weeks of protection are achieved. Active immunity implies that the recipient of the biological will develop specific immunity due to an active response to the introduction of antigenic substances. *(24:329)*

70. **(A)** Protection against measles is recommended for persons 15 months and older. Usually the vaccine is administered as part of the measles, mumps, and rubella virus mixture. However, all individuals born after 1956 are considered susceptible to natural measles and should be revaccinated if they are unable to show immunity to measles. Flugen protects against influenza. Havrix against hepatitis A; Recombivax HB against hepatitis B; and Sabin against poliomyelitis. *(1:1425)*

71. **(A)** Antiserums are prepared by injecting bacteria or viruses into animals and results in the production of specific antibodies. When administered to humans, passive immunity against specific diseases is obtained. *(24:329)*

72. **(B)** The immune gamma globulin is used to prevent or modify several diseases, including measles, infectious hepatitis, German measles, and chickenpox. The immunity is passive, lasting for 1 to 2 months. There are also special forms for individuals exposed to

mumps, pertussis, tetanus, vaccinia, and rabies. *(1:1429)*

73. **(B)** Tuberculin syringes are made of either plastic or glass with a total capacity of 1 mL. Despite their name, they are suitable for measuring small volumes of any liquid. *(13:322)*

74. **(B)** The tuberculin skin test is based on skin hypersensitivity to a specific bacterial protein antigen. Tuberculin can be administered intracutaneously (Mantoux test) or by the multiple puncture method (tine test). The intracutaneous method using purified protein derivative (PPD) is more reliable. Generally, the intermediate strength (5 U/0.1 mL) is used. The first strength (1 U) is generally used for individuals suspected of being highly sensitive, and the second strength (250 U) is exclusively for those who did not react to previous injections of either 1 or 5 units. *(1:1433; 9:36:84)*

75. **(E)** Serum albumin is the protein in plasma that controls blood volume through its water-containing capacity. Normal Human Serum Albumin USP, which is used in the treatment of shock or hemorrhage, is available in either a 6% or 25% sterile solution. *(1:913)*

76. **(B)** The labeling on biologicals is required to specify the recommended storage temperature. With few exceptions, biologicals are stored in a refrigerator at 2 to 8° C. *(24:328)*

77. **(C)** Booster doses of the common toxoids are required to sustain immunity. For example, a 0.5-mL dose of tetanus toxoid should be administered as a routine booster about every 10 years or, as a booster in the management of minor clean wounds, not more frequently than every 6 years. *(1:1427)*

78. **(A)** Diphtheria & Tetanus Toxoid and Pertussis Vaccine (DTP) is administered as a series of four injections starting when the baby is 6 weeks to 2 months of age. Two additional injections are given at 6-week intervals, with a final dose given 1 year later. If needed, a booster injection can be given when the child is 4 to 6 years old. DTP must never be given to children older that 6 years because of serious reactions that may occur. *(1:1428; 24:332)*

79. **(E)** Typhoid fever is a bacterial infection. *(1:1423)*

80. **(C)** Rabies is a viral infection. *(1:1426)*

81. **(B)** Passive immunizations are usually accomplished by the administration of purified and concentrated antibody solutions (antitoxins) derived from humans or animals that have been actively immunized against a live antigen. Active immunizations are usually accomplished by the administration of one of the following: (1) toxoids (eg, A–incorrect), (2) inactivated (killed) vaccines (eg, choices C and E–incorrect), (3) live attenuated vaccines (eg, choice D–incorrect). *(1:1431; 24:328–29)*

82. **(E)** Degradation of either proteins or peptides in solution may occur when denaturation occurs. Changes in temperature, addition of ionic salts, changes in solvent system, freezing, or even vigorous shaking may result in minor structural changes that will reduce the therapeutic activity of the protein. Many of the new "biotech" drugs specify that reconstitution should be accomplished by gentle rolling of the containers between the palms rather than vigorous shaking. *(1:1461; 24:354)*

83. **(C)** Both ipecac syrup and activated charcoal have proved effective in the treatment of many types of drug poisoning. However, they must not be used concurrently because the charcoal will adsorb the active alkaloids present in ipecac syrup. Thus the desired emetic effect may be lost. If both agents are to be administered, it is best to induce vomiting first with the ipecac, then administer the charcoal to absorb remnants of the poison. Activated charcoal is usually administered as a water slurry of 60 to 100 g. Often a mild cathartic such as magnesium sulfate is administered after the charcoal. Some charcoal products already contain either sorbitol or methylcellulose as a laxative. *(2:284)*

(E–incorrect) The "universal antidote" is a mixture of activated charcoal, magnesium oxide, and tannic acid. Only the charcoal in this combination is effective, and its activity is probably reduced by the other two ingredients. *(2:287)*

84. **(B)** Chemicals that are not significantly adsorbed by activated charcoal include boric acid, cyanides, DDT, and ferrous sulfate. *(2:287)*

85. **(D)** Although Alcohol USP (95%V/V ethanol) is usually used in the production of pharmaceuticals, labels stating alcohol concentration are based on 100%V/V ethanol (absolute alcohol). Proof strengths of products are easily calculated by simply doubling the %V/V ethanol concentration. *(1:1404; 23:27)*

86. **(C)** The benzophenones are effective in screening out the harmful (skin burning) UVB wavelengths as well as some of the UVA spectra. The cinnamates will screen the UVB wavelengths and a combination of the two categories of sunscreens are often incorporated into commercial formulas. Methyl salicylate (oil of wintergreen) is included in topical products mainly for its pleasant odor. It does not possess sunscreening properties. However, homomenthyl salicylate (homosalate) is a sunscreen. *(2a:620–24; 19:39–9)*

87. **(C)** The SPF (sun protection factor) is a numeric value that indicates the multiple length of time an individual may be exposed to the sun with minimum erythema as compared to the exposure time without any protection. In this example, 30 minutes × 12 = 6 hours maximum protection that may be expected. Obviously there are many variables that affect the quantity of radiation received on any day. *(2a:619–22; 19:39–41)*

88. **(C)** Colostomy pouches are available in several sizes based on the opening that will surround the stoma on the body. These sizes are designated in inches of diameter. Pouches are designed as either open end, in which the effluent may be drained while the pouch is on the patient, or closed end, for which the pouch must be removed to be either emptied or discarded. There is no difference between pouches worn by males or females but there are pediatric pouches with a smaller capacity. *(1:1863; 2:305)*

89. **(C)** Hygroscopicity is the ability of a substance to attract and retain moisture. Because glycerin will absorb water even in low relative humidities, it is used as a humectant to keep creams and other semisolid formulations from drying out. *(1:1041)*

90. **(C)** Although medicinal oxygen carries the federal legend concerning dispensing, many nonpharmacy sources supply the gas to patients under the concept that they are agents of the prescriber. Because the bulky and unsightly oxygen tanks require frequent refills if used at the normal flow rate of 2 L/min, other systems such as oxygen concentrators are popular substitutes. These concentrators use room air and home electricity. *(1:1854)*

91. **(C)** The term "leaching" is used specifically to designate the release of a container ingredient into the product itself. For example, zinc and accelerators may be leached from rubber closures into a parenteral vial. *(24:139–40)*

(A–incorrect) Adsorption would refer to the binding of a substance onto the surface of the container wall.

(B–incorrect) Diffusion is the passage of a substance through a second substance. For example, volatile oil or dye may diffuse from a solution through the walls of a plastic container.

(D–incorrect) Permeation would denote the solution of a substance in the cell wall followed by passage through the wall.

(E–incorrect) Porosity indicates small holes or passages through which a substance could pass.

92. **(C)** Monoclonal antibodies (MAb) are antibodies derived from single hybrid cells. The resulting product has enhanced selectivity, making it invaluable as a specific diagnostic

agent or drug. Gene splicing refers to those procedures resulting in alterations of the DNA make-up of a microorganism. Using recombinant DNA technology, specific antibodies useful for medical and agricultural applications can be developed. *(1:811; 24:337, 346)*

93. **(B)** Most biotechnological drugs consist of amino acid sequences. Because these proteins have relatively poor stability in the GI tract and have erratic absorption, most of the drugs are intended for parenteral administration. *(13:349; 24:352)*

94. **(E)** The thrombolytic agent urokinase is an enzyme isolated from cultures of human kidney tissue. *(1:819)*

    (A–incorrect) Epoetin (Protropin) is a human growth hormone intended for the long-term treatment of children with growth failure due to insufficient endogenous hormone. A similar product is Lilly's Humatrope. *(24:342–3)*

    (B–incorrect) Erythropoietin is used in dialysis, anemia, and chronic renal failure. *(24:342)*

    (C–incorrect) Humulin is Lilly's human insulin. *(24:320)*

    (D–incorrect) The interferons are used in numerous diseases including AIDS-related Kaposi's sarcoma and multiple sclerosis. *(24:343–44)*

95. **(D)** The increased sensitivity of both types of tests is due to the use of monoclonal antibodies (MAb), which allow earlier determination of the specific hormones involved. Ovulation prediction tests detect surges in luteinizing hormone (LH), which indicate that ovulation is about to occur. Pregnancy determination tests detect an increased level of human chorionic gonadotropin (HCG) hormone that occurs when the egg is fertilized. The fecal occult blood tests are based on the colorimetric detection of hemoglobin. Various chemicals, such as guaiac, tetramethylbenzidine, etc., are used to elicit a characteristic color. The occult blood tests are not very selective or sensitive. *(2:34,36–7)*

96. **(E)** The inclusion of surfactants in topical preparations appears to enhance the penetration of active drugs through the skin. *(24:361)*

    Contact lens solutions may contain surfactants for the cleansing of the lenses before storage or insertion. *(24:414)*

    Nontoxic and nonirritating surfactants such as docusate (dioctyl sodium sulfosuccinate) are used as emollient laxatives because they soften stools. *(2a:232)*

97. **(D)** The hydrophilic–lipophilic balance (HLB) system was originally designed by using combinations of nonionic surfactants in the preparation of a standard emulsion. Although some anionic and cationic emulsifiers have been assigned HLB values, the system's primary use is to classify the hundreds of nonionics that are commercially available. In the HLB system, emulsifiers are given numeric designations between 1 and 20, depending on the relative strength of the hydrophilic and hydrophobic portions of the molecule. Emulsifiers with low HLB values are hydrophobic (lipophilic), whereas emulsifiers with high HLB values are hydrophilic. By mixing two emulsifiers with different HLB values, one may determine the best HLB value in a certain emulsion formula. Generally, an emulsifier with a HLB of less than 9 will produce water in oil (W/O) emulsions, whereas those with values of greater than 11 will produce oil in water (O/W) emulsions. Emulsion systems between 9 and 11 will form either W/O or O/W, depending on other formulation factors. *(1:287)*

98. **(D)** Sorbitan monopalmitate is a sorbitan fatty acid ester, commercially available as Span 40. It is classified as nonionic because the molecules would not have the tendency to migrate to either pole in an electric field. *(1:286)*

    (A–incorrect) (C–incorrect) (E–incorrect) These compounds are anionic surfactants. This designation implies that the large active portion of the surfactant molecule would bear a negative charge and, therefore, would migrate to the anode in an electric field. For example, the stearate portion of triethanolamine stearate is considered the active ion.

(B–incorrect) Cetylpyridinium chloride is a cationic surfactant. The active surfactant portion, cetylpyridinium, has a positive charge and migrates to the cathode.

99. (C) Both ophthalmic and nasal preparations should have only mild buffer capacity so that the organ's natural buffer system can overcome any pH differences. Otherwise, irritation might result. (1:1502)

(A–incorrect) Nasal preparations usually have a pH in the range of 5.5 to 6.5. Often, phosphate buffers are used.

(B–incorrect) Rendering the nasal solution isotonic will decrease potential for damage to the local tissue.

(D–incorrect) The presence of an antimicrobial preservative is important because there may be accidental contamination of the dropper or nasal spray tip. (1:1502)

100. (E) The tablets are enteric coated to avoid gastric irritation. They should not be taken within 1 hour of ingestion of milk or antacids because the enteric coating may be dissolved prematurely. (4:989)

101. (D) InFeD is Iron Dextran Injection USP, a colloidal solution of ferric hydroxide complexed with partially hydrolyzed dextran. It is intended for treatment of confirmed cases of iron-deficiency anemias, particularly among those patients who cannot tolerate or who fail to respond to oral administration of iron. (1:938)

102. (E) Polycarbophil absorbs large quantities of water, allowing the formation of stools. There does not appear to be any effect on the digestive enzymes or nutrients. The drug itself is not absorbed systemically. Polycarbophil is present in Mitrolan and FiberCon. (1:899; 2a:258,287)

(A–incorrect) Activated charcoal possesses good adsorption properties but is seldom used as an antidiarrheal.

(C–incorrect) (D–incorrect) Kaolin and attapulgite are typical examples of adsorbent clays. Attapulgite is a colloidal hydrated magnesium aluminum silicate clay. Studies have indicated that it is an effective adsorbent for alkaloids, toxins, bacteria, and strains of human enteroviruses. However, attapulgite and kaolin are not selective and will also adsorb nutrients and digestive enzymes. Probably their greatest efficacy will be in the treatment of mild functional diarrhea. (2a:258)

103. (C) Perdiem consists of granules containing both a stimulant laxative (senna), and a bulking agent (psyllium). Persons sensitive to phenolphthalein may develop a polychromatic rash. Phenolphthalein-induced rashes vary greatly in size and color. Usually the rash itches or causes a burning sensation. Among the other commercial products containing phenolphthalein are Regular Ex-Lax, Espotabs, and Evac-U-Gen. (2b:143–45,152)

104. (D) Pepto-Bismol contains bismuth subsalicylate. The subsalicylate salt is the preferred insoluble form because the subnitrate may form the nitrite ion in the gut. Absorption of this ion could cause hypotension and possibly methemoglobinemia. Bismuth salicylate is safe when taken orally but should not be consumed by patients sensitive to aspirin. Patients should be counseled that black-stained stools that may occur with bismuth intake are harmless. (2a:258; 2b:158)

105. (E) All three products contain the clay attapulgite, which has been proved to be a more effective adsorbent than kaolin. Another ingredient in Kaopectate and Donnagel is pectin, which is classified as an intestinal absorbent, adsorbent, and protective. The belladonna alkaloids formerly present in Donnagel as antispasmodics have been removed because of the lack of proof for efficacy. (2b:157–58)

106. (D) Phenylpropanolamine (PPA) in combination with behavioral modification and mild caloric restriction and exercise appears to result in weight loss. Although phenylpropanolamine appears to have anorexigenic properties, the dose present in most OTC products (25 mg) is too low. The FDA per-

mits doses of 37.5 mg in immediate-release products and not more than 75 mg in sustained-release products. Higher doses increase the incidence of side effects, such as nervousness, insomnia, hypertension, nausea, and tachycardia. Another OTC drug that is considered effective for weight control is benzocaine. *(2a:432)*

107. **(A)** Actron contains 12.5 mg of ketoprofen. All of the other drug choices contain 200 mg of ibuprofen. *(2b:39)*

108. **(D)** Of the three analgesics, acetaminophen appears the safest for use during pregnancy. Aspirin, as well as all other salicylates, is especially dangerous during the last trimester and when breastfeeding mainly due to increased fetal and maternal morbidity. Ibuprofen may also cause postpartum bleeding and prolonged labor. *(2b:61)*

109. **(D)** Excedrin contains aspirin, caffeine, salicylamide, and acetaminophen, but no buffering agents. All of the other preparations contain aluminum hydroxide, magnesium hydroxide, magnesium carbonate, or some combination of these antacids. *(2b:28)*

110. **(B)** Magnesium salicylate is similar to sodium salicylate in its analgesic activity, but there is the danger of systemic magnesium toxicity, especially in the renal-impaired patient. *(2a:64)*

111. **(E)** The usual adult dose is 30 mg every 8 hours, with a maximum daily dose of 120 mg. Individual doses of 30 mg or higher do not appreciably increase antitussive activity. *(2b:150)*

112. **(C)** Emetrol is a phosphorated carbohydrate solution containing levulose, dextrose, and orthophosphoric acid with a pH adjusted to 1.5. Its effectiveness in preventing or treating motion sickness has not been proved but is considered effective for nausea associated with pregnancy. The Emetrol label states that the oral solution should not be diluted with or accompanied by other fluids. *(2a:291)*

113. **(B)** Calcium carbonate is a rapid, prolonged, potent neutralizer of gastric acid. Some scientists and consumer groups have advocated its use because of its high effectiveness and low cost. However, the listed side effects should warrant curtailment of its use, particularly for chronic therapy. *(2a:206)*

(A–incorrect) Some of the insoluble calcium carbonate is converted to soluble calcium chloride, which is absorbed. Significant amounts of calcium may be absorbed after a few days of antacid therapy.

(D–incorrect) Gastric hypersecretion is believed to be caused by the local effect of calcium on the gastrin-producing cells.

114. **(D)** Calcium carbonate appears to be the antacid of choice when formulating chewable tablets. Although both the Titralac and Rolaid products contain calcium carbonate, Rolaids chewable tablets also contain magnesium hydroxide. Basaljel capsules contain only aluminum hydroxide. Other antacids containing only aluminum hydroxide include Amphojel and ALternaGEL. *(2b:134,139)*

115. **(D)** The generic name for Ayerst's Riopan is magaldrate. The product is a chemical rather than a physical combination of aluminum and magnesium hydroxides. Although this chemical form has a lower neutralizing capacity, it is still considered to be an effective antacid with a low sodium level and does not cause electrolyte imbalance in the body. *(1:888; 2a:208)*

116. **(D)** Both film and sugar coats are water soluble and most will readily disintegrate in the stomach. However, the smooth tablet surface makes the tablet easier to dissolve with less chance of bitter drug powder remaining in the mouth or throat. Enteric coats are intended to slow the disintegration of the tablet until the unit reaches the small intestine. *(1:1616; 24:205–9)*

117. **(E)** The application of film coat, usually by spray techniques, to large batches of tablets is much easier and faster than sugar coating, which usually involves several steps. The

film coat usually adds only 2% to 3% of weight to each tablet and is less likely to chip during handling. *(1:1652; 24:208–9)*

118. **(C)** Tablet friability refers to the ability of tablets to resist breaking or powdering when rolled against each other. This ability to withstand abrasion is important for packaging, handling, and shipping of the tablets. If the powder in a tablet has good cohesiveness and is not compressed with excessive pressure, it is unlikely to crumble, break, or split. *(1:1631; 24:190)*

119. **(A)** Magnesium stearate (as well as other stearates) is included in tablet formulations as a lubricant. *(1:1411; 24:202)*

120. **(C)** Tablet lubricants are characterized by lubricity, as they are usually water insoluble and difficult to wet. The waterproofing property might retard disintegration and dissolution. *(1:1618)*

121. **(D)** Aspartame is a dipeptide that is approximately 200 times sweeter than sucrose. Because it provides less than 1 calorie per dose and does not impart the bitter aftertaste experienced by some people after consuming saccharin, it is a popular sweetening agent in drug products and foods. Its tendency to disintegrate on heating limits potential uses. Patients with phenylketonuria should avoid aspartame because one breakdown ingredient is phenylalanine. *(2a:335,436)*

122. **(D)** Because of individual patient biologic variation and technologic limitations of precise control of drug release, drugs with either short half-lives or low therapeutic indexes are not suited for sustained-release products. Almost all sustained-release products are designed for the treatment of chronic conditions in which acute dosing adjustments are not necessary. Hopefully, sustained release products will improve patient compliance by requiring less frequent dosing. *(24:215)*

123. **(B)** Searle's Covera-HS is formulated into a COER-24 delivery system. The 180 or 240 mg tablets are intended for bedtime dosing to in-

sure maximum plasma levels in the early morning. This time-factor design is intended to take advantage of the body's circadian rhythm because blood pressures tend to be higher when the patient arises in the morning. *(10)*

124. **(B)** Products such as Potassium Chloride Enseals are enteric coated to protect the stomach from irritating substances or to prevent drug decomposition in the stomach. *(10; 24:210,220)*

(A–incorrect) Endurets are sustained-release tablets. Preludin is an example.

(C–incorrect) Extentabs are prolonged-action tablets (for example, Dimetane Extentabs).

(D–incorrect) Filmtabs are tablets coated with a transparent protective coating (for example, Eutron Filmtabs).

125. **(D)** Mannitol possesses characteristics that make it an almost ideal sweetener for chewable tablets. Although not as sweet as sucrose, it has "good body," leaves a cool taste in the mouth, and is not hygroscopic. Mannitol is also easily compressed by wet granulation. *(24:185)*

126. **(B)** Sterile powders of water-unstable drugs are often prepared by lyophilization (freeze-drying). Mannitol may be included in the formula to build up the dry powder, known as the cake. The larger, more visible cake is helpful in that the pharmacist can more readily ascertain when dissolution is completed. *(13:36)*

127. **(A)** Benzyl alcohol is used in many parenterals, especially in Bacteriostatic Sterile Water for Injection as an antimicrobial agent. Although its relative toxicity is low, there are a few reports of hypersensitivity. Also, it is contraindicated for use in premature infants because of incidences of fatal toxic syndrome. *(13:17)*

128. **(D)** Thickening a suspension will slow its sedimentation, but it is still necessary to get the product out of the bottle. A pseudoplastic flow is desirable because it is characterized

by a greater flow rate after the system has been agitated. Thixotropy refers to a reversible sol-gel system; it is characterized by a gel that forms a flowable sol when shaken. On standing, the reformation of the gel will slow particle settling. Caking is undesirable because settling particles form a dense pack in the bottom of the container. It is very difficult to break this cake and to reconstitute the original suspension. *(1:295,298)*

129. **(C)** Inhalation aerosol products may be intended for either localized activity (bronchodilators for asthma) or systemic action (ergotamine for migraine). In either situation, the onset of action will be rapid. When the drug is absorbed through the alveolar–capillary membrane, the first-pass metabolism in the liver is avoided. Because of the limited capacity of aerosol units, especially in the small-chamber metered valves, only a limited amount of drug can be administered. *(1:1676)*

130. **(A)** Epinephrine is the active bronchodilator in such OTC products as Bronkaid Mist and Primatene Mist. Ephedrine is available OTC only in tablet and syrup dosage forms. Metaproterenol aerosol products are by prescription only. *(2a:167–68; 2b:123)*

131. **(B)** An ileostomy results when the entire colon (large intestine) and a portion of the small intestine is removed and the remaining end of the small intestine is attached to the abdominal wall. Because of the narrow diameter of the small intestine, the wall opening (stoma) is not as large when compared to colostomy stomas. The fecal discharge is watery because there has been limited opportunity for water reabsorption. Also there are higher concentrations of enzymes present that may irritate the skin. *(1:1864; 22:208)*

132. **(A)** Diacetylmorphine is commonly known as heroin. It is a Class I controlled substance; this means that it may be used only for experimental work by special permit. *(1:401)*

133. **(A)** The first-degree burn is the mildest injury because only the epidermis is affected.

(C–incorrect) These are characteristics of a second-degree burn, which affects the epidermis and portions of the dermis.

(D–incorrect) A third-degree burn penetrates through the entire skin. Damage may be permanent.

(E–incorrect) These are characteristics of the fourth-degree or char burn. Both the skin and underlying tissues are affected. *(2a:635)*

134. **(C)** Benzocaine is widely used for surface anesthesia of the skin and mucous membranes. It remains on the skin for a long period of time because of its poor water solubility and because it is poorly absorbed. Systemic toxicity is rare. Although the possibility of local sensitization should be considered, the incidence is low considering the frequent use of benzocaine. Although the incidence of hypersensitivity to lidocaine is lower than that of benzocaine, prolonged administration of lidocaine to a large skin area may result in systemic side effects. Lidocaine is present in Medi-Quik Aerosol, Bactine, and Unguentine Plus. *(1:1151)*

Although phenol (carbolic acid) possesses both antiseptic and local anesthetic effects, there is the possibility that it may accentuate tissue damage because of its caustic properties. *(1:1412; 2a:641)*

135. **(D)** Debrisan is not useful in the treatment of nonsecreting wounds. Its action appears to be absorption of fluids and particles that impede tissue repair. The product is available as 0.1- to 0.3-mm spherical beads (4-g packets) that are sprinkled onto secreting wounds. The hydrophilic nature of the beads creates a strong suction force; each gram absorbs about 4 mL of fluid. The beads become grayish yellow when they are saturated with fluid; they should then be washed away by irrigating with sterile water or saline. *(1:881)*

136. **(D)** A topical preparation should contain a minimum of 5% benzocaine. Some studies have indicated that 10% to 20% of the drug is needed. *(2a:641; 4:163)*

137. **(A)** The rectal thermometer bulb has a strong, blunt shape that facilitates insertion

into the rectum and retention by sphincter muscles. The oral bulb is cylindrical, elongated, and thin walled for quick registration of temperature. Rectal thermometers can be used orally. The oral bulb is too easily broken and is not suitable for rectal use. The short, sturdy security bulb represents a compromise intermediate shape. *(1:1860)*

138. **(B)** Because fertilization can occur within only a few hours (perhaps 24) after ovulation, accurate knowledge of this event could permit timing of intercourse to either increase or decrease the possibility of conception. Basal temperature (the lowest temperature of the body during waking hours) typically passes through a biphasic cycle over the course of the menstrual cycle. From an initially low temperature, a midcycle thermal shift occurs to a high level, where it remains until it again becomes low premenstrually. The temperature rise roughly corresponds with the time of ovulation. *(1:1860)*

(A–incorrect) The thermometer is used orally or rectally once daily, immediately on awakening in the morning and before getting out of bed.

(D–incorrect) The scale may be either Fahrenheit or Celsius. The temperature rise is only about 0.5° F, which would be difficult to measure on the usual clinical thermometer. The basal thermometer scale ranges only from 96 to 100° F and is graduated to 0.1°.

139. **(C)** One French unit equals 1 mm on the outside circumference. A catheter with an outside circumference of 20 mm is identified as a 20F or 20Fr size. Sizes range from 10Fr to 34Fr.

(D–incorrect) Although they exist, neither the American nor the English scales for catheter sizing are commonly used.

(E–incorrect) The term "Foley" refers to a type of self-retaining or indwelling urinary catheter. *(1:1867)*

140. **(D)** Although the venoms of some insects are potent, the amounts injected are too small to be toxic. The severity of the sting reaction in some individuals is due to their hypersensi-

tivity to certain proteins in the venom. This results in the anaphylactic shock. *(2a:661)*

141. **(D)** Persons who experience severe anaphylactic reactions to insect sting or bites should carry emergency kits. These kits usually contain antiseptic pads (to clean and disinfect the area), both an antihistamine and epinephrine injection (to counteract the anaphylactic reaction), and tweezers (to remove the stingers). A tourniquet would be of little value because the amount of venom is very small. Self-injectable units of epinephrine, such as EpiPen, are also available for individuals known to be susceptible to stings. *(2a:664)*

142. **(D)** Gauze that has been coated with a layer of emulsified petrolatum serves well as a primary cover over burns even if exudate is present. Not only will the exudate flow through the gauze, the gauze itself will not adhere to the wound. Typical products include J & J's Adaptic. *(19:39-15)*

143. **(D)** Debrox drops are intended to clean cerumen from ears. The carbamide peroxide will effervesce, thereby softening the waxy material, while the glycerin acts as a solvent. *(2b:302)*

144. **(E)** Diffusion of a drug from a vehicle into the skin is often related to the solubility of the drug in the vehicle relative to the solubility in the skin, ie, the partition coefficient. Drugs that are very soluble in a vehicle will tend to remain in the vehicle and will penetrate more slowly than drugs with poorer solubility in the vehicle. *(1:713)*

(A–incorrect) Covering the area to which a topical drug product has been applied will often enhance the rate of drug absorption. Sweat accumulation at the skin–vehicle interface induces hydration of the skin, a condition that facilitates penetration of drugs.

(B–incorrect) Poorer solubility of the drug in PEG ointment than in white ointment may lead to faster diffusion. This is the converse of choice E.

(C–incorrect) The thicker epidermis of the palms results in slower drug penetration than that which occurs on the backs of the hands.

(D–incorrect) Higher drug concentrations will increase the rate of diffusion and penetration. *(1:713; 24:359)*

145. **(E)** White ointment is composed of white wax and white petrolatum, both consisting of hydrophobic aliphatic hydrocarbons. This ointment base has a very low "water number." The water number is defined as the largest amount of water that 100 g of an ointment base will hold at 20° C. *(1:1400)*

146. **(B)** Melatonin is an endogenous hormone produced by the human pineal gland. It appears to shift the circadian rhythm and serves as a sleep aid when taken 1 to 2 hours before bedtime. *(2a:184)*

147. **(E)** Allantoin is included in many topical formulations as a vulnerary (healing agent), which is a substance that stimulates tissue repair. *(1:880)*

148. **(C)** Phenazopyridine (Pyridium) is a urinary tract anesthetic and is available in tablet dosage form. Acetaminophen is inserted for its systemic analgesic properties. Ergotamine Tartrate and Caffeine Suppositories (Cafergot or Wigraine) are helpful in preventing or aborting vascular headaches such as migraine. Prochlorperazine (Compazine) and promethazine (Phenergan) possess antiemetic properties. The suppository dosage form of each allows convenient administration when a patient is actively vomiting or unconscious. *(24:436)*

149. **(D)** The extent of drug release and absorption will vary depending upon the properties of the drug, the suppository base, and the condition of the colon. Oil-soluble drugs will be poorly released from a cocoa-butter base because of their high lipid/water solubility. *(24:425)*

(A–incorrect) The rectal fluid pH is essentially neutral and has a low buffer capacity. Therefore, drugs that can be destroyed by the acidity of the stomach may be successfully administered rectally.

(B–incorrect) Drugs that are absorbed through the colon pass into the lower hemorrhoidal veins and into the general systematic circulation. Avoidance of first-pass exposure to the liver may enhance the effect of those drugs inactivated by the liver. Drugs that are absorbed from the upper intestinal tract pass directly through the portal vein into the liver, where metabolism may occur.

(E–incorrect) The lesser dose frequency and lower propensity for irritation are the reasons certain drugs can be administered rectally but not orally.

150. **(E)** Selected combinations of the polyethylene glycols (PEGs) can be formulated into water-miscible suppositories with a range of consistency. They are easy to insert and do not require refrigeration. *(24:437)*

151. **(A)** Lactose is a readily compressible and water-soluble inert ingredient. It also encourages the growth of Doderlein's bacilli, a microorganism present in the healthy vagina. *(24:438)*

152. **(B)** Semicid inserts contain 100 mg of the spermicide nonoxynol-9. The active ingredient in Norforms vaginal suppositories is the quaternary ammonium germicide benzethonium chloride, which decreases odor-producing microorganisms. Terazole contains terconazole for the treatment of moniliasis. *(2b:50,60; 24:437)*

153. **(C)** When moistened, starch will swell, thus aiding in the disintegration of a tablet. Corn starch in the form of a paste will bind powders during the formation of granules suitable for compression into tablets. *(1:1618–19)*

154. **(E)** Carbomers (Goodrich's Carbopols) are polymers with a number of carboxy groups present. When the pH of a solution containing the carbomer is increased, there will be a significant increase in viscosity. *(1:1396,1518)*

155. **(A)** The disintegration times for uncoated tablets may vary and will be specified in the official monographs. The usual time is 30 minutes. For coated tablets, the time may be

as much as 2 hours, whereas sublingual tablets may have specifications of 3 minutes. *(1:1641)*

156. **(D)** Excessive tablet compression may hinder tablet disintegration into aggregates, thus slowing the dissolution process. Other factors that affect dissolution include drug solubility, particle size, and crystalline structure; however these factors may not influence the disintegration rate. However, there is usually fairly good correlation between tablet disintegration characteristics and dissolution, and disintegration times are a convenient in-house manufacturing control. Increasing drug particle surface area by micronization of drugs such as griseofulvin, chloramphenicol, and sulfadiazine have increased their dissolution rates (decreased dissolution times) and improved absorption. *(1:594–5)*

157. **(A)** Properties of a solution that depend on the number of particles of the solute and are independent of the chemical nature of the solute are termed colligative properties. The magnitude of vapor pressure, freezing-point reduction, boiling-point elevation, and osmotic pressure are all related to the number of particles in solution. *(1:206)*

158. **(A)** Solutions with equal osmotic pressure are isosmotic; they also will be isotonic if separated by a membrane permeable to the solvent but impermeable to the solute. Any of the colligative properties can be used to determine tonicity of solutions. Freezing-point depression values are used most frequently. The freezing point of a 0.9% sodium chloride aqueous solution is –0.52° C; the same as that of human blood and tears. Saline solutions of this concentration are isotonic with these body fluids. More concentrated solutions are hypertonic; less concentrated are hypotonic. *(1:207)*

159. **(D)** Solutions with the same osmotic pressure as blood are usually isotonic with blood. Solutions that have a higher osmotic pressure (ie, hypertonic) will cause water to pass out of the red blood cells. Solutions that have a lower osmotic pressure (ie, hypotonic) will allow water to pass into the cells. This causes them to swell and rupture with a release of hemoglobin (hemolysis). *(1:207; 112:180)*

160. **(C)** A hypertonic solution will draw water from within the cell until an equilibrium is reached with equal pressure on each side of the cell membrane. Because of the loss of volume, the cell will shrink and take on a wrinkled appearance (crenation). *(1:207; 12:180)*

161. **(A)** A sodium chloride equivalent is the weight of sodium chloride that will produce the same osmotic effect as 1 g of the specified chemical. For example, morphine hydrochloride has an E value of 0.15. This indicates that 1 g of morphine hydrochloride produces the same osmotic pressure (and depression of freezing point) in solutions as 0.15 g of sodium chloride. *(1:620; 12:182)*

162. **(C)** Any two solutions that have the same freezing points will have he same osmotic pressure and should be isotonic. Because blood freezes at –0.52° C, any aqueous solution that freezes at this temperature will be isosmotic. The use of freezing-point data for isotonicity adjustment for both ophthalmic and parenteral solutions is common in the pharmaceutical industry because freezing points can be measured easily. *(1:620; 12:181)*

163. **(D)** Aqueous solutions that freeze at the same temperature as blood have the same osmotic pressure as blood (ie, are isosmotic with blood and each other). However, to be isotonic a solution must maintain a certain pressure, or "tone," with the red blood cells. If the chemical in a solution passes freely through the red blood cell membrane, equalized pressure on both sides of the membrane is not possible without changes in the cell volume. Tone will not be maintained, and the solution will not be isotonic, though it might be isosmotic with blood. *(1:619; 12:180)*

164. **(E)** Although it is possible to determine experimentally whether a solution is isosmotic with a 0.9% sodium chloride solution or

blood, one cannot assume that the solution is also isotonic. The pharmacist in product development will adjust a solution to the correct isomotic pressure, then mix the solution with red blood cells to observe whether hemolysis occurs. *(1:619)*

(C–incorrect) *Remington: The Science and Practice of Pharmacy* presents extensive tables of values. *(1:622)*

(D–incorrect) Other chemicals may be used as tonicity adjustors. Concentrations of chemicals that are isosmotic are listed in the Remington or can be calculated by simple proportions. *(1:622)*

165. **(B)** Increasing the contact time between a drug and the cornea will often increase the amount of drug absorption that will occur. *(1:1571)*

166. **(B)** Fluorescein sodium is an ophthalmic diagnostic agent. It is instilled into the eye to delineate scratches and corneal lesions. It would be very dangerous to place a contaminated solution on a damaged cornea through which microorganisms may easily pass. If *Pseudomonas aeruginosa* enters the interior of the eyeball, blindness may occur quickly. Pharmacists should not prepare fluorescein sodium solutions extemporaneously unless sterility can be guaranteed. Pharmaceutical manufacturers supply fluorescein as unit-dose solutions or individual paper strips. *(1:1569)*

167. **(A)** *Acanthamoeba* keratitis has been identified in solutions used by contact lens wearers. These solutions were either home-made or commercial solutions that were recycled. Thermal disinfection is effective in eliminating microbial contamination including *Acanthamoeba*. *(2a:482; 24:414)*

168. **(A)** The combination of benzalkonium chloride and edetate (0.01% of each) is effective against those microorganisms likely to contaminate ophthalmic solutions. These include some strains of *Pseudomonas aeruginosa* that are resistant to benzalkonium chloride alone. *(24:398)*

169. **(C)** Sodium Sulamyd is a brand of sulfacetamide sodium. The label specifies storage in a "cool place," which, according to the USP, has a temperature range between 8 and 15° C. However, storage of Sulamyd Ophthalmic Solution in the refrigerator (2 to 8° C) will not damage the product. *(10)*

170. **(E)** In spite of its name, veegum is not an organic gum but is an inorganic clay. It is water insoluble and would probably be unsuitable for ophthalmic administration since insoluble particles could be deposited in the ocular areas. *(1:1571)*

171. **(D)** Papain and Subtilisin are proteolytic enzymes that aid in the removal of proteinaceous residues that slowly build up on soft lenses during wear. Allergan markets Enzymatic Contact Lens Cleaner as tablets containing papain. Subtilisin is present in Bausch & Lomb's ReNu series of products. A third enzyme that has been used is pancreatin. Once weekly, the soft lenses are soaked overnight in solutions prepared from the previously mentioned products. Hydrogen peroxide is the active ingredient in a number of soft lens disinfecting products. *(2a:142; 2b:298)*

172. **(C)** Sodium bisulfite and sodium metabisulfite are included in pharmaceutical solutions as antioxidants. For example, the oxidation of epinephrine may be retarded by the presence of sodium bisulfite, which is preferentially oxidized. Unfortunately, some individuals are sensitive to the bisulfites and must avoid products containing them. The labels of many wines caution about the presence of bisulfites. *(1:1381)*

173. **(A)** One of the first signs of sensitivity to bisulfites is difficulty in breathing. Also, the patient may experience hives, abdominal pain, and wheezing. *(24:117)*

174. **(A)** Investigators have shown that solutions with a range of sodium chloride concentrations from 0.5% to 1.8% can be tolerated by the eye. Purified water will sting because it has such a low tonicity. *(1:1571)*

175. (C) Because membrane filtration does not involve heat, it is suitable for drug solutions that either are sensitive to heat or have not been studied sufficently concerning their heat stability. The pharmacist may purchase presterilized filter units such as Millipore's Millex through which 15 to 100 mL of solution can be filtered. However, autoclaving is still considered the most reliable sterilization procedure. *(13:68–70)*

176. (A) The capacity of the cul-de-sac is estimated to be not more than 0.03 mL, with a normal tear volume of approximately 0.007 mL. Probably less than 0.02 mL of an ophthalmic solution can be placed successfully in an eye at one time. This volume is less than the nominal 0.05 mL (1 drop) usually requested in prescription directions. This implies that a portion of the dose is lost through drainage or overflow onto the cheek. *(1:1565)*

177. (D) By definition. *(1:221; 12:150)*

178. (C) The Henderson-Hasselbalch equation, or buffer equation for a weak acid and its corresponding salt, is represented by:

$$pH = pKa + \log \frac{salt}{acid}$$

where pKa is the negative log of the dissociation constant of the weak acid and salt/acid is the ratio of the molar concentrations of salt and acid in the system. The volume of the solution is not critical because the chemical concentrations are already expressed in terms of molar concentration. *(12:170)*

179. (E) According to the Henderson-Hasselbalch equation, pH will equal pKa when the expression

$$\log \frac{[salt]}{[acid]} \text{ is equal to zero}$$

This can occur only when the salt/acid ratio equals 1, because the log of 1 is 0. The point at which the salt concentration equals the acid concentration is the half-neutralization point. *(12:170)*

180. (D) For many years, the curie (Ci) has been the basic unit for expressing radioisotope decay. Now the becquerel is recognized as the "official" unit. One becquerel equals one decay per second (dps).

$$1 \text{ curie} = 3.7 \times 10^{10} \text{ bq (dps)}$$

The rad is a quantitative measure of radioactivity. *(24:460)*

181. (B) Decay rate is the rate at which atoms undergo radioactive disintegration. The rate of decay (-dn/dt) is proportional to the number of atoms (n) present at any time (t); thus, radioactive decay is a first-order process. *(1:368)*

182. (B) Although it is desirable to use isotopes with short half-lives to minimize the radiation dose received by the patient, it is evident that the shorter the half-life, the greater the problem of supply. Radioisotope generators, or "cows," have been developed to deal with this problem. A radioisotope generator is an ion-exchange column containing a resin of alumina on which a long-lived parent nuclide is absorbed. Radioactive decay of the long-lived parent results in the production of a short-lived daughter nuclide that is eluted or "milked" from the column by means of an appropriate solvent such as sterile, pyrogen-free saline. *(1:371)*

183. (B) ^{90m}Tc is available commercially as a technetium generator from various manufacturers in which molybdenum ^{99}Mo is the parent nuclide. The half-life of technetium (6 hours) is long enough to allow completion of usual diagnostic procedures for which it is used, yet short enough to minimize the radiation dose to the patient. Lack of a beta component in its radiation further decreases the dose delivered to the patient. The gamma energy is weak enough to achieve good collimation, yet strong enough to penetrate tissue sufficiently to permit deep-organ scanning. *(1:371)*

184. (E) The number of protons in the nucleus of an atom defines its atomic number. This is equal to the number of orbital electrons. The atomic weight or mass number of an element is equal to the number of protons and neutrons in the nucleus. Isotopes are species of nuclides that possess the same number of protons (ie, atomic number) but a different number of neutrons (hence, a different mass number). Isotopes represent the same chemical element, and therefore have the same chemical properties. *(1:365)*

185. (C) Gamma radiation, x-rays, and ultraviolet radiation are forms of electromagnetic radiation and are radiated as photons or quanta of energy. These forms of radiation differ only in wave length and are the most penetrating types of radiation. Gamma rays are the most penetrating of all and can easily penetrate more than a foot of tissue and several inches of lead. *(1:379)*

(A–incorrect) Alpha radiation is particulate radiation consisting of two protons and two neutrons. The range of alpha particles is about 5 cm in air and less than 100 microns in tissue.

(B–incorrect) Beta radiation is also particulate radiation, but exists as two types, the negative electron (negatron) and the positive electron (positron). Both may have a range of over 10 feet in air and up to about 1 mm in tissue.

186. (C) Most alkaloids have a pKa of above 7; therefore, they are weak bases that will form salts with a acid of (eg, pilocarpine hydrochloride, morphine sulfate). *(1:398)*

(D–incorrect) Stereoisomerism is common in alkaloid structures; large differences in therapeutic activity can be expected among isomers.

187. (E) Natural ergot alkaloids are morbid fungus growths on various plants, including rye, wheat, and barley. The ergots are marketed as acid salts (ergotamine tartrate, ergonovine maleate, etc); therefore, they would be stable in acid media. *(1:405)*

188. (E) Values for dissociation constants are always less than 1 and expressed as exponential notations. To provide whole numbers for ease of comparison and calculation, the reciprocal log of the dissociation constant $(1/\log Ka)$ or $(-\log Ka)$ is used to express acid strength. For example, the Ka of acetic acid is 1.75×10^{-5}. The pKa of acetic acid may be calculated as:

$$
\begin{aligned}
pKa &= -\log Ka \\
&= -(\log 1.75 \times 10^{-5)} \\
&= -(\log 1.75 + \log 1 \times 10^{-5}) \\
&= -(0.24 - 5) \\
&= -(-4.76) \\
&= 4.76 \qquad\qquad (12:145,169)
\end{aligned}
$$

189. (C) Hydrochloric acid is classified as a strong acid. Strong acids ionize almost completely into hydronium ions and the corresponding anions. Other strong acids are sulfuric and nitric. These acids do not have pKa values listed because the values would be close to 0. The fact that all of the other acids listed in the question have pKas indicate that they are weaker acids (with less ionization) than hydrochloric acid. *(12:147,154)*

190. (C) Strong acids have larger ionization constants than weak acids. Because the pKa is the reciprocal of the log of the ionization constant, stronger acids have lower pKas than weaker acids. Of the acids listed, boric acid has the highest pKa; thus, it is the weakest of these acids. Salicylic acid, which has the lowest pKa on the list, is the strongest. *(12:146)*

191. (D) A buffer system consists of a weak acid or base and its corresponding strong salt. In preparing a buffer system, one should choose an acid or a base with a pKa close to the desired pH. For example, lactic acid and sodium lactate can be combined to obtain a pH of exactly 4.0. The needed molar concentration of each may be calculated by using the Henderson-Hasselbalch equation. *(1:225; 12:173)*

192. (B) For determining the ratio of a weak acid to its salt present at a given pH, the Henderson-Hasselbalch equation is used.

$$pH = pKa + \log \frac{[disassociated]}{[undisassociated]}$$

If the values for pH and pKa are used in this equation, it can be seen that the ratio of the dissociated form of the drug to the undissociated form will be the antilog of 2, a numeric value of 100. *(24:58)*

193. **(C)** Sustained-release dosage forms are intended to reduce dosing frequency while maintaining relatively consistent blood levels of the drug. The duration of activity of drugs with half-lives between 2 and 8 hours can be extended to obtain convenient once- or twice-daily dosing. Although it would be desirable to increase the therapeutic duration of those drugs with half-lives of less than 2 hours, the required high drug-release rates and high drug concentration in the dosage form reservoir usually preclude sustained-release dosage formulation. Also, individual biologic variation could result in either sub- or hyper-therapeutic blood levels. Drugs with half-lives greater than 8 hours usually have long intervals between dosing, making sustained-release formulations unnecessary. *(1:1665)*

194. **(D)** Valium tablets are available in strengths of 2, 5, and 10 mg. The injection solution is supplied as 2 mL ampules and 10 mL vials, both containing 5 mg/mL concentration of drug. Because of limited water solubility, the injection solution has a mixed solvent system of 40% propylene glycol, 10% ethanol, and water. *(25)*

195. **(A)** Benzoyl peroxide is a very effective agent against acne. All of the products listed contain the chemical except Pernox, which is a lotion containing salicylic acid and polyethylene granules. The granules exhibit an abrasive action. *(2a:574; 2b:362).*

196. **(D)** Salicylic acid is a mild comedolytic agent. It appears to prevent and clear both acne comedones and the inflammation due to acne. The term keratolytic indicates any substance that helps remove superficial skin. *(2a:574)*

197. **(C)** SKB's spansule formulation consists of medicated pellets in a capsule dosage form. Some pellets are uncoated to give almost immediate drug release, whereas other pellets have lipid coatings of various thicknesses. Thus, the initial dose is reinforced with additional drug release over period of time. Another group of products based on the same principle are the sequels such as Artane, Diamox, and Ferro-sequels. *(1:1668; 24:216)*

198. **(A)** Pennwalt's Ionamin capsules contain phentermine, an agent used for dieting. *(1:1669)*

199. **(C)** The OTC product Efidac/24 contains pseudoephedrine for use as a oral nasal decongestant. The weight control agent, phenylpropranol amine is present in Acutrim, also an OTC product. Other osmotic tablets include Procardia XL (nifedipine) and Volmax (albuterol). Because the rate-limiting factor in these tablets is the osmotic pressure, drug release is not affected by GI tract pH. *(1:1668; 10; 24:218)*

200. **(D)** Inderal is available as 20, 40, and 60 mg tablets; long-acting capsules (Inderal LA at 80, 120, and 160 mg); and an injection (1 mL ampules containing 1 mg of drug). *(25)*

201. **(C)** Coumadin is DuPont's brand of warfarin sodium and is available in several strengths for convenient dosage adjustments. Tablets containing 2, 2.5, 5, 7.5, and 10 mg are marketed. *(25)*

202. **(D)** *(25)*

203. **(C)** *(25)*

204. **(C)** The needle hub can be made of plastic or metal. It is fitted onto the syringe body either by a locking system such as the Luer-Lok or by a simple friction fit. *(13:325)*

205. **(A)** The bevel is ground to sharpness, but the back portion (heel) of the bevel is left dull. A dull heel has been shown to decrease the incidence of coring of the rubber closure and the skin. *(13:325)*

206. **(B)** Needle cannulae are made of various grades of steel. Both shaft strength and flexibility are needed. *(13:325)*

207. **(E)** The hole in the shaft is also called the bore. *(13:325)*

208. **(E)** *(10)*

209. **(B)** Although all three products are available as inhalation aerosols, Vanceril contains beclomethasone and Atrovent contains ipratropium. *(10)*

210. **(C)** Principen is an ampicillin. *(10)*

211. **(D)** Hytrin is the antihypertensive agent terazosin. *(10)*

212. **(A)** Both Tylox and Percocet contain oxycodone plus acetaminophen, whereas Vicodon contains a mixture of hydrocodone plus acetaminophen. *(10)*

213. **(B)** *(25)*

214. **(C)** *(25)*

215. **(C)** *(25)*

216. **(E)** *(25)*

217. **(E)** *(25)*

218. **(A)** *(25)*

219. **(C)** *(25)*

220. **(D)** *(25)*

221. **(D)** *(25)*

222. **(B)** *(25)*

223. **(A)** *(25)*

224. **(C)** *(25)*

225. **(D)** Lidocaine (Xylocaine) is a (local) anesthetic available as a cream, an ointment, and an oral spray. Lidocaine HCl is administered by injection as well as topically. *(1:1153,1149)*

226. **(A)** Bupivacaine (Marcaine) is available only for parenteral use. *(1:1148)*

227. **(C)** Procaine (Novocain) is available only for parenteral use. *(1:1150)*

228. **(A)** The antihyperglycemic drug Glucotrol (Glipizide) is also available as a 5 mg tablet. *(10)*

229. **(C)** Ultram (Tramadol) is classified as a central analgesic. *(10)*

230. **(D)** Sporanox (itraconazole) is an oral antifungal agent. *(10)*

231. **(E)** The cholesterol lowering agent Lopid (Gemfibrozil) is marketed as both a 300 mg capsule and a 600 mg tablet. *(10)*

232. **(A)** Toradol (ketorolac) is also available under the tradename of Acular. *(10)*

233. **(B)** The antidepressant Paxil (pamoxetine) is also available as 30 mg tablets. *(10)*

234. **(E)** Azithromycin is classified chemically as a macrolide, and the anti-infective is marketed as Zithromax by Pfizer as 250 mg capsules. *(1:1304)*

235. **(C)** *(10)*

236. **(A)** *(10)*

237. **(D)** *(10)*

238. **(D)** *(10)*

239. **(A)** *(10)*

240. **(E)** *(10)*

241. **(B)** *(10)*

242. **(C)** *(10)*

243. **(D)** *(10)*

244. **(A)** *(10)*

245. **(B)** *(10)*

246. **(E)** *(10)*

247. **(D)** *(10)*

248. **(E)** *(10)*

249. **(A)** *(10)*

250. **(B)** *(10)*

251. **(C)** *(10)*

252. **(A)** *(10)*

253. **(E)** *(10)*

254. **(D)** *(10)*

255. **(B)** *(10)*

256. **(A)** Procainamide *(10)*

257. **(D)** Isosorbide dinitrate *(10)*

258. **(E)** Albuterol *(10)*

259. **(B)** Verapamil *(10)*

260. **(D)** Erythromycin ethylsuccinate *(10)*

261. **(E)** Lithium carbonate *(10)*

262. **(A)** Erythromycin *(10)*

263. **(B)** Nystatin *(10)*

264. **(D)** *(2b:115)*

265. **(A)** *(2b:114)*

266. **(B)** *(2b:114)*

267. **(C)** *(2b:115)*

268. **(E)** *(2b:115)*

269. **(A)** Aluminum hydroxide is a commonly used antacid because of its nonabsorbability, demulcent activity, and ability to adsorb pepsin. It is somewhat slow in respect to onset of action. *(2a:207; 2b:134)*

270. **(C)** Magnesium trisilicate appears to be longer acting than aluminum hydroxide. When it reacts with hydrochloric acid in the stomach, hydrated silicon dioxide, which may coat ulcers, is formed. Gaviscon contains alginic acid, which forms a viscous solution, thereby prolonging contact time. The product is claimed to be effective in the relief of gastroesophageal reflux. *(1:888; 2a:207; 2b:136)*

271. **(B)** Magnesium hydroxide has been mixed with aluminum hydroxide in an attempt to reduce the incidence of constipation attributed to the aluminum ion and reduce the incidence of diarrhea due to the magnesium ion. Most antacid products on the market consist of this combination. *(2a:207; 2b:138)*

272. **(D)** Calcium carbonate is often considered the antacid of choice because of its rapid onset of action, high neutralizing capacity, and relatively prolonged action. Side effects include constipation, which may be prevented by combining calcium carbonate with either magnesium carbonate or magnesium oxide. Prolong use of calcium carbonate may result in the formation of urinary calculi. Also, increased blood levels of calcium have been reported. *(2a:208; 2b:139)*

273. **(B)** *(2:206; 2b:137)*

274. **(A)** *(13:290)*

275. **(B)** *(13:292)*

276. **(E)** *(13:287)*

277. **(D)** *(13:292)*

278. **(D)** *(1:1551)*

279. **(A)** *(1:1551)*

280. **(B)** *(1:1551)*

281. **(C)** *(1:1122)*

282. **(D)** *(1:1121)*

283. **(B)** *(1:1120)*

284. **(A)** *(1:1123)*

285. **(D)** Alcohol USP, sometimes known as grain alcohol, contains 94.9% V/V or 92.3% W/W of C_2H_5OH. The remaining portion is water. *(1:1404)*

286. **(A)** Diluted Alcohol is prepared by mixing equal volumes of Alcohol USP and Purified Water. Because of some volume shrinkage (about 3%), the final strength is somewhat higher than that calculated by simple alligation. *(1:1405)*

287. **(B)** Rubbing alcohol is a form of denatured alcohol containing approximately 70% of absolute alcohol. This product is used as a germicide and an external rubefacient. *(1:1264)*

288. **(D)** *(1:875)*

289. **(A)** *(1:872)*

290. **(E)** *(1:1342)*

291. **(C)** *(1:874)*

292. **(E)** The normal pH range for the blood is 7.36 to 7.40 for venous samples and 7.38 to 7.42 for arterial samples. It is essential that the blood pH remains within the range of 7.35 to 7.45. Normal acid–base balance is generally maintained by three homeostatic mechanisms using endogenous chemical buffers (eg, bicarbonate and carbonic acid), respiratory control, and renal function. An impairment in any of these mechanisms can result in either acidosis or alkalosis. *(1:519)*

293. **(E)** The pH of the lacrimal fluid is approximately 7.4 but varies with certain ailments. The eye can tolerate a pH from 6 to 8 with a minimum of discomfort. The buffering system of the lacrimal fluid is efficient enough to adjust the pH of most ophthalmic solutions.

However, some solutions, particularly those containing strongly acidic drugs, will cause discomfort. *(24:401)*

294. **(B)** The pH of the skin is usually based on measurements of the lipid film that covers the epidermis. Although the value varies greatly between individuals and in various areas of the body, the average value is reported to be 5.5, with a range of 4.0 to 6.5. *(1:1577)*

295. **(A)** The acidic pH (3.5 to 4.2) of the vagina discourages the growth of pathogenic microorganisms while providing a suitable environment for the growth of acid-producing bacilli. *(24:437)*

296. **(B)** *(1:1669)*

297. **(D)** *(1:1668)*

298. **(C)** *(1:1667)*

299. **(A)** *(1:1668)*

300. **(B)** Pennwalt's Tussionex is available in capsules, tablets, and suspension-dosage forms as a long-acting cough suppressant. *(1:1669; 10)*

301. **(E)** Procan SR is a sustained-release form of procainamide HCl. Usually three-times-a-day dosing is needed with this product used as a Class 1A antidysrhythmic drug. *(1:961; 1667)*

302. **(D)** Repetabs are designed to release an initial dose, followed by a second dose from the inner core at a later time. This type of product reduces the number of doses the patient must take during the day. *(1:1668; 24:219)*

303. **(C)** The Durabond principle consists of complexing amine drugs with tannic acid to form the corresponding tannates. These relatively insoluble drug forms are released slowly over a 12-hour period. *(10)*

CHAPTER 4

Pharmaceutical Compounding

Compounding is considered an intrinsic skill of the pharmacist. Although the number of extemporaneously compounded prescriptions is steadily declining, there is a growing demand for hospital pharmacists to prepare parenteral admixtures. The emerging field of home health care has called on both community and institutional pharmacists to prepare sterile chemotherapeutic, analgesic, and nutritional formulations.

This chapter reviews some of the compounding techniques, ingredients, and calculations that the practicing pharmacist may need to use.

Questions

DIRECTIONS (Questions 1 through 79): Each of the numbered items or incomplete statements in this section is followed by answers or by completions of the statement. Select the ONE lettered answer or completion that is BEST in each case.

1. The prescription balance needed for weighing chemicals is currently designated as a Class _____ balance by the NBS.

    (A) I
    (B) II
    (C) III
    (D) P
    (E) Q

2. The USP describes several tests for evaluating prescription balances. These tests include all of the following EXCEPT

    (A) arm ratio
    (B) rest point
    (C) rider and graduated beam
    (D) sensitivity requirement
    (E) shift

Questions 3 through 6 relate to the following prescription:

For: James Latimer	Age: 3
Rx	
Sodium Fluoride	500 µg
M & Ft Cap DTD # LX	
Sig: one cap QD	

3. How many mg of sodium fluoride are required to prepare this prescription?

    (A) 0.5
    (B) 30
    (C) 50
    (D) 300
    (E) 500

4. Problem(s) that the pharmacist should anticipate in preparing this prescription include

    I. caustic nature of sodium fluoride
    II. poor water solubility of sodium fluoride
    III. difficulty in weighing a small quantity of powder

    (A) I only
    (B) III only
    (C) I and II only
    (D) II and III only
    (E) I, II, and III

5. The best choice of a diluent for stock powders, especially when preparing capsules, is

    (A) ascorbic acid
    (B) lactose
    (C) sodium chloride
    (D) starch
    (E) talc

6. The pharmacist fills a #2 capsule and finds that the net weight of the powder is 40 mg less than needed. She may elect to

   I. use a #1 capsule
   II. place additional powder into the head of the capsule
   III. use a #3 capsule

   (A) I only
   (B) III only
   (C) I and II only
   (D) II and III only
   (E) I, II, and III

Answer questions 7 and 8 in reference to the following medication order:

Medication Order—Carefree Hospital

Patient: James Gardner   Room 314

Potassium Pen G   2 Megaunits in 100 mL
mini-bottles q6h ATC for 4 days   2mu(4)xu

Note: The pharmacy has vials containing 5 million units of potassium penicillin G that, when reconstituted with diluent, will contain 750,000 units/mL. The label on the vial states that the powder contains a citrate buffer to maintain a pH of 6 to 6.5.   5mu

7. The total number of bottles needed for Mr. Gardner's therapy will be

   2000mu
   ───────
   100mL

   (A) 3
   (B) 4
   (C) 10
   (D) 12
   (E) 16

8. Which of the following vehicles is (are) suitable for the above order?

   I. D5W (pH = 4.5)
   II. N/S (pH = 6.0)
   III. D2.5W/.45NS (pH = 5.0)

   (A) I only
   (B) III only
   (C) I and II only
   (D) II and III only
   (E) I, II, and III

9. Which of the following procedures should the pharmacist use in preparing the minibottles?

   (A) Remove 2.7 mL of vehicle from the minibottle, then inject 2.7 mL of penicillin solution.
   (B) Inject 2.7 mL of penicillin solution directly into the minibottle.
   (C) Remove 6.7 mL of vehicle from the minibottle, then inject 6.7 mL of penicillin solution.
   (D) Inject 6.7 mL of penicillin solution directly into the minibottle.
   (E) Inject 4 mL of penicillin solution directly into the minibottle.

Questions 10 through 15

Questions 10 through 15 relate to the following parenteral admixture order as received in a hospital pharmacy:

Patient: Claudia Smithen   Room 614
dob 4/28/44

Aminophylline 400 mg + KCl 20 mEq in D5W 500 mL

Infuse over 4 hrs at 1000, 1400, and 1800

---

10. Aminophylline is available in 20-mL ampules (25 mg/mL). How many ampules are needed daily for this order?

    (A) 1
    (B) 2
    (C) 3
    (D) 4
    (E) 5

11. When reviewing this order, the pharmacist should

    (A) inform the prescriber that an incompatibility exists between aminophylline solution and potassium chloride solution
    (B) inform the prescriber that the dose of aminophylline is too high
    (C) inform the nursing staff that the mixture must be protected from sunlight
    (D) inform the prescriber that aminophylline will precipitate when added to D5W
    (E) fill the order as written

12. Correct method(s) for preparing the previously shown admixture include

    I. add the potassium chloride solution to the D5W, followed by the aminophylline solution
    II. add the aminophylline solution to the D5W first, then add the potassium chloride solution
    III. mix the aminophylline solution and the potassium chloride solution, then add this mixture to the D5W

    (A) I only
    (B) III only
    (C) I and II only
    (D) II and III only
    (E) I, II, and III

13. The total amount (mg) of potassium administered in each admixture bottle is:
    [K = 39.1; Cl = 35.5]

    (A) 780
    (B) 1180
    (C) 2340
    (D) 4480
    (E) 2240

14. Which of the following commercial parenteral solutions would be incompatible with the original admixture?

    I. Dobutamine
    II. Morphine
    III. Heparin

(A) I only
(B) III only
(C) I and II only
(D) II and III only
(E) I, II, and III

15. After removing the aminophylline solution from the ampule, the pharmacist should pass the solution through a device such as a filter needle. The filter needle is intended for the removal of

    I. particulate matter
    II. microorganisms
    III. pyrogens

    (A) I only
    (B) III only
    (C) I and II only
    (D) II and III only
    (E) I, II, and III

16. Which of the following laminar flow hoods is (are) considered a suitable working area for preparing the previously mentioned admixture order?

    I. Convergent
    II. Horizontal
    III. Vertical

    (A) I only
    (B) III only
    (C) I and II only
    (D) II and III only
    (E) I, II, and III

17. When preparing a parenteral admixture in a horizontal laminar flow hood, the pharmacist will work

    I. with the hood motor turned off
    II. only in an area within 6 inches of the HEPA filter
    III. in an area at least 6 inches from the edge of the benchtop

    (A) I only
    (B) III only
    (C) I and II only

(D) II and III only

(E) I, II, and III

18. Which of the following would the pharmacist consider as suitable agents for disinfecting a laminar flow hood?

   I. Alcohol 70%

  II. Acetone

 III. Betadine

(A) I only

(B) III only

(C) I and II only

(D) II and III only

(E) I, II, and III

19. The American Society of Health-System Pharmacists (ASHP) has developed a risk level classification with the strictest controls designated as

(A) risk level 1

(B) risk level 3

(C) risk level X

(D) risk level A

(E) risk level F

Questions 20 through 23 relate to the following medication order:

```
┌─────────────────────────────────────────────┐
│ Patient: Constance Morehead      Age: 57      │
│   Room: CCU                                    │
│                                                │
│ Morphine Sulfate  ⟩acidic pH.    60 mg        │
│ Hydroxyzine HCl                  25 mg        │
│                                                │
│ Administer stat                               │
└─────────────────────────────────────────────┘
```

20. Which of the following consultations by the pharmacist to the nurse is (are) appropriate?

   I. The two solutions may be mixed together in a syringe in order to administer a single injection.

  II. The morphine injection may be administered by either the IM or SC route.

III. A precipitate may occur if either drug solution is injected into a heparinized scalp vein infusion set.

(A) I only

(B) III only

(C) I and II only

(D) II and III only

(E) I, II, and III

21. Which of the following steps is INCORRECT when the pharmacist removes 6 mL of solution from a 30-mL multidose vial of morphine sulfate injection (10 mg/mL)?

(A) Draw up 5 mL of air into the syringe.

(B) Place point of syringe needle onto the vial's rubber closure at a 45° angle.

(C) Rotate needle so that the bevel opening is facing upwards.

(D) Raise the needle angle to 90° and insert needle through the rubber closure.

(E) After injecting the air, remove 6 mL of solution and aspirate excess solution into an alcohol swab.

22. When obtaining a 3-mL dose from a 5-mL ampule, which one of the following steps is INCORRECT?

(A) Draw up 3 mL of air into the syringe.

(B) Disinfect the neck of the ampule using an alcohol swab.

(C) Break ampule neck by snapping neck toward the side of the laminar-flow hood.

(D) Place needle tip into solution while holding the ampule almost horizontally.

(E) After drawing up approximately 4 mL of solution, aspirate excess solution into the alcohol swab.

23. A filtering device similar to the filter needle is the filter transfer tube or straw. This device is suitable when the pharmacist wants to

   I. transfer the complete contents of an ampule
   II. transfer a portion of the contents of an ampule
   III. transfer the contents of a vial

   (A) I only
   (B) III only
   (C) I and II only
   (D) II and III only
   (E) I, II, and III

24. The pharmacist will NOT be able to use the filter straw with which of the following parenteral systems?

   I. Abbott's Lifecare
   II. McGaw's Accumed
   III. Travenol's Viaflex

   (A) I only
   (B) III only
   (C) I and II only
   (D) II and III only
   (E) I, II, and III

25. Plastic parenteral bottles and bags differ from glass units in that the plastic units have

   I. an air tube in the unit
   II. a vacuum
   III. two entry ports

   (A) I only
   (B) III only
   (C) I and II only
   (D) II and III only
   (E) I, II, and III

Questions 26 through 28 refer to the following prescription:

For: Daniel Cummins   Age: 16

Rx
Codeine Sulfate   210 mg
Dimenhydrinate   1000 mg
ASA   3000 mg
M & Ft cap #20

Sig: i cap QID prn for pain

NOTE: The pharmacist has 50-mg dimenhydrinate tablets, each weighing 200 mg, and 30-mg codeine sulfate tablets, each weighing 100 mg. Aspirin is available as a powder.

26. Which of the following statements concerning the prescription is (are) true?

   I. The amount of codeine being consumed per day is an overdose.
   II. There is a chemical incompatibility between dimenhydrinate and codeine.
   III. The patient should be cautioned about the possibility of drowsiness from the capsules.

   (A) I only
   (B) III only
   (C) I and II only
   (D) II and III only
   (E) I, II, and III

27. When compounding this prescription, the pharmacist

   I. must use a rubber spatula rather than stainless steel
   II. add lactose to the formula
   III. take into consideration the weight of the excipients in the codeine and dimenhydrinate tablets

   (A) I only
   (B) III only
   (C) I and II only
   (D) II and III only
   (E) I, II, and III

28. The final weight of each capsule will be approximately

(A) 150 mg
(B) 210 mg
(C) 235 mg
(D) 360 mg
(E) 385 mg

Questions 29 through 32

Answer questions 29 through 32 based on the following prescription.

```
Name: James McMaster          Age: 4 yr
                              Wt: 44 lb
Rx
  Ondansetron HCl.        0.15 mg/kg/tsp
  Cherry Syrup                 qs 60 mL

  Sig: 1 tsp before therapy
```

29. How many 4-mg commercial tablets are needed to prepare this order?

(A) 3
(B) 6
(C) 9
(D) 12
(E) 15

30. Which of the following statements concerning compounding this prescription is (are) true?

I. It is necessary to dissolve the crushed tablets in alcohol before adding to the syrup.
II. The pH of the final product should be adjusted to a neutral pH.
III. It is possible to use Ondansetron injectable solution in place of the tablets.

(A) I only
(B) III only
(C) I and II only
(D) II and III only
(E) I, II, and III

31. Ondansetron is available under the tradename of

(A) Kytril
(B) Marinol
(C) Reglan
(D) Zofran
(E) Zoloft

32. Which of the following actions should the pharmacist take when dispensing the original compounded prescription?

I. Place the product in an amber bottle.
II. Place a "Shake Well" label on the bottle.
III. Label the product as a federally controlled drug substance.

(A) I only
(B) III only
(C) I and II only
(D) II and III only
(E) I, II, and III

33. When preparing a liquid oral dosage form, elixirs may be preferred over syrups because elixirs have better solvent properties for

I. weak organic acids
II. weak organic bases
III. flavoring oils

(A) I only
(B) III only
(C) I and II only
(D) II and III only
(E) I, II, and III

Questions 34 through 36

Questions 34 through 36 relate to the following prescription:

```
Rx
  Burow's Solution            15 mL
  White Petrolatum            45 g
```

34. The active ingredient in Burow's solution is

    (A) acetic acid
    (B) aluminum acetate
    (C) aluminum chloride
    (D) alum
    (E) hydrogen peroxide

35. When preparing this prescription, the pharmacist may wish to include

    I. Aquaphor
    II. Alcohol USP
    III. Tween 80

    (A) I only
    (B) III only
    (C) I and II only
    (D) II and III only
    (E) I, II, and III

36. The concentration (% W/W) of Burow's solution in the final preparation will be

    (A) 15
    (B) 16.7
    (C) 20
    (D) 22.5
    (E) 25

37. The process of wetting and smoothing zinc oxide with mineral oil in preparation for incorporation into an ointment base is

    (A) attrition
    (B) levigation
    (C) milling
    (D) pulverization by intervention
    (E) trituration

Questions 38 through 41

Questions 38 through 41 are based on the following order received from a hospital outpatient EENT clinic.

Tetracaine	1.0%
Boric Acid	0.5%
Pur. Water	qs 100%

Dispense 60 mL
Make sterile and label as
            "Ophthalmic Solution TET 1%"

38. Which of the following characteristics concerning tetracaine in the previously mentioned formula is (are) true?

    I. Poor water solubility
    II. Chemically incompatible with boric acid
    III. Not effective as a local anesthetic

    (A) I only
    (B) III only
    (C) I and II only
    (D) II and III only
    (E) I, II, and III

39. Boric acid is present in the formula as a (an)

    I. antioxidant
    II. antimicrobial preservative
    III. buffering agent

    (A) I only
    (B) III only
    (C) I and II only
    (D) II and III only
    (E) I, II, and III

40. How many mg of sodium chloride are needed to adjust the tonicity of the formula? The following "E" values are available: tetracaine HCl = 0.18; boric acid = 0.50; sodium borate = 0.42.

    (A) 260
    (B) 280
    (C) 440
    (D) 540
    (E) 640

41. The most practical method for sterilizing the ophthalmic solution is

(A) autoclaving for 15 minutes
(B) autoclaving for 30 minutes
(C) membrane filtration through 0.2-micron filter
(D) membrane filtration through 5-micron filter
(E) the use of ethylene oxide gas

Questions 42 through 44

Questions 42 through 44 refer to the following prescription:

> **Rx**
> Retinoic acid   0.02%
> Ac. Sal.   2%
> Emulsion base   qs 60 g
>
> Sig: Apply small amount onto spots hs

42. Which of the following statements concerning this prescription is (are) true?

I. Another name for retinoic acid is tretinoin.
II. The amount of aspirin needed is 1.2 g.
III. The term "emulsion base" refers to a brand of ointment base.

(A) I only
(B) III only
(C) I and II only
(D) II and III only
(E) I, II, and III

43. How many grams of 0.05% Retin-A Cream may be used to supply the retinoic acid?

(A) .012
(B) 1.2
(C) 2.4
(D) 15
(E) 24

44. Which of the following should the pharmacist use when compounding this prescription?

I. Pill tile
II. Stainless steel spatulas
III. Alcohol

(A) I only
(B) III only
(C) I and II only
(D) II and III only
(E) I, II, and III

45. A physician requests a 0.1% strength of a steroidal cream that is commercially available as a 0.25% strength in a "vanishing cream" base. Which one of the following ointment bases is the best choice as a diluent for this order?

(A) Cold cream
(B) Hydrophilic ointment
(C) Lanolin
(D) Vaseline
(E) PEG ointment

46. When preparing the ointment in Question 45, the amount of diluent that should be added to 30 g of the 0.25% strength product is

(A) 6.5 g
(B) 12 g
(C) 30 g
(D) 45 g
(E) 75 g

Questions 47 through 50

Questions 47 through 50 refer to the following prescription:

> **Rx**
> Calamine
> Zinc Oxide   aa qs 15 g
> Resorcinol   2 g
> Glycerin   15 mL
> Alcohol 70%   30 mL
> Pur. Water   ad 120 mL
>
> Sig: Use as directed TID

47. The final dosage form of this prescription is best described as a (an)

    (A) colloidal solution
    (B) elixir
    (C) O/W emulsion
    (D) W/O emulsion
    (E) suspension

48. Calamine powder is a mixture of zinc oxide and

    (A) aluminum oxide
    (B) F &D red #28
    (C) triethanolamine
    (D) cochineal
    (E) ferric oxide

49. When preparing the prescription, the pharmacist will

    I. use 15 g of calamine
    II. dissolve the resorcinol in the alcohol
    III. triturate calamine and zinc oxide together and wet with glycerin

    (A) I only
    (B) III only
    (C) I and II only
    (D) II and III only
    (E) I, II, and III

50. Which of the following auxiliary labels should the pharmacist attach to the container when dispensing the previously mentioned product?

    I. For External Use Only
    II. Shake Well
    III. Keep in a Cool Place

    (A) I only
    (B) III only
    (C) I and II only
    (D) II and III only
    (E) I, II, and III

51. The following prescription is received:

Rx	
Norfloxacin	2%
Propylene Glycol	10 mL
MC 1500	1.5%
Purified Water	qs 100 mL
Sig: Apply to inflamed areas BID	

When preparing this prescription, the pharmacist should

    I. disperse 1.5 g of methylcellulose 1500 in hot water
    II. use the contents from five 400-mg Noroxin tablets
    III. wet the Norfloxacin powder with the propylene glycol

    (A) I only
    (B) III only
    (C) I and II only
    (D) II and III only
    (E) I, II, and III

52. A prescription calls for 10% urea in Aquaphor base. Which of the following is the best technique to make a pharmaceutically elegant product?

    (A) Dissolve urea in water then incorporate into the Aquaphor.
    (B) Dissolve urea in alcohol then incorporate into the Aquaphor.
    (C) Finely powder the urea and incorporate directly into the Aquaphor.
    (D) Dissolve urea in small amount of mineral oil and incorporate into the Aquaphor.
    (E) Melt the Aquaphor and dissolve the urea in the hot liquid.

Questions 53 through 55

Questions 53 through 55 refer to the following formula:

Progesterone	20 mg
PEG 400	60%
PEG 6000	40%

To make one vaginal suppository

53. Which of the following statements is (are) true with respect to the previously shown formula?

    I. The weight of the individual suppository must be determined experimentally.
    II. It is necessary to prepare the formula suppositories using a mold.
    III. The volume density of the progesterone must be calculated.

    (A) I only
    (B) III only
    (C) I and II only
    (D) II and III only
    (E) I, II, and III

54. The ideal weight for a vaginal suppository will be approximately

    (A) 1 g
    (B) 2 g
    (C) 5 g
    (D) 10 g
    (E) 15 g

55. Which of the following suppository bases melt rather than dissolve when inserted into the rectum?

    I. Cocoa butter
    II. Witepsols
    III. PEGs

    (A) I only
    (B) III only
    (C) I and II only
    (D) II and III only
    (E) I, II, and III only

56. A lotion formula calls for Coal Tar Solution. Which of the following statements concerning Coal Tar Solution is NOT true?

    (A) Alcohol is used as the solvent.
    (B) L.C.D. is another name for the solution.
    (C) The solution is for external use only.
    (D) Solution is usually diluted 1:9 with water or ointment base.
    (E) The solution contains only coal tar and a volatile solvent.

Questions 57 through 60

Answer questions 57 through 60 based on the following prescription:

Rx	
Ephedrine Sulfate	2%
Menthol	0.5%
Camphor	
Methyl Salicylate	aa 0.2%
Mineral Oil	qs 30mL

Sig: gtt ii both sides TID

57. This prescription is intended to be administered into the

    I. nose
    II. eyes
    III. ears

    (A) I only
    (B) III only
    (C) I and II only
    (D) II and III only
    (E) I, II, and III

58. Which of the following ingredients will NOT dissolve in the prescribed solvent?

    I. Ephedrine sulfate
    II. Menthol
    III. Methyl salicylate

    (A) I only
    (B) III only
    (C) I and II only
    (D) II and III only
    (E) I, II, and III

59. Which is NOT true for camphor?

   I. Forms a eutectic mixture with menthol
   II. Can be powdered by rubbing with a small amount of alcohol or ether
   III. Dissolves readily in water

   (A) I only
   (B) III only
   (C) I and II only
   (D) II and III only
   (E) I, II, and III

60. Methyl salicylate is also known as

   (A) camphorated oil
   (B) peppermint oil
   (C) salicylamide
   (D) oil of wintergreen
   (E) sweet oil

61. Salicylic acid is employed in topical products as a (an)

   (A) antioxidant
   (B) chelating agent
   (C) buffer
   (D) keratolytic
   (E) emollient

62. Alcohol is suitable as a solvent for menthol or aspirin when preparing which of the following dosage forms?

   I. Lotions
   II. Ointments
   III. Suppositories

   (A) I only
   (B) III only
   (C) I and II only
   (D) II and III only
   (E) I, II, and III

63. Which one of the following diluents is LEAST suitable for reconstituting single-dose vials?

   (A) Bacteriostatic Sterile Water for Injection (BSWFI)
   (B) D5W injection

(C) N/S Injection
(D) 1/2 N/S Injection
(E) Sterile Water for Injection (SWFI)

64. When dispensing Amphotericin, which of the following statements is (are) true?

   I. The original powder may be reconstituted only with SWFI.
   II. The resulting liquid is a colloidal solution.
   III. The solution is intended to be infused into a patient within 60 minutes.

   (A) I only
   (B) III only
   (C) I and II only
   (D) II and III only
   (E) I, II, and III

Questions 65 through 78

Answer the following series of questions based on the availability of the following parenteral solutions and hospital medication order:

Patient: Danielle Howell	Room: Main 218
Aminosyn II 8.5%	
D50W	aa 500 mL
Potassium Chloride	40 mEq
Sodium Chloride	20 mEq
Potassium Phosphate	40 mEq
MVI-12	1 vial
Zinc Chloride	2 mg
Insulin	40 units
Calcium Gluconate	10 mL

Infuse above TID for 6 days. Add 500 mL Liposyn III 10% once daily.

Available to the pharmacist are the following parenteral solutions:

Aminosyn II 8.5%	500-mL full bts
Dextrose 50% injection	500-mL full bts
Calcium Chloride 10%	10-mL vials
Calcium Gluconate 10%	10-mL vials
Intralipid 10%	250-mL bottles
Magnesium Sulfate (0.8 mEq/mL)	20-mL vials
MTE-4	10-mL vials
Potassium Chloride inj (20 mEq)	20-mL vials
Potassium Phosphate (4.4 mEq K/mL)	10-mL vials
Sodium Chloride inj (2.5 mEq/mL)	30-mL vials

65. The TPN formula is best prepared by

    (A) adding the D50W to the Aminosyn bottle
    (B) adding the Aminosyn to the D50W bottle
    (C) transferring both the Aminosyn and the D50W to an empty, sterile infusion bag
    (D) hanging the Aminosyn and the D50W solutions separately on the patient
    (E) piggybacking the D50W into the Y-tubing of the Aminosyn administration set

66. Which of the following options are available to the pharmacist if D50W solutions were out of stock?

    I. Use 360 mL of D70W
    II. Increase the amount of amino acids solution to obtain the same calories
    III. Use 200 mL of D70W + 300 mL of D20W

    (A) I only
    (B) III only
    (C) I and II only
    (D) II and III only
    (E) I, II, and III

67. A potential problem is the incompatibility between

    (A) potassium chloride and calcium gluconate
    (B) potassium chloride and insulin
    (C) potassium phosphate and calcium gluconate
    (D) potassium phosphate and zinc chloride
    (E) insulin and zinc chloride

68. To avoid the possibility of a precipitate, the pharmacist may choose to

    I. place the calcium gluconate and potassium phosphate into separate, alternate containers
    II. use sodium phosphate rather than potassium phosphate
    III. use calcium chloride rather than calcium gluconate

    (A) I only
    (B) III only
    (C) I and II only
    (D) II and III only
    (E) I, II, and III

69. Potassium phosphate has been included in the formula as a (an)

    (A) source of phosphorus
    (B) source of potassium
    (C) buffer
    (D) antioxidant
    (E) stabilizer

70. The prescribing physician should be encouraged to order the potassium phosphate using concentration expressions of

    (A) milliequivalents
    (B) milligrams
    (C) milliliters
    (D) millimoles
    (E) milliosmoles

71. It is convenient and accurate for the pharmacist to measure the insulin required for this order by using a

   I. tuberculin syringe

   II. low-dose insulin syringe

   III. a 10-mL regular syringe

(A) I only

(B) III only

(C) I and II only

(D) II and III only

(E) I, II, and III

72. The pharmacist may consider contacting the physician to inform him that

   I. approximately half of the insulin will be adsorbed onto the walls of the glass container

   II. a strength of insulin is needed

   III. insulin is available as both a solution and a suspension

(A) I only

(B) III only

(C) I and II only

(D) II and III only

(E) I, II, and III

73. The addition of Liposyn to the TPN

   I. causes the final solution to be cloudy

   II. is intended to prevent EFAD

   III. will adversely affect the osmolarity of the already hypertonic solution

(A) I only

(B) III only

(C) I and II only

(D) II and III only

(E) I, II, and III

74. Other names given to TPN solutions that contain the intravenous fat emulsions include

   I. MCT

   II. TNA

   III. 3 in 1s

(A) I only

(B) III only

(C) I and II only

(D) II and III only

(E) I, II, and III

75. Which of the following metals is NOT included in M.T.E.-4 or multiple trace element solutions?

(A) Chromium

(B) Copper

(C) Iron

(D) Manganese

(E) Zinc

76. Another trace metal that the physician is likely to include in the TPN is

(A) lithium

(B) sodium

(C) selenium

(D) silicon

(E) fluoride

77. If the physician changes the 500 mL of D50W to D60W, how many additional kilocalories will be received daily?

(A) 170

(B) 510

(C) 850

(D) 1020

(E) 3060

78. To reduce the amount of chloride ion being consumed, the physician requests that the acetate salts of potassium and sodium be used. What minimum information must the pharmacist have for these changes?

   I. The molecular weights of both acetate salts

   II. The valences of the ions

   III. The concentrations of the salt solutions in mEq/mL

(A) I only

(B) III only

(C) I and II only

(D) II and III only

(E) I, II, and III

79. A dermatologist requests a prescription for Tetracycline HCl 4% in sufficient Lubriderm lotion to make 45 g. How many 500-mg capsules of the antibiotic are needed for compounding this order?

(A) 1

(B) 3

(C) 4

(D) 8

(E) 16

DIRECTIONS (Questions 80 through 90): Each group of items in this section consists of lettered headings followed by a set of numbered words or phrases. For each numbered word or phrase, select the ONE lettered heading that is most closely associated with it. Each lettered heading may be selected once, more than once, or not at all.

Questions 80 through 86

(A) Hydrocarbon (oleaginous)

(B) Absorption (anhydrous)

(C) Emulsion (W/O type)

(D) Emulsion (O/W type)

(E) Water-soluble

80. Cold cream

81. Hydrophilic petrolatum

82. Lanolin

83. Petrolatum

84. Polyethylene glycol

85. Hydrophilic ointment

86. Aquaphor

Questions 87 through 90

(A) Cold cream

(B) Hydrophilic ointment

(C) Hydrophilic petrolatum

(D) PEG ointment

(E) White petrolatum

87. For an ophthalmic drug

88. For an antibiotic with limited stability

89. For absorbing a large quantity of water

90. To aid in hydrating the skin

Answers and Explanations

1. **(C)** The prescription torsion balance designated by NBS as Class III must have a sensitivity requirement (SR) of not greater than 10 mg. This SR allowance is greater than the 6 mg requirement for the former Class A balance. Most Class III balances have a maximum capacity of 60 g rather than the usual 120 g for the Class A. The pharmacist should check the serial plate on the back of the balance to ascertain the limits of the balance. Obviously a balance with a SR of 6 mg is more accurate than one with a SR of 10 mg. The USP/NF specifies that more accurate balances such as certain electronic balances may be used. *(1:69)*

2. **(B)** The rest point is simply the point at which the balance indicator needle stops. It may be easily shifted by adjusting the leveling screws of the balance. On an undamped balance, the rest point is determined by observing the equidistant swing of the indicator to confirm equilibrium. *(1:70; 18c)*
   (A–incorrect) This test confirms that the two arms of the balance are equal in length.
   (C–incorrect) The rider test confirms the accuracy of the calibrated beam or dial at both the 500-mg and 1-g positions.
   (D–incorrect) The sensitivity is reflected by the minimum weight that will shift the indicator point one unit or mark on the indicator plate. This shift is considered the smallest change that an operator can consistently observe. Therefore, it is the smallest discernible weighing error. The SR specified for Class III is 10 mg and for the Class A balance is 6 mg.
   (E–incorrect) The shift tests check the balance construction, especially the arm and lever components.

3. **(B)** 500 mcg is equivalent to 0.5 mg. Because 60 capsules were requested

   $$0.5 \text{ mg} \times 60 \text{ capsules} = 30 \text{ mg}$$

   (23:61)

4. **(B)** The minimum quantity that can be weighed accurately on the Class III (Class A) prescription balance with an error of not more than 5% is 120 mg (assuming a SR of 6 mg). In order to weigh the required 30 mg of sodium fluoride, a stock powder of NaF is needed. In this problem, mixing 120 mg of NaF with 360 mg of diluent and using 120 mg of this stock powder will deliver the required 30 mg of sodium fluoride. Because of its strong ionic bonds, sodium fluoride is not caustic. A stainless steel spatula can be used for the weighing procedure. Sodium fluoride has good water solubility. *(1:69,884; 23:32–33)*

5. **(B)** Lactose is a relatively inert water-soluble substance that also packs well into capsules. An alternative would be the use of starch. For the sodium fluoride prescription, the pharmacist will have to include additional lactose to raise the content of capsule to a quantity that is weighable and convenient to pack into capsules. For example, a net weight of 300 mg may be selected arbitrarily. *(24:171)*

6. **(A)** Empty capsules are sized by a numbering system, the largest being a #000 and the smallest a #5. If the #2 capsule is too small, the pharmacist should try the next largest, the #1. The correct capsule filling procedure is to place powder only into the body or base of the empty capsule. It is not good technique to place powder into the head of the cap be-

cause the fit of the head onto the body may not be tight. *(1:1642; 24:170–73)*

7. **(E)** The direction of q6h ATC indicates that a minibottle will be hung every 6 hours around the clock. Therefore, 4 bottles daily × 4 days = 16 bottles. *(23:40)*

8. **(E)** The citrate buffer system is intended to readily adjust the pH of each listed vehicle to a pH range in which the penicillin is stable. Although the Dextrose 5% Injection has a pH of 4.5, it has virtually no buffering capacity and does not influence the pH of admixtures. Some hospitals prefer to use dextrose solutions as the vehicle for most admixtures to limit the sodium intake by patients. Other hospitals use normal saline (NS) injection to avoid supplying the calories present in dextrose solutions. *(13:243; 21:843)*

9. **(B)** There is no need to remove vehicle solution when adding small volumes of drug additives. The final volume will always vary because the manufacturer places some excess of solution into each unit. To calculate the mL of penicillin solution required:

$$\frac{750,000 \text{ units}}{1 \text{ mL}} = \frac{2,000,000 \text{ units}}{x \text{ mL}}$$

$$x \text{ mL} = 2.7 \text{ mL}$$

(23:192)

10. **(C)** Each 20-mL ampule of aminophylline contains 500 mg of drug. Because the individual admixture order requires 400 mg, the pharmacist will have to open an ampule for each admixture and remove 16 mL of solution. Even if the pharmacist is preparing all three admixtures at one time, three ampules (48 mL total) will still be needed for the order. *(23:61)*

11. **(E)** Aminophylline injection has an alkaline pH (8.6–9.0), whereas potassium chloride solutions are essentially neutral (pH of 4–7) and have no buffering capacity. Therefore, a mixture of these two solutions will not represent either a physical or chemical incompatibility resulting in a precipitate. Aminophylline so-

lutions are not sensitive to light, nor is the dose requested unrealistic. *(21:55)*

12. **(C)** Because no incompatabilities exist between the aminophylline and the potassium chloride, either could be added first to the D5W container. It would be impractical and time consuming to mix the two solutions first in a syringe and then add them to the D5W. Also there would be an increased possibility of inaccurate measurements. For example, if only 9 mL of KCl solution was drawn up instead of the correct 10 mL, 17 mL rather than 16 mL of aminophylline solution may be drawn into a syringe to make the desired volume of 26 mL. *(21:62)*

13. **(A)** Each admixture container will contain 20 mEq of KCl or 20 mEq each of potassium and chloride ion. To determine the mg of potassium present, use the relationship

$$\text{mg (potassium)} = \frac{(20 \text{ mEq}) (39.1)}{1}$$

$$x = 780 \text{ mg, ANS}$$

[39.1 = atomic wt of potassium; 1 = valence of K]

(23:157)

14. **(C)** The pH of the original admixture is likely to be alkaline due to the presence of aminophylline. Therefore, the addition of solutions with acidic pHs may result in a chemical reaction and precipitation. Both dobutamine and morphine are weak organic bases that are combined with acids to form water-soluble compounds. Dobutamine HCl solutions have a pH of 2.5–5.5 and morphine sulfate solutions have pHs ranging from 2.5 to 6. Because heparin sodium solutions have higher pHs (5–8), they will be compatible with aminophylline solutions. *(21:61,369, 526,537)*

15. **(A)** The pore size of filter needles is approximately 5 microns, which is too coarse for removing either pyrogens or bacteria. Instead, the filter needle is intended to remove larger particulate matter such as glass fragments that may have fallen into the ampule during the breaking of the ampule's neck. *(13:84)*

16. **(C)** Air in the horizontal laminar flow hood flows directly toward the operator, thereby preventing contaminants from entering the admixtures being prepared. This hood provides maximum protection for the parenteral admixture. Vertical hoods have downward air flow, which increases the risk of product contamination but protects the operator from droplets of product solution. These hoods should be used only for the preparation of products that pose a significant risk to the operator; for example, carcinogenic or mutagenic chemotherapeutic drugs. The newest concept for hood design is the convergent flow, which combines both vertical and horizontal flow. *(13:59)*

17. **(B)** As the air passing through the HEPA filter nears the edge of the benchtop, it becomes more turbulent, thus defeating the purpose of the horizontal or convergent laminar flow hood. For this reason, many horizontal laminar flow hoods have a line drawn 6 inches from the edge as a reminder to work further inside the hood. Usually hoods are left running 24 hours a day or are turned on and left running throughout the workday. Work should not commence until the hood has been running for at least 15–30 minutes. It is inadvisable to work within 6 inches of the HEPA filter because air flow may be partially blocked. *(13:60–63)*

18. **(A)** Alcohol 70% or isopropyl alcohol 70% are the two disinfectant solutions usually used to disinfect laminar flow hoods before compounding admixtures. Both are effective antimicrobial agents and will evaporate within a few minutes. Acetone is never used because it is flammable and dangerous if inhaled. Betadine is an effective antimicrobial agent as a skin antiseptic or hand wash but would leave a residual build-up if used in hoods. It also is not very volatile. *(1:1404)*

19. **(B)** Improvements in quality control for the preparation of sterile products by pharmacies have been advocated by several health groups including the ASHP and FDA. The ASHP "Risk Level Classification" describes compounding, storage, and stability standards that should be followed. Of the three risk levels, level 3 is the strictest. Clean room standards have also been proposed to assure tight standards, especially when manipulating unsterile ingredients. *(24:313)*

20. **(E)** Both morphine sulfate and hydroxyzine HCl solutions will have acidic pHs and are therefore expected to be compatible when mixed together in a syringe. However, if either solution is placed directly into a heparinized lock or infusion set, there may be a precipitate because heparin sodium has a higher pH. *(21:590,761–66)*

21. **(E)** It is preferable to aspirate excessive solution and air bubbles while the needle is still in the vial. This prevents accidental contamination of the hood and personnel. Also, it is inadvisable to waste 1 mL of drug solution, especially a controlled substance. It is necessary to inject a volume of air equal to the volume of solution to be withdrawn. Otherwise, a vacuum would occur in the vial, making it difficult to remove liquid. *(13:84)*

22. **(A)** There is no reason to inject air into the opened ampule because no vacuum will form when an ampule is opened and solution is removed. All ampules are intended as single-dose units and should be discarded after opening. *(13:84)*

23. **(A)** The filter straw consists of a plastic tube attached to a needle containing a 5-micron filter. The tube end is placed into an opened ampule, and the needle then inserted into the glass parenteral bottle. The vacuum inside the glass bottle will pull over the entire contents of the ampule. It is impossible to obtain an accurate partial dose, and it is essential that the receiving container have a vacuum. *(13:336)*

24. **(E)** None of the listed parenteral systems of large-volume parenteral (LVPs) containers have vacuums present. *(1:1551; 13:132)*

25. **(B)** Parenteral plastic bottles and bags are characterized by the presence of two entry ports or sleeves. One port is covered with a

latex-type cap through which the pharmacist or nurse can inject solutions into the unit. When the unit is to be administered to the patient, the spike of the administration set is inserted into the second port. This second port does not have a latex cap. Advantages of the plastic units include their lighter weight and resistance to breakage as compared to glass. They also will collapse as solution flows out, thus precluding the need for a method to add air as the solution exits. Glass bottles require either an air tube or air filter. *(13:131–39)*

26. **(B)** Both codeine and dimenhydrinate have a tendency to produce drowsiness as a side effect. Codeine is a weak organic base whereas dimenhydrinate is a combination of diphenhydramine and 8-chlorotheophylline. No chemical reaction between the two drugs would be expected. The amount of codeine consumed per dose is 10 mg or 40 mg daily. This is within the therapeutic dosage range for a 10-year-old child. *(1:1199)*

27. **(B)** If only pure chemicals were available, the weight of powder in each capsule would be 210 mg (4210 mg divided by 20 caps). However, if the pharmacist has to use commercial tablets when preparing this prescription, the contributory weight of the additional ingredients (excipients) present in the tablets must be included in the calculations. Although lactose is a popular diluent when making capsules, the high weight of each capsule precludes its use. Weighing the aspirin with a rubber spatula is not necessary because aspirin is not as reactive as salicylic acid. *(13:195–97)*

28. **(E)** The total amount of ingredients may be calculated as follows:

Drug	Total Weight of Powder	
Codeine	7 tabs each weighing 100 mg =	700 mg
Dimenhydrinate	20 tabs each weighing 100 mg =	4000 mg
Aspirin	powder weighing	3000 mg
	Total weight =	7700 mg

7700 mg divided into 20 capsules = 385 mg each *(13:195–97)*

29. **(C)** The weight of the child in kg =

$$44\,\text{lb} \times \frac{1\,\text{kg}}{2.2\,\text{lb}} = 20\,\text{kg}$$

Each teaspoon dose will contain

$$.15\,\text{mg} \times 20\,\text{kg} = 3\,\text{mg}$$

number of doses =

60 divided by 5 mL = 12 doses
12 doses × 3 mg/dose = 36 mg;

therefore 9 tablets are needed.

(23:67)

30. **(B)** Ondansetron HCl injection is available in vials containing 2 mg/mL. The solution contains both methyl and propyl paraben preservatives that will protect the prescription from microbial growth. Because ondansetron HCl has good water solubility, it is inadvisable to include alcohol in the prescription. As the pH of solutions of the drug is increased, a precipitate may occur. It is best to use acidic vehicles such as orange juice, Coca-Cola, or cherry syrup. *(3; 20:187)*

31. **(D)** Zofran is often prescribed during chemotherapy especially with cisplatin therapy to reduce the severity of nausea and vomiting. Kytril (granisetron), Marinol (dronabinol), and Reglan (metoclopramide) are also antinauseants, whereas Zoloft is an antidepressant. *(3; 25)*

32. **(C)** Because ondansetron is somewhat sensitive to intense light, the prescription product, as well as almost all prescription liquids, should be dispensed in a light-resistant container such as an amber bottle. It is advisable to place a Shake Well label on the container because tablet excipients may settle out. Ondansetron is not a controlled substance. *(3; 20:187)*

33. **(E)** Elixirs may be defined as clear, sweetened, usually flavored hydroalcoholic solutions intended for oral use. Ethanol, commonly at a 20 to 25% V/V concentration is

included and serves as a good solvent for most weak organic acids and bases. The water in the elixir is a good solvent of the salts of weak organic acids and bases. Although water will keep the ionized drug in solution, alcohol will dissolve any un-ionized drug formed if there is a change in solution pH. Problems caused by sucrose competing for water molecules in either syrups or elixirs have been solved by using the newer artificial sweeteners. Flavoring oils, which are usually mixtures of terpenes, possess good alcohol solubility. *(1:1506; 24:247)*

34. **(B)** Burow's solution is officially known as Aluminum Acetate Topical Solution. It is classified as a topical astringent dressing. *(1:871; 24:386)*

35. **(A)** Aqueous solutions such as Burow's solution cannot be incorporated directly into oleaginous bases such as petrolatum or white petrolatum. Aquaphor is an adjuvant that will absorb aqueous solutions and is miscible with petrolatum. Although smaller amounts could be used, 15 g of Aquaphor will readily pick up the required amount of Burow's solution. The amount of white petrolatum must be decreased by 15 g to assure the correct concentration of Burow's solution in the final preparation. Alcohol is seldom included in semisolid ointments or creams because it is likely to evaporate slowly. It is more likely to be included in lotion formulas. *(20:373)*

36. **(E)** The prescription requires 15 mL of Burow's solution plus 45 g of white petrolatum (of which the pharmacist replaced 15 g with Aquaphor). Because Burow's solution is essentially an aqueous solution, one may assume its specific gravity is close to that of water (ie, 1.0). Therefore, the total weight of the final ointment prescription will be 60 g, and 15 g divided by 60 g equals 25% W/W. *(1:86,871)*

37. **(B)** Incorporating powders into ointment bases may be eased by first wetting the powders with a small amount of liquid that is miscible with the main vehicle. The wetted powder is rubbed with a spatula on an oint-ment tile to form a paste. Usually, mineral oil is employed when the vehicle is oleaginous. Glycerin or propylene glycol may be used for more hydrophilic bases. *(1:1588; 24:376)*

38. **(A)** Tetracaine is a weak organic base with poor water solubility (1 g in 1 L of water). The hydrochloride salt, which is very soluble (1 g needs less than 1 mL of water), should be used. Boric acid, which is a very weak acid, is chemically compatible with both tetracaine free base and the HCl salt. Tetracaine, epinephrine (Adrenalin), and cocaine combinations are used as local anesthetics and are known as "TAC Topical Solutions." *(1:1151; 20:246)*

39. **(D)** Boric acid is an effective buffer in ophthalmic solutions because it will maintain a slightly acidic pH, but when placed in the eye, it is quickly neutralized by the buffers in the lacrimal fluid. Boric acid has weak antimicrobial activity. *(1:1407)*

40. **(B)** This problem may be solved using the "E" values for the chemicals.

Drug	Wt. of Drug	×	"E" values		Equiv. Amt. of NaCl
Tetracaine	600 mg		0.18	=	108 mg
Boric Acid	300 mg		0.50	=	150 mg
				Total =	258 mg

60 mL of solution × 0.9% NaCl
$$= 540 \text{ mg of NaCl } 540 - 258 \text{ mg}$$
$$= 282 \text{ mg of NaCl to adjust for tonicity}$$
(1:620–21; 23:149)

41. **(C)** Membrane filtration represents one of the most convenient sterilization methods available to the pharmacist performing extemporaneous compounding. It involves the passing of solutions through a 0.2 micron filter using one of the commercially available sterile filter units such as Millipore's Millex or Swinnex units. The method does not involve heat, therefore there is little decomposition of heat labile drugs as might occur with autoclaving. Ethylene oxide gas is not practical for solutions because it would have

to penetrate the solution and residues may be left behind. *(1:1478; 13:350)*

42. **(A)** Tretinoin is the official name for retinoic acid. The drug is commercially available under the tradename of Retin-A. The designation of Ac. Sal. refers to salicylic acid, not aspirin (acetylsalicylic acid). The term emulsion base is nondescript. It could refer to a number of ointment bases, including those with either W/O or O/W characteristics. Clarification of the type of ointment base desired should be made. Before compounding this prescription, the pharmacist should contact the prescriber concerning the inclusion of a keratolytic agent such as salicylic acid in a topical preparation containing tretinoin, a compound that exhibits keratolytic activity as a side effect. *(1:879; 19:37–3; 20:235)*

43. **(E)** An easy method for determining the amount of 0.05% cream is:

$$60 \text{ g} \times .02\% = .012 \text{ g of pure retinoic acid}$$

$$\frac{0.012 \text{ g}}{x \text{ g}} = \frac{0.05 \text{ g}}{100 \text{ g}}$$

$$.05 \text{ x} = 1.2$$

$$x = 24 \text{ grams of } .05\%$$

(23:117)

44. **(A)** Incorporating powders or liquids into relatively small amounts of ointment base is best accomplished on a pill tile (also known as an ointment tile). Because of the caustic nature of salicylic acid, rubber spatulas should be used rather than stainless steel, which would discolor. *(1:879,1588)*

45. **(B)** Hydrophilic ointment is an O/W emulsion base containing sodium lauryl sulfate, petrolatum, and stearyl alcohol. Of the listed bases, it is closest to a vanishing cream base because such a system is characterized by the presence of an O/W stearate emulsion. *(24:378)*

46. **(D)** Let Q_1 and C_1 represent the quantity and concentration desired and Q_2 and C_2 represent the original quantity and strength:

$$[Q_1] [C_1] = [Q_2] [C_2]$$
$$[x \text{ g}] [0.01\%] = [30 \text{ g}] [0.25\%]$$
$$x = 75 \text{ g (total amount of ointment}$$
$$\text{that can be prepared)}$$

75 g – 30 g (original amount of 0.25% ointment available) = 45 g (amount of diluent ointment base needed)

(1:89)

47. **(E)** A suspension must be prepared because there are water-insoluble powders present in the prescription. An emulsion is not possible because there is no oil indicated in the formula. *(1:1515,1519)*

48. **(E)** Calamine consists of 99% zinc oxide and 1% ferric oxide. The ferric oxide imparts a pink color to the mixture, which is more cosmetically acceptable than the white zinc oxide. *(1:872)*

49. **(D)** The designation "aa qs" translates as "of each enough to make 15 g." Therefore, 7.5 g of calamine and 7.5 g of zinc oxide are needed. The water-insoluble powders, calamine and zinc oxide, should be triturated together in a mortar and pestle, then wetted with the glycerin. Resorcinol is soluble in both water and alcohol, but it is more convenient to dissolve it in the alcohol and dilute the powder paste with the liquid. Finally, add portions of purified water to rinse out the mortar while placing the suspension into a precalibrated wide-mouth bottle. *(1:1515, 1519)*

50. **(C)** Most of the ingredients in this preparation are intended for topical use only. Although the suspension may not separate or settle immediately, it may do so after a few days. It is standard procedure to place "Shake Well" labels on all suspension formulas. None of the ingredients decompose in the presence of moderate heat; therefore, a "Store in a Cool Place" label is not required. *(24:381)*

51. **(E)** The easiest way to hydrate methylcellulose is to add the powder to hot water and al-

low the powder to hydrate for 10 to 15 minutes before adding cold water. Five ofloxacin (Floxin) 400 mg tablets are crushed and wetted by the addition of propylene glycol. The thickened methylcellulose solution can then be added to the powder and suffcent purified water added to make 100 mL. *(1:1312,1515)*

52. **(A)** Urea has good solubility in water. The resulting solution can readily be incorporated into the Aquaphor. *(24:373)*

53. **(C)** Because the exact density of the PEG 400/6000 mixture is not known, the pharmacist must prepare a trial batch in a mold to determine the weight of an individual suppository. In this prescription, the volume occupied by 20 mg of progesterone is insignificant, and it is not necessary to determine its volume density. However, one must realize that larger quantities of drugs will contribute to the bulk volume of the suppository. In these situations, one must prepare a trial suppository that includes the active drug to calculate its bulk density. For example, boric acid has been prescribed at a dose of 600 mg per suppository. Progesterone has been extemporaneously incorporated into vaginal suppositories for the maintenance of pregnancy in luteal phase dysfunction. The usual dose has been 25 mg. *(1:1594; 24:429–435)*

54. **(C)** Vaginal suppositories or pessaries are traditionally larger in size and weight (5 grams) than rectal suppositories (2 grams). However, a regular rectal suppository mold could be used if the larger vaginal mold is not available. For many suppostory formulas, a water-soluble base such as the polyethylene glycol (PEG) or glycerinated gelatin are preferred over oil bases such as cocoa butter. *(1:1591–93; 24:437)*

55. **(C)** Cocoa butter, a mixture of triglycerides, has been used for more than 100 years as a suppository base. A disadvantage of cocoa butter is its inability to absorb aqueous solutions. It melts at slightly below body temperature, and its melting point might be affected by drugs. The Witepsol series of bases consists of natural triglycerides of saturated fatty acids with carbon chains between 12 and 18. Another series of suppository bases that melt is the Wecobees, triglycerides of coconut oil. Although cocoa butter suppositories can be hand rolled or prepared by fusion in molds, the other two bases are intended for mold use. Different molecular weight PEGs can be blended and formed into suppositories by fusion using molds. PEG suppositories do not melt in the body; instead, they slowly dissolve in the limited amount of water in the colon. *(1:1593; 24:427)*

56. **(E)** The solution also contains Polysorbate 80. This nonionic surfactant is included to disperse the water-insoluble components of coal tar, which will precipitate when the highly alcoholic solution is mixed with an aqueous preparation.
(B–incorrect) The Latin name of coal tar solution is Liquor Carbonis Detergens (L.C.D.). *(20:74; 24:386)*

57. **(A)** This prescription uses mineral oil as the solvent. It is not suited for administration into the eye. Ephedrine is used as a topical decongestant when administered by the intranasal route. The product would be ineffective if placed in the ear. *(1:989; 24:420)*

58. **(A)** Ephedrine sulfate is water soluble. It is best to receive the prescriber's permission to use ephedrine base, which is soluble in nonpolar solvents such as mineral oil. *(1:989)*

59. **(B)** Camphor is soluble in alcohol or organic solvents but is only slightly soluble in water (1 g in 800 mL). *(1:874)*

60. **(D)** Methyl salicylate can be used in small quantities as a flavoring or perfuming agent. It is also included in many topical products such as rubbing alcohol, gels, and liniments as a counterirritant. *(1:1387; 2a:80)*

61. **(D)** Salicylic acid is a keratolytic, which means that it helps to dissolve and loosen keratin. This is a useful property in the treatment of conditions such as psoriasis in which

the skin becomes hyperkeratotic, that is, the keratin layer thickens. *(1:879)*

62. **(A)** Because of the volatility of alcohol, it is not suitable in dosage forms from which it may slowly evaporate. If ingredients were dissolved in alcohol and incorporated into either ointments or suppositories, crystals of the ingredients would slowly appear on the surface of the dosage unit. However, one would expect alcohol to remain within the lotion formula until placed on the skin. *(1:1404)*

63. **(A)** Product inserts are the best sources of information concerning appropriate diluents for a given drug powder. However, BSWFI should not be used for reconstituting single-dose units because the preservative present would serve no useful purpose, and large amounts of the preservative could increase the incidence or severity of toxicity. The use of BSWFI may be appropriate if a powder in a multidose vial is being reconstituted. *(13:423; 24:292)*

64. **(C)** Amphotericin B is available in vials containing 50 mg of drug as a powder. Because of the colloidal nature of the product, only sterile water for injection without preservatives is suitable as a reconstituting vehicle. Other vehicles such as normal saline may cause a precipitate. Amphotericin B is administered by slow intravenous infusion over a 2–6 hour period. *(21:74)*

65. **(C)** Because the pharmacist only has the D50W and Aminosyn II packaged in 500-mL bottles, it is most convenient to transfer each solution aseptically to an evacuated glass bottle or plastic bag. *(3)*

66. **(A)** The amount of dextrose requested may be calculated by:

$$500 \text{ mL} \times 50\% = 250 \text{ g dextrose}$$
$$200 \text{ mL} \times 70\% = 140 \text{ g dextrose}$$
$$300 \text{ mL} \times 20\% = 60 \text{ g dextrose then,}$$
$$[Q_1][C_1] = [Q_2][C_2]$$
$$[500 \text{ mL}][50\%] = [x \text{ mL}][70\%]$$

$$x = 360 \text{ mL}$$

(23:117–19)

67. **(C)** Many calcium salts, such as the phosphate and carbonate, have limited water solubility. When calcium salts and phosphate salts are included in the same admixture, it is possible that the very insoluble calcium phosphates may form. The pharmacist must recognize the potential danger of infusing such solutions into patients. Several reference sources list the limits of each salt that is compatible with the other. However, the precipitate may form slowly and would be invisible if a fat emulsion is included in the TPN. *(19:35–11; 21:160)*

68. **(A)** It is often possible to reduce the incidence of a precipitation if the potassium phosphate is dissolved or mixed with the vehicle first followed by the calcium solution, which is added slowly while stirring. The pharmacist could also alternate the calcium and the phosphate solutions in the series of TPN containers. However, he or she should inform the prescriber and double the amount of ion added each time. *(21:160)*

69. **(A)** Phosphorus is an essential mineral for the body and is readily available in the phosphate ion. When the potassium ion is required, the chloride or acetate salts are used. *(13:215–16)*

70. **(D)** Most electrolytes are ordered in terms of milliequivalents. The exception is phosphate. Commercially available potassium phosphate injections consist of a mixture of monobasic (potassium) and dibasic (dipotassium) phosphates. Because body phosphate requirements are usually expressed in terms of millimoles (mM) per kg per day and the available solutions are mixtures of the two salts, it is more convenient to express the phosphate additive in terms of mM/L rather than mEq/L. The average adult needs 10–15 mmol of phosphorus per day. *(13:216; 19:28–23)*

71. **(C)** Low-dose insulin syringes are calibrated to contain 0.5 mL (50 units) of insulin. The 40 units of insulin (0.4 mL) could also be measured accurately using the tuberculin syringe, which has the capacity of 1 mL. The smallest calibrations on 10-mL syringes will not allow accurate enough measurements of 0.4 mL. *(13:322)*

72. **(A)** When low concentrations of insulin are included in LVPs, the percentage of insulin adsorbed onto the walls of the containers and also onto the administration sets is significant. One can expect at least 50% insulin loss when only 20 units are added to the container. *(13:265)*

    The other answers are incorrect. Because the insulin dosage is expressed in units, the strength of the insulin is not needed. Most likely the U-100 solution will be used. Only insulin solution is given intravenously; the suspension forms are intended for subcutaneous administration.

73. **(C)** Liposyn is a fatty acid emulsion with a physical appearance similar to that of milk. When included in TPN solutions, the resulting product will be somewhat cloudy. The intent of the Liposyn is to correct or prevent fatty acid deficiencies by providing linoleic and linolenic acids, which are present in either soybean or safflower oil. The fat emulsions also provide calories. For example, every mL of the 10% strength contributes 1.1 kcal, and a mL of the 20% provides 2.0 kcal. Because the fat emulsions have been adjusted for tonicity, they do not adversely affect the osmolarity of TPN solutions. *(19:35–9; 21:435)*

74. **(D)** Multicomponent admixtures that contain dextrose, amino acids, and fat oil emulsions are referred to as total nutrition admixtures (TNAs), or 3 in 1s. Although these combinations simplify administration of calories and protein, the cloudy nature of the product precludes examination of the product for fine precipitants. The designation MCT has been used to represent medium

chain triglycerides, which may be used in patients suffering from malabsorption. *(19:35–9; 21:47; 24:327)*

75. **(C)** There are several sterile solutions that contain the most popular trace metals likely to be requested for TPNs. Iron is not included mainly because of compatibility problems. *(3)*

76. **(C)** Selenium deficiencies may cause muscle pain and tenderness and cardiomyopathy. *(3; 19:35–10)*

77. **(B)** An increase in concentration from 50% to 60% dextrose will mean an additional 50 g of dextrose per bottle or 150 g per day. (500 mL × 10% × 3 bts daily). Because every gram of dextrose provides 3.4 calories, 150 g × 3.4 kcal/g = 510 kilocalories. *(19:35–9; 23:177)*

78. **(B)** Milliequivalent expressions allow direct comparisons of ions when different salt forms are being used. In other words, 40 mEq of sodium acetate will contain the same weight of sodium as will 40 mEq of sodium chloride. *(23:156)*

79. **(C)** The tetracycline strength requested is 4% and 500-mg capsules are available.

$$445 \text{ g} \times 4\% = 1.8 \text{ g or } 1800 \text{ mg of drug}$$

$$\frac{1800 \text{ mg tetracycline}}{x \text{ capsules}} = \frac{500 \text{ mg tetracycline}}{1 \text{ capsule}}$$

$$x = 3.5 \text{ or } 4 \text{ capsules}$$

When preparing this prescription, the pharmacist should carefully empty four capsules and weigh the powder obtained. Then a proportion equation is set up:

$$\frac{3.5}{\text{wt to use}} = \frac{4}{\text{total wt in 4 caps}}$$

The powder from the capsules can be mixed easily with the Lubriderm lotion. Lubriderm is an W/O emulsion base with good emollient activity. Tetracycline is still used both topically and orally for treatment of acne.

Oral dosing is 500 mg once a day. *(1:1311; 19:37–5; 23:195–98)*

80. **(C)** Cold cream is a W/O emulsion base with good emollient properties *(24:374)*

81. **(B)** Hydrophilic petrolatum is an anhydrous preparation that will absorb significant amounts of water forming a W/O emulsion. It contains cholesterol as the emulsifying agent. *(1:1586)*

82. **(C)** *(1:1586)*

83. **(A)** *(1:1585)*

84. **(E)** *(1:1587; 24:374)*

85. **(D)** *(1:1586; 24:374)*

86. **(B)** Large quantities of liquids may be incorporated into Aquaphor. *(1:1586; 24:373)*

87. **(E)** White petrolatum is a bland base with a very low incidence of irritation to the eye. Also, because of the absence of water, it has low susceptibility to microbial growth. *(24:409)*

88. **(E)** The decomposition of most antibiotics is initiated with the presence of water. White petrolatum is anhydrous and is relatively inert. *(1:1585)*

89. **(C)** Of all the bases listed, hydrophilic petrolatum will absorb the greatest quantity of water. *(1:1586)*

90. **(E)** The occlusive characteristics of petrolatum will prevent further water loss through the stratum corneum. Thus, the skin will remain more hydrated. *(1:1585)*

CHAPTER 5

Biopharmaceutics and Pharmacokinetics

Biopharmaceutics is a scientific discipline concerned with the relationship between the physicochemical properties of a drug in a dosage form and the biologic response observed after its administration. It includes the study of the release of the drug from its dosage form. Pharmacokinetics is the study of the absorption, distribution, metabolism, and elimination (ADME) of drugs. As more quantitative and sophisticated assay techniques have been developed, a better understanding of the therapeutic pathways for drugs has emerged. This chapter tests the reader's knowledge of the principles of biopharmaceutics and pharmacokinetics, which is fundamental to the rational selection of quality drug products, the determination of appropriate dose and dosing schedules, and the monitoring of therapy.

Questions

DIRECTIONS (Questions 1 through 75): Each of the numbered items or incomplete statements in this section is followed by answers or by completions of the statement. Select the ONE lettered answer or completion that is BEST in each case.

1. The term "biologic availability" or "bioavailability" refers to the relative amount of drug that reaches the

   (A) small intestine
   (B) stomach
   (C) systemic circulation
   (D) liver
   (E) kidneys

2. The relative bioavailability of a drug product can be determined by comparing which of the following values to similar control drug values?

   I. Areas under the curve (AUC)
   II. Total drug urinary excretion
   III. Peak blood drug concentrations

   (A) I only
   (B) III only
   (C) I and II only
   (D) II and III only
   (E) I, II, and III

3. Which of the following is the first process that must occur before a drug can become available for absorption from a tablet dosage form?

   (A) Dissolution of the drug in the GI fluids
   (B) Dissolution of the drug in the GI epithelium

   (C) Ionization of the drug
   (D) Dissolution of the drug in the blood
   (E) Disintegration of the tablet

4. Which of the following may be the rate-limiting step for drug absorption from an orally administered drug product?

   I. Disintegration of the unit
   II. Dissolution of the active drug
   III. Diffusion of active drug through the intestinal wall

   (A) I only
   (B) III only
   (C) I and II only
   (D) II and III only
   (E) I, II, and III

5. The rate of dissolution may be described by which one of the following equations or laws?

   (A) Fick's Second Law
   (B) Henderson-Hasselbalch Equation
   (C) Noyes-Whitney Equation
   (D) Poiseuille's Law
   (E) Stoke's Law

6. The area under the serum concentration–time curve represents the

   (A) biologic half-life of the drug
   (B) amount of drug that is cleared by the kidneys
   (C) amount of drug in the original dosage form

(D) amount of drug absorbed

(E) amount of drug excreted in the urine

7. The AUC can be described as being

I. a theoretic value

II. a measure of drug concentration–time curve

III. a value with units of weight and time/volume

(A) I only

(B) III only

(C) I and II only

(D) II and III only

(E) I, II, and III

8. The AUC of a drug can be determined from a graph by using which of the following methods?

I. Law of diminishing returns

II. Rule of nines

III. Trapezoidal rule

(A) I only

(B) III only

(C) I and II only

(D) II and III only

(E) I, II, and III

9. The "F" value for a drug product is ideally compared to its

(A) absolute bioavailability

(B) dosing rate

(C) clearance rate

(D) relative bioavailability

(E) route of administration

10. Determine the F value for a drug available as a 100-mg capsule with a calculated AUC of 20 mg/dL/h when a 100-mg IV bolus of the same drug exhibits an AUC of 25 mg/dL/h.

(A) 0.2

(B) 0.4

(C) 0.8

(D) 1.25

(E) 20

11. What is the F value for an experimental drug tablet based on the following data?

Drug Dosage		
Form	Dose	AUC (μg/mL/h)
Tablet	100 mg po	20 ✓
Solution (control)	100 mg po	30
Injection (control)	50 mg IV push	40

(A) 0.25

(B) 0.38

(C) 0.50

(D) 0.66

(E) 0.90

12. Drug products can also be evaluated by comparing curves of serum concentration vs time (ie, blood level curves). The most important parameters for comparison that can be obtained from such curves are

(A) peak concentration, biologic half-life, elimination rate constant

(B) biologic half-life, time of peak concentration, absorption rate constant

(C) peak concentration, time of peak concentration, total AUC

(D) average serum concentration, AUC, biologic half-life

(E) absorption rate constant, AUC, elimination rate constant

13. The peak of the serum concentration vs time curve approximates the

(A) point in time when the maximum pharmacologic effect occurs

(B) point in time when absorption and elimination of the drug have equalized

(C) maximum concentration of free drug in the urine

(D) time required for essentially all of the drug to be absorbed from the GI tract

(E) point in time when the drug begins to be metabolized

14. Differences in bioavailability are most frequently observed with drugs administered by which of the following routes?

    (A) Subcutaneous
    (B) Intravenous
    (C) Oral
    (D) Sublingual
    (E) Intramuscular

15. Two different oral formulations of the same drug having equal areas under their respective serum concentration–time curves

    (A) deliver the same total amount of drug to the body and are, therefore, bioequivalent
    (B) deliver the same total amount of drug to the body but are not necessarily bioequivalent
    (C) are bioequivalent by definition
    (D) are bioequivalent if they both meet USP disintegration standards
    (E) are bioequivalent if they both meet USP dissolution standards

16. If an oral capsule formulation of the drug A produces a serum concentration–time curve having the same area under the curve as that produced by an equivalent dose of drug A given IV, it can generally be concluded that

    (A) the IV route is preferred to the oral route
    (B) the capsule formulation is essentially completely absorbed
    (C) the drug is very rapidly absorbed
    (D) all oral dosage forms of drug A will be bioequivalent
    (E) there is no advantage to the IV route

17. In vitro dissolution rate studies for drug products are useful for evaluating bioavailability only if they can be correlated with

    (A) disintegration rates
    (B) in vivo studies in humans
    (C) in vivo studies in at least three species of animals
    (D) the chemical stability of the drug
    (E) USP disintegration limits

18. According to pH partition theory, a weakly acidic drug will most likely be absorbed from the stomach because

    (A) the drug will exist primarily in the un-ionized, more lipid-soluble form
    (B) the drug will exist primarily in the ionized, more water-soluble form
    (C) weak acids are more soluble in acid media
    (D) the ionic form of the drug facilitates dissolution
    (E) weak acids will further depress pH

19. Which of the following statements concerning the blood protein albumin is (are) true?

    I. Blood levels are approximately 3.5 to 5.0 g/liter.
    II. It is a very site-specific binding agent.
    III. It will bind acidic drugs.

    (A) I only
    (B) III only
    (C) I and II only
    (D) II and III only
    (E) I, II, and III

20. Reducing drug particle size to enhance drug absorption is limited to those situations in which the

    (A) absorption process occurs by active transport
    (B) absorption process is rate-limited by the dissolution of drug in GI fluids
    (C) drug is very water soluble
    (D) drug is very potent
    (E) drug is irritating to the GI tract

21. Drugs whose absorption have been significantly increased by micronization include

    I. griseofulvin
    II. nitrofurantoin
    III. potassium chloride

    (A) I only
    (B) III only
    (C) I and II only

(D) II and III only

(E) I, II, and III

22. Drugs that are absorbed from the GI tract are generally

(A) absorbed into the portal circulation and pass through the liver before entering the general circulation

(B) filtered from the blood by the kidney, then reabsorbed into the general circulation

(C) absorbed into the portal circulation and are distributed by an enterohepatic cycle

(D) not affected by liver enzymes

(E) stored in the liver

23. For two drug products to be considered "pharmaceutic equivalents," the products must

   I. have the same active drug (therapeutic moiety)

   II. consist of the same salt

   III. contain the same excipients

(A) I only

(B) III only

(C) I and II only

(D) II and III only

(E) I, II, and III

24. Requirements for drug products to be considered "pharmaceutic alternatives" include having the same

   I. active drug or precursor

   II. dosage form

   III. salt or ester

(A) I only

(B) III only

(C) I and II only

(D) II and III only

(E) I, II, and III

25. Gastric emptying is slowed by all of the following EXCEPT

(A) vigorous exercise

(B) fatty foods

(C) hot meals

(D) hunger

(E) emotional stress

26. For many drugs, bioavailability can be evaluated using urinary excretion data. This is based on the assumption that

(A) bioavailability studies can be done only on drugs that are completely excreted unchanged by the kidneys

(B) drug levels can be measured more accurately in urine than in blood

(C) a drug must first be absorbed into the systemic circulation before it can appear in the urine

(D) all of the administered dose can be recovered from the urine

(E) only drug metabolites are excreted in the urine

27. Estimating bioavailability from urinary excretion data is less satisfactory than estimates based on blood level data because accurate urinary excretion studies require

   I. complete urine collection

   II. normal or near-normal renal function

   III. that the drug be completely excreted unchanged by the kidney

(A) I only

(B) III only

(C) I and II only

(D) II and III only

(E) I, II, and III

Questions 28 and 29 are to be answered using the following data.

Product by Company	Dosage Form	Dose Administered	Cumulative Urinary Amount (mg)
A	Parenteral injection	10 mg IV	9.4
A	Tablet	20 mg po	12.0
B	Tablet	20 mg po	8.2
B	Capsule	15 mg po	6.8

28. The absolute bioavailablity of Company B tablets is best estimated to be

    (A) 25%
    (B) 40%
    (C) 44%
    (D) 68%
    (E) 87%

29. True statements concerning Company B dosage forms when compared to the standard Company A include

    I. the relative bioavailability of Company B tablets is 68%
    II. the relative bioavailability of Company B capsules is 57%
    III. Company B products could be considered to be bioequivalent to Product A tablets.

    (A) I only
    (B) III only
    (C) I and II only
    (D) II and III only
    (E) I, II, and III

30. The excretion of a weakly acidic drug (eg, pKa of 3.5) will be more rapid in alkaline urine than in acidic urine because

    (A) all drugs are excreted more rapidly in alkaline urine
    (B) the drug will exist primarily in the un-ionized form, which cannot be reabsorbed easily
    (C) the drug will exist primarily in the ionized form, which cannot be reabsorbed easily
    (D) weak acids cannot be reabsorbed from the kidney tubules
    (E) active transport mechanisms function better in alkaline urine

31. If a fixed dose of a drug that is eliminated by first-order kinetics is administered at regular intervals, the time required to achieve a steady-state plasma level depends only on the

    (A) dose of the drug

    (B) volume of distribution of the drug
    (C) half-life of the drug
    (D) dosing interval
    (E) fraction of dose absorbed (bioavailability)

32. The biologic half-life of a drug

    (A) is a constant physical property of the drug
    (B) is a constant chemical property of the drug
    (C) is the time for one-half of the therapeutic activity to be lost
    (D) may be decreased by giving the drug by rapid IV injection
    (E) depends entirely on the route of administration

33. A specific drug has a first-order biologic half-life of 4 hours. This half-life value will

    (A) be independent of the initial drug concentration
    (B) increase when the concentration of the drug increases
    (C) decrease when the concentration of the drug increases
    (D) decrease if the patient has renal impairment
    (E) be the same whether the drug level is determined in the blood or by observing the pharmacologic action

34. The biologic half-life of a drug that is eliminated by first-order kinetics is represented mathematically by _____ where k is the first-order rate constant for elimination.

    (A) $1/k$
    (B) $\log k$
    (C) $0.693/k$
    (D) $2.303/k$
    (E) peak serum concentration/2k

35. Assuming complete absorption and an elimination half-life of 4 hours, how many mg of a drug will remain in the body 12 hours after administering a 400-mg dose? Assume linear pharmacokinetics (ie, first order).

(A) <10
(B) 25
(C) 50
(D) 100
(E) 200

36. The biologic half-life of many drugs is often prolonged in newborn infants because of

(A) a higher degree of protein binding
(B) microsomal enzyme induction
(C) more complete absorption of drugs
(D) incompletely developed enzyme systems
(E) incompletely developed barriers to the distribution of drugs in the body

37. A certain drug appears to be eliminated from the body at a rate constant of 20% per hour. Estimate the drug's half-life assuming first-order kinetics.

(A) 1 hour
(B) 2.5 hours
(C) 3.5 hours
(D) 5 hours
(E) 10 hours

38. The volume of distribution of a drug is

I. a mathematic relationship between the total amount of drug in the body and the concentration of drug in the blood
II. a measure of an individual's blood volume
III. a measure of an individual's total body volume

(A) I only
(B) III only
(C) I and II only
(D) II and III only
(E) I, II, and III

39. The volume of distribution (V_d) of a particular drug will be

(A) greater for drugs that concentrate in tissues rather than in plasma

(B) greater for drugs that concentrate in plasma rather than in tissues
(C) independent of tissue concentration
(D) independent of plasma concentration
(E) approximately the same for all drugs in a given individual

40. A knowledge of V_d for a given drug is useful because it allows us to

(A) estimate the elimination rate constant
(B) determine the biologic half-life
(C) calculate a reasonable loading dose
(D) determine the best dosing interval
(E) determine the peak plasma concentration

41. Estimate the plasma concentration of a drug when 50 mg is given by IV bolus to a 140-lb patient if her volume of distribution is 1.6 L/kg.

(A) 0.1 mg/L
(B) 0.5 mg/L
(C) 1 mg/L
(D) 5 mg/L
(E) 31 mg/L

Questions 42 through 46

The following graph represents drug blood level curves. Answer the next five questions based upon this graph.

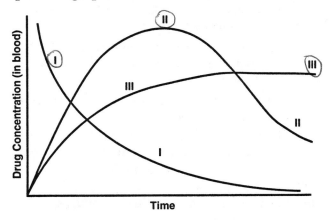

42. Curve I represents the blood level concentration of a drug administered by

    I. the oral route
    II. intramuscular injection
    III. intravenous injection

    (A) I only
    (B) III only
    (C) I and II only
    (D) II and III only
    (E) I, II, and III

43. The upward slope of curve II could represent

    I. increased absorption of drug from a capsule dosage form
    II. absorption of drug from an intramuscular injection
    III. absorption of drug from a sustained-release tablet

    (A) I only
    (B) III only
    (C) I and II only
    (D) II and III only
    (E) I, II, and III

44. Which one of the following statements concerning the graph is completely true?

    (A) Once the peak in curve II has been reached, no further drug absorption is likely to occur.
    (B) Doubling the administered dose will double the height of curve II.
    (C) The Y axis (concentration of drug in the blood) should be expressed as a log function.
    (D) The X axis (time) should be expressed as a log function.
    (E) The curves in lines II and III indicate that the absorption rate (K_a) is greater than the elimination rate (K_e).

45. Curve III would best illustrate a drug administered by

    (A) intravenous push
    (B) intravenous infusion
    (C) intramuscular injection

    (D) intrathecal injection
    (E) either intravenous push or infusion

46. The time needed to reach optimum drug blood levels (the plateau portion of curve III) during constant-rate intravenous infusion is

    (A) directly proportional to the rate of infusion
    (B) inversely proportional to the rate of infusion
    (C) independent of the rate of infusion
    (D) independent of the biologic half-life
    (E) not related to either the infusion rate or the biologic half-life

47. Compartmental models are often used to illustrate the various principles of pharmacokinetics. A compartment is best defined as

    (A) any anatomic entity that is capable of absorbing drug
    (B) a kinetically distinguishable pool of drug
    (C) specific body organs or tissues that can be assayed for drug
    (D) any body fluid—such as blood or urine—that may contain drug
    (E) any component of the blood, including blood proteins, that would have a tendency to absorb drug

48. At diffusion equilibrium, the concentrations of a drug in the various body compartments (body fluids, tissues, organs) are usually NOT equal because

    (A) all body compartments are not equal in size and weight
    (B) those compartments closest to the absorption site(s) will absorb most of the drug
    (C) the CNS is a body compartment that usually does not accumulate drugs
    (D) most drugs end up in the urine
    (E) the various body compartments are not equally accessible to the drug, nor do they have equal affinities for it

49. The pharmacokinetic parameter known as clearance is essentially the

- (A) rate at which the plasma is cleared of all waste materials and foreign substances (eg, drugs)
- (B) volume of blood that passes through the kidneys per unit of time
- (C) volume of blood that passes through the liver per unit of time
- (D) rate at which a drug is removed (cleared) from its site of absorption
- (E) volume of blood that is completely cleared of drug per unit of time

50. A knowledge of the clearance (Cl) of a given drug is useful because it allows the

- (A) calculation of the maintenance dose required to sustain a desired average steady-state plasma concentration
- (B) determination of the volume of distribution
- (C) determining the ideal dosing interval
- (D) decision whether a loading dose is necessary
- (E) determination if the drug is metabolized or excreted unchanged

51. The difference between peak and trough concentrations is greatest when a drug is given at dosing intervals

- (A) much longer than the half-life
- (B) about equal to the half-life
- (C) much shorter than the half-life
- (D) equal to the half-life times serum creatinine
- (E) equal to the time it takes to reach peak concentration following a single oral dose

52. Which of the following pharmacokinetic parameters is (are) likely to decrease in the geriatric population when compared to the average population?

- I. Renal elimination
- II. Drug metabolism
- III. Volume of distribution

- (A) I only
- (B) III only
- (C) I and II only
- (D) II and III only
- (E) I, II, and III

53. In dosing drugs that are primarily excreted by the kidneys, one must have some idea of the patient's renal function. A calculated pharmacokinetic parameter that gives us a reasonable estimate of renal function is the

- (A) blood urea nitrogen (BUN)
- (B) serum creatinine (Sr_{Cr})
- (C) creatinine clearance (Cl_{Cr})
- (D) urine creatinine (U_{Cr})
- (E) free water clearance (Cl_{fw})

54. If the rate of elimination of a drug is reduced because of impaired renal function, the effect on the drug half-life and the time required to reach steady-state plasma levels (steady-state concentrations–C_{ss}) will

- (A) both increase
- (B) both decrease
- (C) be an increase in half-life and a decrease in the time to reach C_{ss}
- (D) be a decrease in half-life but an increase in the time to reach C_{ss}
- (E) be negligible

55. When comparing a highly protein-bound drug to its less- or nonprotein-bound analog, the highly bound drug will probably have

- I. faster metabolism rate
- II. a longer biologic half-life
- III. delayed elimination from the body

- (A) I only
- (B) III only
- (C) I and II only
- (D) II and III only
- (E) I, II, and III

56. Which one of the following drugs does NOT bind to plasma protein to any significant extent?

    (A) allopurinol (Zyloprim)
    (B) amitriptyline (Elavil)
    (C) lidocaine (Xylocaine)
    (D) propranolol (Inderal)
    (E) warfarin (Coumadin)

57. The metabolism of drugs generally results in

    (A) less acidic compounds
    (B) more acidic compounds
    (C) compounds having a higher oil/water partition coefficient
    (D) more polar compounds
    (E) compounds with lower aqueous solubility

58. The pharmacist may suspect that a drug undergoes a significant first-pass effect when

    I. the average oral dose is significantly higher than the parenteral bolus dose
    II. the drug is marketed in a sustained-release dosage form
    III. the drug is contraindicated when renal impairment is present

    (A) I only
    (B) III only
    (C) I and II only
    (D) II and III only
    (E) I, II, and III

59. All of the following drugs are believed to undergo significant first-pass hepatic biotransformation EXCEPT

    (A) phenytoin
    (B) lidocaine
    (C) morphine
    (D) nitroglycerin
    (E) propranolol

60. When converting a patient from theophylline to aminophylline, a dose adjustment

    (A) is not needed
    (B) with an increase of 20% is suggested
    (C) with an increase of 50% is suggested
    (D) with a decrease of 20% is suggested
    (E) with a decrease of 50% is suggested

61. The transfer of most drugs across biologic membranes occurs by

    (A) active transport from a region of high concentration to one of low concentration
    (B) active transport from a region of low concentration to one of high concentration
    (C) passive diffusion from a region of high concentration to one of low concentration
    (D) passive diffusion from a region of low concentration to one of high concentration
    (E) facilitated diffusion regardless of concentration gradient

62. The equation that describes the process of "passive transport" is

    (A) Fick's Law
    (B) Henderson-Hasselbalch equation
    (C) Noyes Whitney equation
    (D) Stoke's Law
    (E) Hoftmeister Rule

63. The rate of diffusion of drugs across biologic membranes is most commonly

    (A) independent of the concentration gradient
    (B) directly proportional to the concentration gradient
    (C) dependent on the availability of carrier substrate
    (D) dependent on the route of administration
    (E) directly proportional to membrane thickness

64. When graphed, nonlinear pharmacokinetics are characterized by data that

    (A) does not yield a straight line at any time
    (B) exhibits a straight line only when plot-

ted as log/log functions

(C) follows zero-order kinetics

(D) follows first-order kinetics

(E) will have a negative slope

65. Which one of the following statements concerning carrier-mediated transport is NOT correct? Carrier-mediated transport systems

(A) consume energy

(B) may be adversely affected by certain chemicals

(C) are structure specific

(D) reach equilibrium faster than passive transport systems

(E) can become saturated

66. When the active transport system described in the Question 65 becomes saturated, the rate process will be

(A) zero order

(B) pseudo–zero order

(C) first order

(D) pseudo–first order

(E) second order

67. The term "prodrug" refers to a

(A) chemical substance that is part of the synthesis procedure in preparing a drug

(B) compound that liberates an active drug in the body

(C) compound that may be therapeutically active but is still under clinical trials

(D) drug that has only prophylactic activity in the body

(E) drug that is classified as being "probably effective"

68. Which of the following drugs is (are) classified as prodrugs?

I. Clorazepate (Tranxene)

II. Enalapril (Vasotec)

III. Lisinopril (Zestril)

(A) I only

(B) III only

(C) I and II only

(D) II and III only

(E) I, II, and III

69. The rectal route of administration may be preferred over the oral route for some systemic-acting drugs because

(A) the drug does not have to be absorbed

(B) absorption is predictable and complete

(C) a portion of the absorbed drug does not pass through the liver before entering the systemic circulation

(D) inert binders, diluents, and excipients cannot interfere with absorption

(E) the dissolution process is avoided

70. If a drug appears in the feces after oral administration,

(A) the drug cannot have been completely absorbed from the GI tract

(B) the drug must not have completely dissolved in the GI fluids

(C) the drug must have complexed with materials in the GI tract

(D) parenteral administration of the drug may determine the contribution of the biliary system to the amount of drug in the feces

(E) parenteral administration of the drug will be useful to determine the bioavailability of the oral formulation

71. Drugs that are poorly lipid soluble, polar, or extensively ionized at the pH of blood generally

(A) penetrate the CNS very slowly and may be eliminated from the body before a significant concentration in the CNS is reached

(B) penetrate the CNS very slowly but are centrally active in much lower concentration

(C) achieve adequate CNS concentrations only if given IV

(D) must be metabolized to a more polar form before they can gain access to the CNS

(E) can gain access to the CNS if other drugs are used to modify blood pH

72. Increasing which of the following is (are) desirable when developing new antibiotics?

    I. The minimum inhibitory concentration
    II. The tendency for protein binding
    III. The minimum toxic concentration

    (A) I only
    (B) III only
    (C) I and II only
    (D) II and III only
    (E) I, II, and III

73. Which of the following properties of a drug may preclude its formulation into a sustained-release dosage form?

    I. Half-life <2 hours
    II. Erratic absorption from the GI tract
    III. Low therapeutic index

    (A) I only
    (B) III only
    (C) I and II only

    (D) II and III only
    (E) I, II, and III

74. Which one of the following peroral dosage forms is likely to exhibit the longest lag time?

    (A) Delayed-release tablet
    (B) Elixir (20% alcohol)
    (C) Enteric coated tablet
    (D) Osmotic tablet
    (E) Sustained-release capsule

75. The pharmacokinetic symbol f_u most closely relates to

    (A) drug concentration found in the plasma
    (B) amount of active drug released from a dosage form
    (C) protein binding characteristics of a drug
    (D) drug elimination in the urine
    (E) drug metabolism

Answers and Explanations

1. **(C)** For most drugs, a dose-response relationship can be correlated with the amount of drug that gains access to the general circulation. In many cases, the amount of drug that is present in the blood (blood level) directly relates to the intensity and duration of the pharmacologic effect. The relative amount of drug that is biologically available compared to the total amount of drug in the dosage form administered is a measure of bioavailability. Usually, bioavailability is expressed as the fraction or percentage of the administered drug that is absorbed. The term "absolute bioavailability" compares the amount of drug absorbed with the "gold standard" of the amount present in the blood after administration by an IV bolus. *(15:34)*

2. **(C)** The availability of a drug from a specific formulation is compared to a reference standard that is administered at the same dose level. The standard for oral drugs is usually a solution of the pure drug. The relative bioavailability is then calculated by dividing either the AUC of the drug or the total amount of the drug excreted in the urine by respective values for the reference standard. The absolute bioavailability can be calculated by comparing similar data for the drug product to an IV bolus dose. *(17:196)*

3. **(E)** The surface area of a drug is so limited in the intact tablet that dissolution of drug from the intact tablet is negligible except for very water-soluble drugs. Therefore, although a drug must dissolve before it can be absorbed, a tablet must generally disintegrate before the drug can dissolve. *(17:136)*

4. **(E)** The rate-limiting step is considered the slowest step in the kinetics of drug absorption. For some drugs, especially tablet dosage forms, the slow release of the drug from the dosage form may be due to slow tablet disintegration due to excessive tablet hardness or excessive amounts of water-insoluble lubricant. Once disintegration has occurred, a poorly water-soluble drug may only slowly dissolve, thus limiting absorption. If a drug has high water solubility and the tablet has disintegrated rapidly, the rate-limiting step may be the ability of the drug to diffuse through the GI tract wall. *(17:136)*

5. **(C)** Terms in the Noyes-Whitney Equation reflect the rate at which a drug dissolves from the surface of a solid mass followed by diffusion through the stagnant layer that surrounds the solid particle. The Noyes-Whitney Equation is a modified form of Fick's First Law used to describe diffusion. *(17:138)*

6. **(D)** Because the serum concentration–time curve is a quantitative representation of the concentration of drug in the serum over a specific period of time, the AUC is a mathematic function of the amount of drug that has entered the blood. The total AUC, then, represents the amount of drug that has been absorbed. By comparing the AUCs of two formulations of the same drug, we can determine the relative amount of drug that is available from each formulation. *(17:195)*

7. **(D)** The AUC can be calculated mathematically by the use of equations or evaluation of a graph when concentration (drug W/V)

is plotted on the Y axis and time is plotted on the X axis. Units for AUC are weight and time/volume. *(17:14)*

8. **(B)** By employing the mathematic technique known as the trapezoidal rule, one may calculate an AUC. The AUC is subdivided into individual segments and the area of each is determined. By totaling these areas, an accurate estimate of the total AUC is obtained. *(17:180)*

9. **(A)** F values are calculated for drugs in their dosage forms by comparing AUCs, or total amount of drug excreted, to the control reference of an IV bolus dose, as outlined in Question 2. An ideal F value would be 1.0, which indicates complete absorption of the drug and no losses from other mechanisms such as hepatic first-pass effect. The F value is also known as the bioavailability factor. *(17:196; 23:201)*

10. **(C)** As outlined in Question 9, the F value can be estimated by using the equation

$$F = \frac{AUC_{cap}}{AUC_{iv}} = \frac{20}{25} = 0.8$$

Because in this example the comparison of AUCs relates to the absolute standard of an IV bolus dose, the drug's absolute bioavailability was calculated. If the comparison had been to another standard, such as to an oral solution or another product of the same drug, the F value would be the relative bioavailability. *(17:197)*

11. **(A)** This problem is similar to Question 10, except that a correction factor is necessary because different doses of the drug were administered. *(17:197)*

12. **(C)** Peak concentrations and times of peak concentrations can be easily read from the graph. AUCs involve complex calculations. *(1:609; 17:35)*

13. **(B)** Prior to the peak time, the rate of absorption is greater than the rate of elimination, and the curve ascends. After the peak, the rate of elimination is greater than the rate of absorption, and the curve descends. If these rates are equal for some time interval, the curve will show a plateau rather than a distinct peak. *(1:607; 17:172)*

14. **(C)** Differences in bioavailability of various drug products might be anticipated with any route of administration that requires the drug to be absorbed into the blood compartment. The oral route is most often involved because it is the most common route of administration and the drug must pass through the GI lumen, gut wall, and the hepatic circulation system before reaching general circulation. *(15:123; 17:153)*

15. **(B)** Although equal areas indicate that the same total amount of drug was made available to the body, the areas alone give no information regarding the rate at which the drugs were made available. Two formulations of a drug can yield radically different serum concentrations vs time curves that have approximately equal areas. It should be emphasized that the concept of bioequivalence involves not only the amount of drug that is available, but also the rate at which it becomes available. *(1:607)*

16. **(B)** If the areas under the respective curves are equal, it can be concluded that the total amount of drug delivered to the body by each dosage form was equal. Because the intravenous administration did not involve an absorption process, the fact that the same amount of drug administered in a capsule formulation delivered the same total amount of drug indicates that the absorption of the drug from the oral capsule was essentially complete. *(1:609)*

17. **(B)** Although in vitro dissolution rate studies may be useful in quality control procedures to evaluate batch-to-batch variability, they are of little value in bioavailability evaluations unless they can be correlated with in vivo studies in humans. More commonly, when several formulations of a particular

drug are found to be biologically inequivalent through studies in humans, in vitro dissolution studies are performed to establish the basis of their inequivalence. *(17:146)*

18. **(A)** The ionic equilibrium that is established in the acid contents of the stomach will favor a relatively higher concentration of unionized drug in solution. The unionized molecule, because of the absence of a charge, is more lipid soluble than the ionic species and will be able to cross biologic membranes more easily. If the drug reaches the more alkaline contents of the intestines before absorption is complete, the higher pH will then favor the ionic form of the drug, which has considerably less lipid solubility and is much less readily absorbed. It should be pointed out, however, that because of the extremely large surface area of the intestine, weakly acidic drugs can be absorbed from the intestine in spite of the unfavorable ion/molecule ratio. *(15:114,120)*

19. **(B)** Albumin will bind numerous drugs that have an acid functional group. Because of its nonspecificity and high blood levels (3.5% to 5%), the loading doses of some drugs must be high to at least partially saturate the protein binding sites. *(1:181–82; 15:143,271–72)*

20. **(B)** Making a drug dissolve faster (eg, by particle size reduction) will not increase the rate of its absorption if the absorption process itself is the rate-limiting step in the overall transport of the drug from its intact dosage form to the blood. Furthermore, there are some circumstances in which particle size reduction may actually reduce the amount of drug absorbed. For example, for drugs such as penicillin G that are unstable in gastric fluids, more rapid dissolution would enhance degradation by increasing residence time of dissolved drug in the stomach and thereby result in reduced availability. *(17:159)*

21. **(C)** Both griseofulvin and nitrofurantoin have been formulated into dosage forms as micronized powders. Such poorly water-soluble drugs will dissolve faster due to the increase in surface area with subsequent absorption. Potassium chloride readily dissolves in water. Reducing its particle size will not significantly enhance its dissolution or absorption. *(1:595; 17:159)*

22. **(A)** Drugs are generally absorbed from the GI tract through capillaries that empty into the portal vein. This vessel carries the absorbed drugs to the liver, where they are subjected to varying degrees of metabolism before they are carried into the general circulation. This initial passage through the liver is therapeutically significant, primarily for drugs that are metabolized to a less active or inactive form by the liver. *(17:315)*

23. **(C)** Pharmaceutic equivalents are considered to be drug products that are almost identical in all aspects and are expected to exhibit almost identical therapeutic activity. Bioavailablity data submitted to the FDA must show that similar values for onset of action, duration, peak concentrations, and time for peak concentration are obtained. One of the few variables allowed is the choice of excipients. These excipients or "inactive ingredients," include binders, diluents, lubricants, and so on. Naturally the manufacturers must include data proving that these excipients do not adversely affect the performance of their product. *(24:73)*

24. **(A)** Drug products considered to be pharmaceutic alternatives are allowed greater variations from each other. Although they must contain the same active drug or its precursor, they may consist of different dosage forms, strengths, or contain a different salt of the drug. *(24:73)*

25. **(D)** Gastric emptying appears to be an exponential process with a normal half-life of between 20 and 60 minutes. However, many factors can influence the rate of this process. It is slowed by the A, B, C, and E choices and is speeded by hunger, mild exercise, cold meals, dilute solutions, and lying on the right side. Because some drugs and some dosage forms (eg, enteric-coated tablets) are absorbed at rather specific sites along the GI tract, alterations in the rate of gastric empty-

ing may lead to erratic and unpredictable absorption. For example, if an acid-labile drug that is preferentially absorbed from a portion of the small intestine is consumed as an enteric-coated tablet, a greatly reduced gastric emptying rate may permit the tablet to dissolve in the stomach and be degraded by the acid fluids of the stomach. Similarly, if the gastric emptying rate is greatly increased, the tablet may not dissolve before it reaches its primary site of absorption. *(17:126)*

26. **(C)** After a drug gains access to the systemic circulation, it may be metabolized to varying degrees and/or be excreted unchanged. For most drugs and their metabolites, the kidneys are the primary organ of excretion. The presence of a drug and/or its metabolites in the urine must be preceded by the presence of drug in the blood. When an appreciable amount of drug is excreted in the urine, it is often possible to use urinary excretion data—such as cumulative amount of drug in the urine and maximum urinary excretion rate—to evaluate the systemic availability of various drug formulations. *(17:200)*

27. **(C)** Urinary excretion studies require complete urine collection so that the total quantity of drug that is excreted in the urine can be determined. Normal or near-normal renal function is also a prerequisite for accurate urinary excretion studies because sufficiently impaired renal function can alter the composition of various body fluids that, in turn, can alter the pharmacokinetic properties of many drugs. Although urinary excretion studies are usually conducted on drugs that are primarily excreted unchanged by the kidney, it is not necessary that a drug be completely excreted unchanged by the kidney. *(17:56)*

28. **(C)** The best measure of absolute bioavailability is considered to be AUC data obtained after a bolus IV injection of a drug. Because AUC data is not available for these drug products, the next best comparison will be the use of cumulative drug amounts found in the urine. Because the IV injection dose was 10 mg whereas the oral tablet dose was 20 mg, a correction factor of 2 × is needed. Cu-

mulative amount if 20 mg had been injected will be 9.4 × 2 = 18.8. Dividing 8.2 mg by 18.8 mg = 0.44, or 44%. *(17:197)*

29. **(A)** Relative bioavailability of Company B's tablet when compared to Company A's tablet will be 8.2 mg divided by 12 mg = 0.68, or 68%. To determine the relative bioavailability of Company B's capsule, one must correct for the fact that the capsule dose was 15 mg. That is, determine the mg of drug that would accumulate in the urine if a 20 mg capsule dose was administered.

$$\frac{15\text{-mg cap}}{6.8 \text{ mg (in urine)}} = \frac{20 \text{ mg}}{x \text{ mg (in urine)}}$$
$$x = 9.1 \text{ mg}$$

Relative bioavailability will equal 9.1 divided by 12 mg = 0.76, or 76%. Neither Company B's tablet or capsule can be considered bioequivalent to Company A's tablet because neither is within 80% of the cumulative amount of drug in the urine. This 80% guideline has been accepted by the FDA for determining bioequivalency of similar drug products. *(17:197)*

30. **(C)** Just as shifting the ionic equilibrium in favor of the ionic species reduces the probability that a weakly acidic drug will be absorbed from the alkaline fluids of the intestines, it also reduces the probability that the drug will be reabsorbed from the renal tubules into the blood. Consequently, a greater fraction of drug in the tubules cannot be reabsorbed and will be excreted in the urine. *(15:176; 17:271)*

31. **(C)** For any drug that is eliminated by first-order kinetics, the time required to achieve steady-state plasma levels is dependent only on the biologic half-life of that drug in a given individual. As a drug is repeatedly administered in constant dosage and at constant time intervals (that are short enough to preclude complete elimination of the drug), the elimination rate of the drug increases as the concentration of drug in plasma increases. The tendency of a drug to accumulate on repeated dosing is, therefore, bal-

anced by increased amounts of drug being eliminated. Eventually, a steady state will be reached in which the amount of drug absorbed will equal the amount of drug being eliminated. The time to reach steady state corresponds to about four to five half-lives and is more completely described in the following table:

Time Plasma (Half-Lives)	Concentration (% of Steady-State Level)
1	50
2	75
3	88
4	94
5	97
6	98
7	99

(17:337; 19:2–5)

32. **(C)** Generally, when a particular drug has a half-life of 6 hours, there is reasonable certainty that in spite of as much as a one- to twofold intersubject variation, the mean biologic half-life in any group of subjects will approximate 6 hours. Alterations in biologic half-life can be expected when a particular drug is primarily excreted unchanged by the kidneys. The presence of renal impairment slows the process of excretion and thereby increases the biologic half-life of the drug in the blood. *(1:605; 24:92)*

33. **(A)** Most drugs have biologic half-lives that follow first-order kinetics. A basic characteristic of first-order kinetics is that the rate constants for metabolism or excretion are independent of the initial drug concentration. That is, a specific fraction of drug will be lost in a given time period. Doubling the drug concentration will not change the rate constant, even though the amount of drug lost in a given time period would increase.
(D–incorrect) Renal impairment may affect the biologic half-life of drugs eliminated by the kidneys. However, the half-life would be expected to increase (not decrease), because the drug remains in the circulation for longer periods of time.

(E–incorrect) Two methods for determining half-life are (1) to determine drug blood levels with respect to time and (2) to quantify with respect to time actual biologic responses to the drug. Ideally, the half-life values by each method should be identical. However, they will be identical only when there is a direct and measurable relationship between drug blood concentrations and the biologic response. *(17:27)*

34. **(C)** *(1:728; 24:92)*

35. **(C)** One-half (200 mg) of the administered dose will be eliminated in 4 hours. Of the remaining 200 mg, one-half (100 mg) will be eliminated in the second 4-hour period. In the next 4-hour span, an additional 50 mg of drug will be lost. Therefore, after 12 hours (or three half-lives), only 50 mg of drug remains. If graphed as log drug remaining (Y axis) versus time (X axis), the data will appear as a straight line (first-order kinetics). *(1:593; 23:206)*

36. **(D)** The metabolic pathways of newborn infants are incompletely developed at birth; most notably, the oxidative and conjugative mechanisms that are known to metabolize many drugs. The reduced capacity to metabolize certain drugs will therefore result in prolonged biologic half-lives of these drugs in newborn infants. Because of inadequate metabolic inactivation, the plasma concentration of chloramphenicol is higher in infants younger than 2 weeks of age than in older infants. *(17:416; 19:96–5)*

37. **(C)** A rate constant of 20% per hour refers to a fraction loss of 0.2 per hour. The equation for determining half-lives for first-order reactions is

$$t_{50} = \frac{0.693}{k} = \frac{0.693}{0.2} = 3.5 \text{ hours}$$

(23:306)

38. **(A)** Volume of distribution (V_d) is an "apparent volume" measured in terms of a reference compartment, usually the blood, because of the accessibility of this compartment

to sampling. Because the drug dose is known and the blood concentration can be determined, the V_d may be calculated by:

$$V_d = A_b/C_b$$

where
A_b = total amount of unchanged drug in the body, and
C_b = concentration of drug in the blood.

Knowledge of the Vd for a particular drug permits calculation of the total amount of drug in the body (Ab) at any time by measuring the drug concentration in the blood (because Ab = Vd) accumulation in specific body areas. Also, because only the unbound fraction of drug is available for biotransformation and excretion, protein-bound drugs have a tendency to remain in the body longer (ie, delayed elimination and longer half-lives). *(1:726; 17:48)*

39. **(A)** Following a given dose of a drug, the greater its concentration in various tissue compartments, the smaller its concentration in plasma. Therefore, according to the relationship $A_b = V_d \times C_b$ (see commentary for Question 38), the V_d of a particular drug will be greater for those drugs that tend to concentrate in tissues as opposed to plasma. *(1:726; 15:20–22)*

40. **(C)** Because the V_d is a parameter that allows accountability for all of the drug in the body, it can be used to calculate the loading dose that would rapidly result in a desired plasma concentration (C_p).

$$\text{Loading Dose} = \frac{(V_d)(C_p)}{(S)(F)}$$

where S = portion of the salt form that is active drug and
F = fraction of dose absorbed. *(19:2–3)*

41. **(B)** One can easily picture that the drug blood concentration (C_o) will be equal to the amount of drug (LD) administered or absorbed divided by the body volume (V_d) in which it is distributed.

$$C_o = \frac{LD}{V_d} \text{ or } LD = (C_o)(V_d)$$

In this problem:

Step 1: 140 lb × 1 kg/2.2 lb = 64 kg (body wt)

Step 2: V_d = 64 kg × 1.6 L/kg = 102 L

Step 3: 50 mg = (C_o)(102 L)

Step 4: C_o = 0.5 mg/L, ANS

(6:25; 23:205)

42. **(B)** Curve I shows an initial high concentration of drug in the blood with a steadily decreasing concentration. This curve is characteristic of drugs administered by rapid intravenous injection. *(17:156)*

43. **(E)** Any of the listed dosage forms could exhibit blood level curves similar to curve II. The first portion of the curve shows an increasing concentration of drug in the blood. This pattern would be expected whenever there is steady drug absorption (ie, when absorption is greater than elimination), either from the GI tract or from a tissue injection site. Curve III is also a good representation for a sustained-release product as it illustrates a plateau effect. *(17:156)*

44. **(E)** For any drug to exhibit high blood levels it must be absorbed at a rate significantly greater than the rate by which it is eliminated. That is, K_a must be greater than K_e, at least in the early period of its therapeutic curve. Obviously the manufacturer bases dosing amounts on the relative speed and extent of absorption versus how quickly the drug is being eliminated. *(15:36–37)*
(A–incorrect) Blood levels of drug increase until a peak occurs where the rate of absorption equals the rate of elimination. Drug absorption will usually continue to occur even after the peak blood concentration has been reached. However the blood level curve is then declining, because the rate of elimination is greater than the rate of absorption.
(B–incorrect) Because most of the factors affecting pharmacokinetics are first order, doubling a drug dose will seldom double the

height of a blood level curve. However, the total area under the drug curve can be expected to double, because the AUC is directly proportional to the dose.

(C–incorrect) The pharmacokinetics of most drugs follow a first-order pattern. Therefore, if the concentration of drug in the blood is plotted as a log function on the Y axis, a straight line will be obtained rather than a curve, as shown on the graph.

(D–incorrect) The time factor is a constant variable plotted at regular intervals (hours, days, etc). It is very seldom expressed as a log function.

45. **(B)** Administration of drugs by intravenous infusion, which implies slow flow into a vein, will result in a plateau effect in respect to drug blood levels. The resulting steady-state levels are directly proportional to the infusion rate.

(A–incorrect) An intravenous push (bolus dose) will give a curve similar to curve I on the graph.

(D–incorrect) The blood level curve for an intrathecal (spinal) injection will probably resemble curve II as the drug slowly diffuses into the blood. *(15:68)*

46. **(C)** The time in which the optimum drug blood level is obtained is independent of the infusion rate. It is dependent only on the biologic half-life of the particular drug. The time required to reach the plateau (steady state) is approximately four to five half-lives. At the blood concentration plateau, the K_e equals the infusion rate. *(15:69)*

47. **(B)** Although various organs, tissues, and fluids in the body can be considered to be compartments for a specific drug, a compartment does not necessarily have to be an anatomic entity. Any body site or fluid that appears to contain drug may be described as a compartment or "pool" in the model. *(17:39; 24:89–91)*

48. **(E)** *(6:20–21:17:41)*

49. **(E)** This is the definition of total systemic (whole body) clearance, which is the sum of all the separate clearances (ie, renal, hepatic, etc). *(19:2–5)*

50. **(A)** When the clearance (Cl) of a drug is known, the maintenance dose required to sustain a desired average steady-state plasma concentration can be calculated by:

$$\text{Maintenance dose} = \frac{(\text{Cl})\,(\text{C}_p)\,(\tau)}{(\text{S})\,(\text{F})}$$

Where C_p = average steady-state plasma concentration
τ = dosing interval
S = portion of salt that is active drug
F = fraction of dose absorbed

(19:2–5)

51. **(A)** Drugs (eg, aminoglycosides) given at intervals that are much longer than one half-life are almost completely eliminated from the body before the next dose is given. This results in a large difference between peak and trough drug concentrations, thus timing of blood samples(s) becomes crucial to interpretation of results. At the other extreme, drugs given at intervals that are much shorter than one half-life (eg, phenobarbital) are slowly cleared from the body; consequently, their peak-to-trough concentration differences are relatively small. *(19:2–6)*

52. **(E)** Decreased efficiency in renal function occurs in approximately 70% of the geriatric population. Also, both blood circulation and hepatic function decrease in many of the elderly. Because both extracellular and other body fluids may decrease in volume, reported volume of distributions in some geriatric patients may be lower than expected. *(2a:26)*

53. **(C)** Drug elimination by the kidneys can often be correlated with blood urea nitrogen (BUN), serum creatinine (Sr_{Cr}), and creatinine clearance (CL_{cr}). The BUN and Sr_{Cr}, however, are less useful indices of renal function than the CL_{cr} because they are influenced by other factors (eg, state of hydration, age, etc). For example, as patients age, both the production and clearance of creatinine decrease. Therefore, an elderly patient with a normal serum creatinine of 1 mg/dL may

have a CL_{cr} of much less than 100 mL/min (normal CL_{cr} is 100 to 120 mL/min for a 70-kg adult). There are a number of methods used to calculate CL_{cr}. An example of a useful equation is

$$CL_{cr} \text{ (for a male)} = \frac{(40 - \text{age}) \text{ (weight)}}{72 \text{ (Sr}_{Cr})}$$

Units include age in years, weight in kilograms, and serum creatinine measurements in mg/dL. For females, the calculated CL value is reduced by multiplying by 0.85. (19:2–7)

54. **(A)** If the biologic half-life of a drug increases in patients with impaired renal function, the time required to reach steady-state plasma levels will also be increased. This time factor is only dependent on the biologic half-life of a given drug in a given individual. (17:472)

55. **(D)** Only the unbound fraction of a drug is available for biotransformation and excretion. Protein-bound drugs have a tendency to remain in the body longer because they do not readily enter hepatocytes for metabolism by the liver. Protein-bound drugs are larger molecules and cannot as readily diffuse through the renal glomeruli for eventual excretion, thus their half-lives will be longer. (17:91–94; 24:85)

56. **(A)** When administered in therapeutic doses, allopurinol does not appear to bind to plasma proteins. The pharmacist should carefully monitor drug therapy when two or more drugs that exhibit significant protein-binding properties are prescribed. Relatively small changes in the degree of protein binding caused by competition for binding sites can result in significant changes in plasma concentration of free drug and in the intensity of the clinical response. (1:745)

57. **(D)** Drug metabolites are usually more polar and less lipid soluble than the parent compound. Because of these changes, metabolites are usually not as tightly nor as extensively protein bound. They are ionized to a greater degree and are less likely to cross biologic membranes than the parent compound. Drug metabolism, therefore, is generally a process that inactivates a drug and changes it to a form that can be excreted more easily and rapidly. For some drugs, however, metabolism may result in activation of an inactive substance, or an active substance may be transformed into (an) active metabolite(s). In these cases, either further biotransformation takes place to inactivate the metabolite(s), or it (they) is (are) excreted unchanged. (1:717)

58. **(A)** The term "first pass" refers to the first passage of drug molecules through a designated organ such as the lungs or the liver. Biotransformation will often occur at this site, thereby altering the absolute bioavailability of a drug. Commercial preparations of such drugs are formulated to contain sufficient quantities of drug to compensate for loss due to first-pass biotransformation. Although acetylsalicylic acid does not appear to undergo a significant first-pass hepatic biotransformation, some drug loss does occur in the intestinal lumen or during absorption through the GI mucosa. (17:320)

59. **(A)** Only 5% of phenytoin is metabolized in the liver; most of the drug is excreted unchanged. When significant amounts of a drug are metabolized by the liver immediately after absorption through the GI tract wall (first-pass effect), manufacturers may compensate by increasing the dose present in oral dosage forms. For example, propranolol is available as 40- and 80-mg tablets, whereas the parenteral form is 2-mL ampules containing 2 mg/mL. (19:2–3; 24:78)

60. **(B)** The water solubility of theophylline is enhanced by combining it with ethylenediamine, forming the drug aminophylline. Because the active moiety, theophylline, contributes 80% of the molecular weight of aminophylline, a correction factor is needed to convert between the two drugs when predicting therapeutic activity. This conversion factor is often referred to as the "S" factor, and is expressed as a fraction. The S value for

aminophylline is 0.8, whereas the S value for oxtriphylline (Choledyl) is 0.65. *(1:971–73; 19:19–24)*

61. **(C)** Although some drugs are absorbed from the gastrointestinal tract by active transport mechanisms against a concentration gradient or by facilitated diffusion with a concentration gradient, most drugs are passively absorbed from a region of high concentration to a region of low concentration (ie, with a concentration gradient). *(17:113)*

62. **(A)** Fick's First Law states that the rate of diffusion is directly related to the diffusion coefficient and the surface area of the membrane and inversely proportional to the thickness of the membrane. The driving force in the equation is the concentration gradient, because the greater the difference in concentrations on each side of the membrane, the greater the amount of drug diffusing (first-order kinetics). *(17:113; 24:57)*

63. **(B)** The greater the difference between the drug concentrations on each side of a biologic membrane, the greater the rate of transfer from the side having the higher concentration to the side having the lower concentration. *(17:113)*

64. **(C)** Linear pharmacokinetics is characterized by straight line relationships when plotted as a log function (Y axis) versus time (X axis). Certain drugs deviate from this straight line, especially when their doses are increased or multidoses are given. Such drugs are described as following dose-dependent or nonlinear pharmacokinetics. The classic example is a drug that demonstrates capacity-limited (saturation) metabolism. *(17:375)*

65. **(D)** As the name implies, carrier-mediated or active transport involves active participation of a membrane in transferring molecules from one side to the other. The "carrier," such as an enzyme in the membrane, aids in transporting the molecules of drug across the membrane. Because this transfer process is continuous, it can work against a concentration gradient and continue until all of the

drug has been transported. Therefore, equilibrium does not occur.

(A–incorrect) Active transport requires energy. Facilitated diffusion is a carrier-mediated transport process that does not require energy.

(B–incorrect) Certain chemicals, known as poisons, can reduce active transport, probably by destroying or inactivating the drug carriers.

(C–incorrect) Carriers are often very specific in respect to the drug they will transport. Only a certain chemical structure or similar chemical structures may be actively transported by a given carrier.

(E–incorrect) Because of the chemical specificity and limited capacity of carriers, active transport systems may become saturated. When this occurs, the active transport rate becomes a constant value until the drug concentration is reduced. *(6:4,23; 17:116)*

66. **(A)** A characteristic of a zero-order process or reaction is a constant rate of change. When the active transport system is saturated, there are not enough carriers to handle the large number of transferable molecules. Therefore, the carriers work at maximum capacity, transferring molecules at a constant rate until the drug concentration is reduced to less than the capacity of the carrier system. At this time, the number of molecules transferred will be a fraction of those present for transfer (ie, a first-order rate will exist). *(1:725)*

67. **(B)** In order to take advantage of certain desirable characteristics, some drugs are marketed as prodrugs. These are chemical modifications of biologically active drugs and may not be active themselves. However, the active form of the drug is liberated in the body by biotransformation. Prodrugs may possess better water solubility, be more stable, have a less objectionable taste, or give higher blood levels than the parent compound. *(17:307; 24:86)*

68. **(C)** Clorazepate (Tranxene) is rapidly decarboxylated in the acidic stomach to an active metabolite that possesses antiepileptic properties. Enalapril (Vasotec) is hydrolyzed to

enalaprilate, which is the active angiotensin-converting enzyme (ACE) inhibitor for hypertension. However, lisinopril (Zestril) does not undergo metabolism, and instead is excreted unchanged in the urine. Other drugs, such as verapamil (Calan) form a large number of metabolites. *(10; 24:87)*

69. **(C)** Although it is desirable for certain drugs rapidly metabolized by the liver to bypass absorption into the portal circulation, the value of using the rectal route for this purpose is limited. This is due to the fact that whereas the blood supply to the rectum is drained by three principal veins, only the middle and inferior hemorrhoidal veins actually bypass the liver. The superior hemorrhoidal vein enters the portal circulation via the inferior mesenteric vein. *(17:156:24:425)*

70. **(D)** If an orally administered drug appears in the feces, it might be desirable to determine whether this is the result of incomplete absorption or secretion of the drug into the GI tract via biliary excretion. The clinical significance of biliary excretion or enterohepatic cycling of the drug depends on the fraction of the dose excreted in the bile. By administering the drug parenterally, this fraction can be determined. *(15:168; 17:328–29)*

71. **(A)** The "blood–brain barrier" appears to behave as a lipoid membrane toward foreign compounds. This barrier may be due to a sheath of glial cells surrounding the capillaries of the brain. The rate of entry of a drug can often be correlated with its oil/water partition coefficient and degree of ionization at plasma pH. *(17:82)*

72. **(B)** Antimicrobials with poor lipid solubility have difficulty in penetrating the blood–brain barrier. The minimum inhibitory concentration is the concentration of antibiotic that prevents the growth of microorganisms. The lower the value, the more effective the antibiotic is in respect to the concentration needed. Increasing the minimum toxic con-

centration will increase the safety of the drug and decrease the incidence of side effects. Binding of drug to plasma protein is generally undesirable, because the bound fraction of drug is unavailable for therapeutic activity. *(17:472; 19:56–2; 24:215)*

73. **(E)** All of these drug characteristics are probably undesirable for a sustained-release dosage form. For a successful sustained-release product, the rate-limiting step must be drug release from the dosage form. If the drug has poor solubility, the dissolution rate may become the rate-limiting step. In this case, the patient may not absorb the quantity of drug needed for desired blood levels and therapeutic activity. Drugs with very long half-lives do not need to be formulated for sustained-release, because they will be biologically present for a long period of time. Intelligent dosing, such as every 12 or 24 hours (depending on the actual half-life), ensures sufficient blood levels. The release of drug from most sustained-release dosage forms is subject to individual biological variations. This patient-to-patient variability may result in the release of two or three times the normal dose in a particular patient. Therefore, a dangerous situation may develop if very large amounts of very potent drugs are formulated as sustained-release products. Conversely, a drug with a very short half-life is also a poor candidate for sustained release. A very large amount of drug would have to be included in the dosage form, and rapid release of the drug would be necessary. *(17:230–32; 24:215)*

74. **(C)** The lag time is the time delay between drug administration and the beginning of absorption, usually reflected in the appearance of drug in the plasma. Enteric-coated tablets are intended for disintegration in the small intestine, which could slow absorption for several hours. Both delayed-release and sustained-release tablets are usually designed to begin some drug release shortly after administration. *(15:36)*

75. (C) The binding of drugs to body proteins is an important concept when considering dosing and possible drug displacement from binding sites due to other drugs. The symbol. f_u, refers to the fraction of a specific drug that is not bound. A value of 0.8 indicates that 80% of the drug is available, whereas 20% is protein bound. *(1:181)*

CHAPTER 6

Pharmaceutical Care

Pharmaceutical care is a term many have found difficult to define. A U.S. Supreme Court Justice, when challenged to define pornography, is said to have replied that although he could not define it, he was sure he could recognize it if he saw it. One definition of pharmaceutical care states that it is "the responsible provision of drug therapy for the purpose of achieving definite outcomes that improve a patient's quality of life."[1] With this example in mind, we have assembled a series of questions for this chapter that we believe fall under the category of Pharmaceutical Care—that is, they relate to patients, diseases, drugs, information, and pharmacists.

[1] C. D. Hepler and L. M. Strand. *Opportunities and responsibilities in pharmaceutical care.* Amer J Hosp Pharm 47:533–543, 1990.

Questions

DIRECTIONS (Questions 1 through 210): Each of the numbered items or incomplete statements in this section is followed by answers or by completions of the statement. Select the ONE lettered answer or completion that is BEST in each case.

1. Which of the following drugs is generally considered the drug of choice in treating status epilepticus?

   (A) Phenobarbital
   (B) Ethosuximide (Zarontin)
   (C) Diazepam (Valium)
   (D) Paraldehyde
   (E) Phenytoin (Dilantin)

2. A syndrome strongly resembling systemic lupus erythematosus (SLE) is an adverse reaction associated with the use of

   (A) pirbuterol (Maxair)
   (B) reserpine
   (C) diazoxide (Hyperstat IV)
   (D) methyldopa (Aldomet)
   (E) hydralazine (Apresoline)

3. The antihypertensive effect of guanethidine (Ismelin) is inhibited by

   (A) erythromycin (E-mycin)
   (B) nalbumetone (Relafen)
   (C) hydrochlorothiazide (HydroDIURIL)
   (D) probenecid (Benemid)
   (E) amitriptyline (Elavil)

4. In terms of its major pharmacologic effect, metoprolol (Lopressor) is most similar to

   (A) isoproterenol (Isuprel)
   (B) metaproterenol (Alupent)
   (C) guanethidine (Ismelin)
   (D) hydrochlorothiazide (HydroDIURIL)
   (E) timolol (Blocadren)

5. When dispensing a new prescription, for which of the following drugs should the pharmacist advise the patient that he or she may experience a large fall in blood pressure following the first dose?

   (A) Terazosin (Hytrin)
   (B) Fosinopril (Monopril)
   (C) Clonidine (Catapres)
   (D) Reserpine (Serpasil)
   (E) Propranolol (Inderal)

6. A common measure in assessing the degree of immunodeficency in acquired immunodeficiency syndrome (AIDS) patients is the determination of levels of

   (A) ACTH
   (B) *Pneumocystis carinii* organisms
   (C) thrombocytes
   (D) CD4 cells
   (E) erythrocyte sedimentation rate (ESR)

7. In the treatment of acute hypertensive crisis, diazoxide (Hyperstat IV) is administered

   (A) orally
   (B) intramuscularly
   (C) rapidly, by intravenous (IV) injection
   (D) by slow infusion over 1–4 hours
   (E) by slow infusion for 6–24 hours

8. A physician has decided on a course of tetracycline therapy for a patient with renal impairment. Which of the following drugs is LEAST likely to accumulate in the patient's blood?

   (A) Demeclocycline
   (B) Oxytetracycline
   (C) Minocycline
   (D) Doxycycline
   (E) Tetracycline

9. Which of the following antihypertensive agents would probably be the BEST choice to use in a severely depressed hypertensive patient?

   (A) Reserpine (Serpasil)
   (B) Clonidine (Catapres)
   (C) Guanethidine (Ismelin)
   (D) Methyldopa (Aldomet)
   (E) Ramipril (Altace)

10. Which of the following agents has NOT been suggested as an agent to use to eradicate *Helicobacter pylori* from the gastrointestinal (GI) tract?

    (A) Ketoconazole
    (B) Bismuth subsalicylate
    (C) Metronidazole
    (D) Clarithromycin
    (E) Tetracycline

11. Cholestyramine (Questran) will probably interfere with the GI absorption of

    I. chlorothiazide
    II. warfarin
    III. phenobarbital

    (A) I only
    (B) III only
    (C) I and II only
    (D) II and III only
    (E) I, II, and III

12. A clinically noticeable drug interaction resulting from the displacement of drug A by drug B from common plasma protein–binding sites is most often seen when

    (A) drug A has a high association constant (K) for binding the protein
    (B) drug B has a low association constant (K) for binding the protein and is given in large doses
    (C) drug B has a high association constant (K) for binding the protein and is given in large doses
    (D) drug B is more toxic than drug A
    (E) drug B is rapidly absorbed

13. The metabolism of which of the following compounds is altered in patients taking anticonvulsants?

    (A) Pyridoxine
    (B) Tyramine
    (C) Riboflavin
    (D) Folic acid
    (E) Tyrosine

14. Which of the following agents would be likely to affect the platelet aggregation of an adult?

    I. NAPAP (Tylenol)
    II. Acetylsalicylic acid (ASPIRIN)
    III. Naproxen sodium

    (A) I only
    (B) III only
    (C) I and II only
    (D) II and III only
    (E) I, II, and III

15. A microorganism that is particularly dangerous to the eye is

    (A) *Aspergillus niger*
    (B) *Bacillus subtilis*
    (C) *Escherichia coli*
    (D) *Streptococcus thermophilus*
    (E) *Pseudomonas aeruginosa*

16. Purulent boils in the ear are usually caused by species of

(A) *Staphylococcus*
(B) *Candida*
(C) *Pseudomonas*
(D) *Aspergillus*
(E) *Streptococcus*

17. The treatment of choice for herpes simplex infection of the eyelids and conjunctiva is

(A) thiabendazole (Mintezol)
(B) bacitracin (Baciguent)
(C) amphotericin B (Fungizone)
(D) idoxuridine (Stoxil)
(E) mupirocin (Bactroban)

18. Which of the following antifungal agents is ineffective against *Candida* organisms?

(A) Nystatin (Mycostatin)
(B) Clotrimazole (Lotrimin)
(C) Tolnaftate (Tinactin)
(D) Ciclopirox olamine (Loprox)
(E) Miconazole (Micatin)

19. Methotrexate has been shown to be of clinical use in the management of

(A) venereal warts
(B) seborrhea
(C) acne
(D) ringworm infections of the skin
(E) psoriasis

20. Important potential complications of corticosteroid therapy include

I. dissemination of local infection
II. masking symptoms of an infection
III. increased susceptibility to infection

(A) I only
(B) III only
(C) I and II only
(D) II and III only
(E) I, II, and III

21. The primary advantage of piroxicam (Feldene) over most other nonsteroidal anti-inflammatory drugs (NSAIDs) is that it

(A) is relatively inexpensive
(B) acts by a different mechanism of action that may be additive to other NSAIDs
(C) may be given on a once-a-day schedule
(D) has a cytoprotective effect
(E) has essentially no GI side effects

22. Which of the following NSAIDS would be of particular use in an arthritic patient who has difficulty remembering to take his or her medication during the day?

(A) Tolmetin (Tolectin)
(B) Fenoprofen (Nalfon)
(C) Ibuprofen (Motrin)
(D) Oxaprozin (Daypro)
(E) Diclofenac sodium (Voltaren)

23. When dispensing the fluorouracil solutions Fluoroplex or Efudex, the pharmacist should give the patient all of the following advice and warnings EXCEPT

(A) apply with a nonmetallic applicator or fingertips
(B) avoid prolonged exposure to sunlight
(C) cover infected area with an occlusive dressing after application
(D) avoid exposure to ultraviolet (UV) light
(E) burning sensation and inflammation may occur

24. Which of the following best describes the condition known as hypoprothrombinemia?

(A) The development of transient ischemic attacks (TIAs).
(B) Blood clot formation in a peripheral blood vessel.
(C) A low level of iron in the blood.
(D) A reduced capability for blood to clot.
(E) A decrease in the production of red blood cells by the bone marrow.

25. The rapid reversal of anticoagulant-induced hemorrhage is best accomplished by the administration of

   I. phytonadione (AquaMEPHYTON)
   II. menadiol sodium diphosphate (Synkayvite)
   III. fresh blood or plasma

   (A) I only
   (B) III only
   (C) I and II only
   (D) II and III only
   (E) I, II, and III

26. A patient complains of a reddish discoloration of his or her urine. Which of the following drugs would most likely produce such an effect?

   (A) Aluminum hydroxide
   (B) Methenamine
   (C) Sulfamethoxazole
   (D) Isoniazid
   (E) Phenazopyridine

27. Menotropins (Pergonal, Humegon) is used clinically in the treatment of

   (A) psoriasis
   (B) depression
   (C) nausea
   (D) infertility
   (E) dysmenorrhea

28. The e.p.t. Quick Stick Test, the home pregnancy test marketed by Parke-Davis, assays for the presence of

   (A) estradiol
   (B) estrogen
   (C) progesterone
   (D) prolactin
   (E) human chorionic gonadotropin

29. The clinical investigation of a new drug consists of four phases. Phase I of the clinical testing involves administering the drug

   (A) by select clinicians to healthy volunteers
   (B) to animals for toxicity studies

   (C) to animals to determine the effectiveness of the drug
   (D) by select clinicians to patients suffering from the disease
   (E) by general practitioners to patients suffering from the disease

30. Which of the following best describes the common clinical manifestations of hypoparathyroidism?

   (A) Hypocalcemia and hyperphosphatemia
   (B) Hypocalcemia and hypophosphatemia
   (C) Hypercalcemia and hypophosphatemia
   (D) Hypercalcemia and hyperphosphatemia
   (E) Hypercalcemia and hypochlorhydria

31. Tubocurarine should NOT be used in patients who are taking

   (A) aspirin
   (B) morphine
   (C) amikacin
   (D) levodopa
   (E) reserpine

32. Myxedema is what kind of state?

   (A) Hyperthyroid
   (B) Hypoparathyroid
   (C) Hypothyroid
   (D) Hyperparathyroid
   (E) Hypopituitarism

33. Enuresis refers to

   (A) gout
   (B) urinary tract infection
   (C) urinary retention
   (D) diminished stature
   (E) bedwetting

34. Which of the following should NOT be used in patients who are allergic to aspirin?

   (A) Stadol
   (B) Darvocet-N
   (C) Excedrin PM
   (D) Fiorinal
   (E) Wygesic

35. Which of the following phrases best defines the clinical disorder known as hemochromatosis?

    (A) A lack of circulating antibodies
    (B) Diminished circulating blood volume
    (C) Abnormally shaped red blood cells
    (D) Excessive storage of iron by the body
    (E) Absence of pigmentation in circulating red blood cells

36. A reversible cholestatic hepatitis with fever and jaundice has been observed as an adverse drug reaction in patients taking erythromycin

    (A) estolate (Ilosone)
    (B) ethylsuccinate (EES Granules)
    (C) base (E-Mycin tablets)
    (D) stearate (Erythrocin Filmtab)
    (E) gluceptate (Ilotycin)

37. The most important indication for vancomycin (Vancocin) is in the treatment of serious infections that do NOT respond to other treatment and that are caused by which of the following organisms?

    (A) Pneumococcal
    (B) Streptococcal
    (C) Staphylococcal
    (D) Gonococcal
    (E) Pseudomonal

38. Famotidine (Pepcid) inhibits gastric acid secretion as a result of what kind of activity?

    (A) Antihistaminic
    (B) Proton pump inhibition
    (C) Anticholinergic
    (D) Buffer generation
    (E) *Helicobacter pylori* inhibition

39. Benzylpenicilloyl–polylysine is a substance used to

    (A) stabilize crystalline penicillin G preparations
    (B) counteract allergic reactions to penicillin
    (C) reduce the renal secretion of penicillin

    (D) reduce copper levels in the blood
    (E) skin test patients for penicillin allergy

40. A tricyclic amine that is used as an antiviral agent is

    (A) desipramine (Norpramin, Pertofrane)
    (B) amantadine (Symmetrel)
    (C) tromethamine (Tham)
    (D) cytosine arabinoside (Cytarabine, Cytosar)
    (E) idoxuridine (Herplex)

41. Which of the following agents are indicated for the treatment of the human immunodeficiency virus (HIV) infection?

    I. Ifosfamide
    II. Cytarabine
    III. Didanosine

    (A) I only
    (B) III only
    (C) I and II only
    (D) II and III only
    (E) I, II, and III

42. A patient complains about a headache that is localized in the periorbital area and seems to be worse in the morning than the afternoon. Which of the following would be the best way to characterize the headache?

    (A) Sinus
    (B) Vascular–migraine
    (C) Muscle contraction
    (D) Eye strain
    (E) Tumorigenic

43. The purpose of combined drug treatment in tuberculosis (TB) is to

    I. increase the tuberculostatic effects of the drugs
    II. delay the emergence of drug resistance
    III. reduce the duration of active therapy

    (A) I only
    (B) III only
    (C) I and II only

(D) II and III only

(E) I, II, and III

44. Patients taking the antitubercular drug rifampin (Rifadin) should be told that the drug

(A) may cause diarrhea

(B) may cause them to sunburn more easily

(C) may produce nausea and vomiting if alcoholic beverages are consumed

(D) may impart an orange color to their urine and sweat

(E) should be swallowed whole (ie, not chewed) to prevent staining of the teeth

45. A patient using ticlopidine (Ticlid) should be monitored for the development of

(A) pseudomembranous enterocolitis

(B) gynecomastia

(C) xerophthalmia

(D) respiratory impairment

(E) abnormal bleeding

46. A penicillin derivative that is most closely related to ampicillin but has a much greater activity against *Pseudomonas* is

(A) methicillin (Staphcillin)

(B) ticarcillin (Ticar)

(C) nafcillin (Unipen)

(D) dicloxacillin (Dynapen)

(E) oxacillin (Prostaphlin)

47. Antibiotic-induced pseudomembranous colitis is most commonly treated with

(A) attapulgite (Kaopectate)

(B) loperamide (Imodium)

(C) vancomycin (Vancocin)

(D) gentamicin (Garamycin)

(E) sulfasalazine (Azulfidine)

48. Cushing syndrome is a condition associated with

(A) hyperthyroidism

(B) adrenal hyperplasia

(C) hypothyroidism

(D) obsessive–compulsive disorder

(E) polyuria

49. The aminoglycoside antibiotics are

I. metabolized by the liver

II. suitable for long-term treatment of chronic urinary tract infections (UTIs)

III. bactericidal for a wide range of gram-positive and gram-negative microorganisms

(A) I only

(B) III only

(C) I and II only

(D) II and III only

(E) I, II, and III

50. Which one of the following cephalosporins is available in both oral and parenteral dosage forms?

(A) Cefaclor (Ceclor)

(B) Cefazolin (Ancef, Kefzol)

(C) Loracarbef (Lorabid)

(D) Cephradine (Velosef)

(E) Cefotaxime (Claforan)

51. A disadvantage of using cromolyn sodium in asthma treatment is

(A) its brief duration of action

(B) its nephrotoxicity

(C) that it may cause tachyphylaxis

(D) that it is ineffective in treating acute attacks

(E) that it causes cardiac stimulation

52. An asthmatic patient who is currently taking terbutaline (Brethine) 5-mg tablets (TID), prednisone 5 mg (QID), and Proventil Inhaler (PRN) presents you with a prescription for Vanceril Inhaler. The directions on the prescription are "one inhalation PRN breathing difficulty." The most appropriate action for you to take is to

    (A) fill the prescription
    (B) inform the prescriber that Vanceril (beclomethasone) is a prophylactic drug that should be taken regularly
    (C) inform the prescriber that the prednisone should be discontinued before Vanceril therapy is initiated
    (D) advise the patient to stop using the Proventil Inhaler
    (E) advise the prescriber to discontinue the terbutaline tablets

53. A common name for the antidiuretic hormone elaborated by the posterior pituitary gland is

    (A) norepinephrine
    (B) vasopressin
    (C) luteotropic hormone
    (D) renin
    (E) secretin

54. Which of the following is true of lithium carbonate (Eskalith, Lithane)?

    (A) Usually given to adult patients in single daily doses
    (B) May only be administered by the intramuscular (IM) route
    (C) Onset of action occurs within 2 hours of the first administered dose
    (D) Should be administered with a diuretic to minimize edema formation
    (E) Indicated in the treatment of severe manic–depressive psychoses

55. Patients on lithium carbonate therapy should be advised

    (A) not to restrict their normal dietary salt intake
    (B) to stop taking the drug if they experience drowsiness
    (C) to limit water intake
    (D) not to take the drug during the manic phase of their cycle
    (E) not to take the drug with food

56. Hemolytic anemia due to erythrocyte deficiency of glucose-6-phosphate dehydrogenase (G6PD) would most likely be precipitated by

    (A) phenytoin (Dilantin)
    (B) pyridoxine HCl
    (C) isoniazid (INH)
    (D) primaquine
    (E) gentamicin (Garamycin)

57. The anticoagulant action of heparin is monitored by the

    (A) complete blood count
    (B) bleeding time
    (C) prothrombin time (PT)
    (D) activated partial thromboplastin time (APTT)
    (E) antiplatelet clotting time

58. Two hours after receiving the last dose of heparin (9000 units IV), a male patient begins bleeding from the gums after brushing his teeth. What is the most appropriate therapeutic action?

    (A) Inject 10 mg of phytonadione (Aqua-MEPHYTON) IV
    (B) Inject 10 mg of phytonadione (Aqua-MEPHYTON) IM
    (C) Inject 30 mg of protamine sulfate IV
    (D) Swab a small amount of epinephrine 1:100 onto the gum tissue to produce local vasoconstriction
    (E) Wait for the anticoagulant effect to subside

59. A 40-year-old woman with a history of deep-vein thrombosis (DVT) is stabilized on 5 mg of warfarin daily. The administration of which of the following medications to this patient would result in increased chance of hemorrhage?

  (A) Acetaminophen (Tylenol) 650 mg q4h
  (B) Captopril (Capoten)
  (C) Milk of magnesia 30 mL hs
  (D) Diazepam (Valium) 5 mg QID
  (E) Cimetidine (Tagamet) 300 mg QID

60. Which of the following would be considered to be a blood sugar concentration within normal limits for a fasting adult?

  (A) 100 mg/dL
  (B) 200 mg/dL
  (C) 300 mg/dL
  (D) 400 mg/dL
  (E) 500 mg/dL

61. Which of the following drugs can interfere with the diagnosis of pernicious anemia?

  (A) Pyridoxine
  (B) Folic acid
  (C) Thiamine
  (D) Ascorbic acid
  (E) Menadione

62. Rebound hyperacidity is most likely to occur when a patient uses which of the following antacids?

  (A) Magnesium hydroxide
  (B) Aluminum hydroxide
  (C) Calcium carbonate
  (D) Aluminum phosphate
  (E) Magaldrate

63. A white cell differential count is a laboratory procedure that

  (A) determines the relative proportions of the various white blood cells
  (B) determines the relative proportions of white cells to red cells

  (C) differentiates between iron-deficient and folic acid-deficient anemia
  (D) differentiates immature from mature white blood cells
  (E) differentiates normal from abnormal white blood cells

64. A patient who has recently suffered a myocardial infarction (MI) will most likely have elevated serum levels of

  (A) catechol o-methyl transferase
  (B) amylase
  (C) acid phosphatase
  (D) alkaline phosphatase
  (E) creatine kinase (CK)

65. The hematocrit (HCT) measures the

  (A) total number of blood cells per volume of blood
  (B) percentage of red blood cells per volume of blood
  (C) number of red blood cells per volume of blood
  (D) weight of hemoglobin per volume of blood
  (E) weight of red blood cells per volume of blood

66. Which of the following is NOT a white blood cell (or leukocyte)?

  (A) Basophil
  (B) Eosinophil
  (C) Monocyte
  (D) Lymphocyte
  (E) Reticulocyte

67. A unit-dose package is one that contains

  (A) precisely enough medication to complete a dosage regimen
  (B) solid dosage forms only
  (C) a premixed drug in an IV infusion solution
  (D) the exact dose of a drug ordered for a given patient
  (E) a 24-hour supply of a specific drug that is sent to a nursing unit

68. Which of the following agents is/are capable of producing an antipyretic action in humans?

    I. Naproxen sodium
    II. Acetylsalicylic acid
    III. Acetaminophen

    (A) I only
    (B) III only
    (C) I and II only
    (D) II and III only
    (E) I, II, and III

69. Which of the following is specific for the measurement of glucose?

    (A) Benedict's solution
    (B) Acetest tablets
    (C) Clinitest tablets
    (D) Clinistix
    (E) Ketostix

70. Zollinger-Ellison syndrome can be best treated with which of the following agents?

    (A) Proton pump inhibitors
    (B) Antimetabolites
    (C) Cytoprotectants
    (D) HMG-CoA reductase inhibitors
    (E) Quinidine

71. Intermittent IV therapy is used to

    I. avoid anticipated or potential stability or compatibility problems
    II. reduce the potential of thrombophlebitis
    III. promote better diffusion of some drugs into the tissues because of a greater concentration gradient

    (A) I only
    (B) III only
    (C) I and II only
    (D) II and III only
    (E) I, II, and III

72. Parenterally administered electrolytes are usually ordered in

    (A) equivalents
    (B) milliequivalents (mEq)
    (C) milligrams percent (mg %, or mg/dL)
    (D) millimoles
    (E) micrograms (μg)

73. Which of the following statements is/are true of aspirin?

    I. It should not be used during the last trimester of pregnancy.
    II. Low doses of aspirin may increase plasma uric acid levels.
    III. High doses of aspirin may decrease plasma uric acid levels.

    (A) I only
    (B) III only
    (C) I and II only
    (D) II and III only
    (E) I, II, and III

74. Which of the following reference sources would be appropriate to use to find an American equivalent of a British drug?

    (A) *Facts and Comparisons*
    (B) *The Royal Compendium*
    (C) *USPDI*
    (D) *AHFS Drug Information*
    (E) *Martindale's Extra Pharmacopoeia*

75. Generally, drug literature abstracts are most appropriately used to

    (A) provide the individual requesting the information with written documentation
    (B) provide detailed answers to specific questions
    (C) answer general questions
    (D) provide a rapid response to questions
    (E) identify those articles likely to contain the desired information

76. Kernicterus is a drug-induced disorder that may occur in the neonate following therapy with which of the following drugs?

    (A) Sulfisoxazole (Gantrisin)
    (B) Ranitidine (Zantac)
    (C) Phenytoin (Dilantin)

(D) Gentamicin (Garamycin)

(E) Promethazine (Phenergan)

77. Generally, the presence of impaired renal function or overt renal failure in a patient reduces the requirement(s) for

   I. drugs that are directly excreted or whose active metabolites are excreted by the kidneys

   II. drugs that are reabsorbed from the kidney tubules

   III. all drugs

   (A) I only

   (B) III only

   (C) I and II only

   (D) II and III only

   (E) I, II, and III

78. A patient who is a slow acetylator of isoniazid is characterized by

   (A) a predisposition to aspirin hypersensitivity

   (B) peripheral neuropathy that is resistant to pyridoxine therapy

   (C) slow metabolism and reduced therapeutic response

   (D) slow metabolism and enhanced therapeutic response

   (E) slow metabolism but normal therapeutic response

79. Cold sores (fever blisters) are most commonly caused by

   (A) *Staphylococcus aureus*

   (B) *Streptococcus viridans*

   (C) herpes simplex

   (D) *Pseudomonas aeruginosa*

   (E) candidiasis

80. Patients receiving doses of plantago (psyllium) should be advised to

   (A) avoid dairy products

   (B) take the medication with food

   (C) mix the product with water and let stand for 30 minutes before administering

(D) avoid driving or operating heavy machinery within 1 hour of taking the medication

(E) take the product with lots of water

81. The cation most prevalent in the extracellular fluid of the human body is

   (A) potassium

   (B) chloride

   (C) sodium

   (D) phosphate

   (E) magnesium

82. A child who swallows an overdose of a fluoride-containing multivitamin product should be treated with

   (A) acetylcysteine (Mucomyst)

   (B) dilute calcium hydroxide solution

   (C) docusate sodium

   (D) neostigmine bromide

   (E) atropine sulfate

83. The blood concentration of which of the following cations would normally rise if a patient became hypophosphatemic?

   (A) Phosphorus

   (B) Magnesium

   (C) Calcium

   (D) Iron

   (E) Potassium

84. Pyrantel pamoate (Antiminth) is

   I. available only as an oral suspension

   II. indicated for the treatment of ringworm

   III. taken for 7 days

   (A) I only

   (B) III only

   (C) I and II only

   (D) II and III only

   (E) I, II, and III

85. Large overdoses of acetaminophen are likely to cause

    (A) tinnitis
    (B) seizures
    (C) pseudomembranous enterocolitis
    (D) renal tubular necrosis
    (E) hepatic necrosis

86. An adult patient who ingested 30 acetaminophen tablets (325 mg/tab) 6 hours ago should be treated with/by

    (A) careful observation for signs of central nervous system (CNS) toxicity
    (B) *N*-acetylcysteine
    (C) activated charcoal
    (D) ipecac syrup
    (E) glutathione

87. Which of the following statements is (are) correct descriptions of sulfasalazine (Azulfidine)?

    I. Used in treating ulcerative colitis and regional enteritis
    II. Poor absorption from GI tract
    III. Available as oral tablets and IM injection

    (A) I only
    (B) III only
    (C) I and II only
    (D) II and III only
    (E) I, II, and III

88. Asthmatic patients with a documented allergy to aspirin should NOT receive

    (A) propoxyphene (Darvon)
    (B) acetaminophen (Tylenol)
    (C) nalbuphine (Nubain)
    (D) pentazocine (Talwin)
    (E) ibuprofen (Motrin)

89. Patients who have a history of penicillin allergy should also be suspected of exhibiting a possible allergy to

    (A) sulfonamides
    (B) aminoglycosides

    (C) tetracyclines
    (D) cephalosporins
    (E) fluoroquinolones

90. Which of the following agents would be most dangerous to use in a patient already receiving high doses of gentamicin?

    (A) Tetracycline HCl
    (B) Torsemide (Demadex)
    (C) Fosinopril (Monpril)
    (D) HydroDIURIL
    (E) Pentobarbital sodium

91. A patient arriving in a hospital emergency room suffering from severe hypertensive crisis would most likely be treated initially with

    (A) guanethidine (Ismelin)
    (B) methyldopa (Aldomet)
    (C) reserpine (Serpasil)
    (D) minoxidil (Loniten)
    (E) nitroprusside sodium (Nitropress)

92. An infant with nasal congestion could be treated safely with a (an)

    (A) infant nasal inhaler
    (B) topical pseudoephedrine product
    (C) nonsedating antihistamine
    (D) Epi-Pen device
    (E) infant nasal aspirator

93. Which of the following antihypertensive drugs should be administered by slow IV infusion?

    (A) Minoxidil (Loniten)
    (B) Clonidine (Catapres)
    (C) Hydralazine (Apresoline)
    (D) Prazosin (Minipress)
    (E) Nitroprusside (Nitropress)

94. Food containing tyramine should NOT be part of the diet of patients taking which of the following agents?

    (A) Cefixime (Suprax)
    (B) Hydralazine (Apresoline)

(C) Phenelzine (Nardil)

(D) Methyldopa (Aldomet)

(E) Acetazolamide (Diamox)

95. Which of the following symptoms would be LEAST likley to be exhibited by a patient suffering from diabetes mellitus?

(A) Weight loss

(B) Excessive thirst

(C) Glycosuria

(D) Urinary retention

(E) Weakness

96. Which of the following agents would most logically be given to a patient suffering from hypoparathyroidism? $\downarrow Ca^{2+} \uparrow PO_4$

(A) Alpha-tocopherol

(B) Pantothenic acid

(C) Phytonadione

(D) Nicotinamide

(E) Ergocalciferol

97. Which of the following therapeutic agents is specifically contraindicated for use in patients who have bronchial asthma?

(A) Sotalol (Betapace)

(B) Quinapril (Accupril)

(C) Procainamide (Pronestyl)

(D) Digoxin

(E) Chlorpromazine (Thorazine)

98. Which of the following phenothiazines is LEAST likely to produce extrapyramidal side effects?

(A) Chlorpromazine (Thorazine)

(B) Thioridazine (Mellaril)

(C) Prochlorperazine (Compazine)

(D) Perphenazine (Trilafon)

(E) Trifluoperazine (Stelazine)

99. Which of the following potential adverse effects of the phenothiazines is thought to be irreversible?

(A) Akathisia

(B) Muscular rigidity

(C) Tardive dyskinesia

(D) Orthostatic hypotension

(E) Tremor

100. Which of the following agents can be classified as an antagonist of angiotensin II receptors?

I. Benazepril (Lotensin)

II. Gemfibrozil (Lopid)

III. Losartan (Cozaar)

(A) I only

(B) III only

(C) I and II only

(D) II and III only

(E) I, II, and III

101. The antiemetic effect of which of the following drugs is the result of increased gastric emptying?

(A) Amitriptyline (Elavil)

(B) Benzotropine (Cogentin)

(C) Olsalazine (Dipentum)

(D) Baclofen (Lioresal)

(E) Metoclopramide (Reglan)

102. Which of the following agents is/are indicated for the treatment of Parkinson's disease?

I. Selegiline (Eldepryl)

II. Bromocriptine (Parlodel)

III. Amantadine (Symmetrel)

(A) I only

(B) III only

(C) I and II only

(D) II and III only

(E) I, II, and III

103. Patients diagnosed with Alzheimer's disease may be treated with which of the following agents?

   I. Carbamazepine (Tegretol)
   II. Gabapentin (Neurontin)
   III. Tacrine (Cognex)

   (A) I only
   (B) III only
   (C) I and II only
   (D) II and III only
   (E) I, II, and III

104. Patients receiving metformin (Glucophage) for the treatment of diabetes mellitus should be monitored for the development of

   (A) agranulocytosis
   (B) hearing loss
   (C) lactic acidosis
   (D) respiratory alkalosis
   (E) ankylosing spondylitis

105. A pharmacist tells a young mother about clinical (fever) thermometers and advises her to report to the pediatrician both the degrees of temperature and whether the temperature was taken rectally or orally. This is good advice because

   (A) oral temperature is about 1° Fahrenheit (1° F) higher than rectal temperature
   (B) oral thermometers have degree calibrations that differ from rectal thermometers
   (C) rectal temperature is about 1° F higher than oral temperature
   (D) the normal temperature (marked with an arrow) is 99.6° F on the rectal thermometer and 98.6° F on the oral one
   (E) the bulb on the rectal thermometer is round and contains more mercury than in the thin cylindrical bulb of the oral thermometer

106. The best emergency advice that a pharmacist could give an individual who has just suffered a minor burn is to

   (A) apply butter to the burn
   (B) immerse the burned area in cold water
   (C) contact a physician immediately
   (D) immerse the burned area in warm water followed by cold water
   (E) apply Vaseline to the burn

107. Angle-closure glaucoma is present in approximately what percentage of the total glaucoma population?

   (A) 10%
   (B) 25%
   (C) 50%
   (D) 75%
   (E) 95%

108. Which of the following is (are) effect(s) associated with the use of pilocarpine ophthalmic products?

   I. Mydriasis
   II. Cholinergic agonism
   III. Pupillary constriction

   (A) I only
   (B) III only
   (C) I and II only
   (D) II and III only
   (E) I, II, and III

109. The number 20 in Ocusert Pilo-20 refers to the

   (A) rate of release of drug from the Ocusert
   (B) strength of the preparation as a percentage
   (C) strength of the preparation in milligrams
   (D) duration of action of one Ocusert System in days
   (E) number of dosage units (Ocuserts) per original container

110. Which of the following should NOT be administered to a patient being treated for narrow-angle glaucoma?

   (A) Physostigmine
   (B) Pilocarpine

(C) Homatropine — mydriasis

(D) Phospholine iodide

(E) Carbachol

111. Advantage(s) of levobunolol (Betagan) over pilocarpine for the reduction of elevated intraocular pressure include(s)

   I. longer duration of activity

   II. little or no effect on visual acuity or accommodation

   III. little or no effect on pupil size

(A) I only

(B) III only

(C) I and II only

(D) II and III only

(E) I, II, and III

112. All of the following drugs are used to treat patients with open-angle glaucoma EXCEPT

(A) carbachol

(B) atropine

(C) demecarium

(D) physostigmine

(E) betaxolol

113. Epinephrine is a useful drug for lowering intraocular pressure in open-angle glaucoma because it

(A) increases outflow of aqueous humor and inhibits the formation of aqueous humor

(B) causes miosis

(C) causes mydriasis

(D) inhibits carbonic anhydrase

(E) dilates blood vessels in the eye

114. Scabies is a contagious skin disease caused by a

(A) mite

(B) fungus

(C) flea

(D) protozoa

(E) tick

115. Psoriasis is characterized by

(A) granulomatous lesions

(B) nodules

(C) small, water-filled blisters

(D) small red vesicles

(E) silvery gray scales

116. A patient with a documented allergy to morphine should NOT receive which one of the following analgesics?

(A) Meperidine (Demerol)

(B) Codeine

(C) Pentazocine (Talwin)

(D) Methadone (Dolophine)

(E) Butorphanol (Stadol)

117. Which one of the following is NOT a transdermal nitroglycerin patch?

(A) Minitran

(B) Nitro-Dur

(C) Nitrol

(D) Deponit

(E) Nitrodisc

118. The purpose for including vitamin C in oral iron supplements is to

(A) correct the vitamin C deficiency that accompanies iron deficiency

(B) enhance iron absorption

(C) prevent GI side effects of iron

(D) prevent the unabsorbed iron from darkening the stool

(E) increase the rate of formation of hemoglobin

119. Which of the following antihypertensive agents is available in a transdermal patch dosage form?

(A) Penbutolol

(B) Guanethidine

(C) Terazosin

(D) Lisinopril

(E) Clonidine

120. Ideally, an antacid should raise the pH of the stomach contents to a value of approximately

(A) 3.5
(B) 5.5
(C) 6.5
(D) 7.5
(E) 9.5

121. Which of the following agents is classified as a dopa decarboxylase inhibitor?

(A) Carbidopa
(B) Dopamine
(C) Tyrosine
(D) Dipyridamole
(E) Haloperidol

122. A patient with Parkinson's disease has been receiving levodopa (1 g four times daily) with fairly good response but excessive side effects. The patient's physician wishes to switch from levodopa to Sinemet. An approximate dose of Sinemet would be

(A) one 10/100 tablet daily
(B) one 10/100 tablet four times daily
(C) one 25/250 tablet daily
(D) one 25/250 tablet four times daily
(E) four 25/250 tablets four times daily

123. A patient is being treated effectively for Parkinson's disease with levodopa. Suddenly, all therapeutic benefits of the levodopa are lost and the adverse effects also disappear. Which one of the following facts obtained from a medication history would most likely explain this phenomenon?

(A) The patient has forgotten to take two doses of the medication.
(B) The patient began using an OTC multivitamin product.
(C) Trihexyphenidyl was added to the drug regimen for 1 week.
(D) Antacids were taken occasionally.
(E) The patient regularly consumed alcoholic beverages.

124. Which one of the following antiparkinson agents would be least likely to product anticholinergic adverse effects?

(A) Benztropine mesylate (Cogentin)
(B) Trihexyphenidyl HCl (Artane)
(C) Ethopropazine HCl (Parsidol)
(D) Pergolide mesylate (Permax)
(E) Procyclidine HCl (Kemadrin)

125. Which of the following drugs is associated with the "gray syndrome" in infants?

(A) Chloramphenicol
(B) Ciprofloxacin
(C) Demeclocycline
(D) Amphotericin B
(E) Kanamycin

126. Stomatitis refers to an inflammation of the

(A) eyelid
(B) oral mucosa
(C) stoma formed by intestinal surgery
(D) stomach wall
(E) tongue

127. An obese individual would most likely be suffering from

(A) polymorphism
(B) hypotonia
(C) polyphagia
(D) polyhydrosis
(E) nystagmus

128. Hypertrophy refers to

(A) an abnormal increase in the number of cells in a tissue
(B) an enlargement or overgrowth of an organ
(C) excessive perspiration
(D) increased motor activity
(E) excessive sensitivity of the skin

129. Dyspnea refers to

(A) restlessness
(B) difficulty in swallowing
(C) impairment of digestive function
(D) painful or difficult urination
(E) difficult or labored breathing

130. All of the following terms relate directly to body muscles EXCEPT

(A) myalgia
(B) myocardia
(C) myoclonus
(D) myopia
(E) myositis

131. Ischemia refers to

(A) a red, inflamed patch of skin
(B) excessive collection of blood in an area
(C) a jaundice condition
(D) nodules usually located on the back
(E) a deficiency of blood in a part of the body

132. Stenosis refers to

(A) hardening of tissues with a loss of elasticity
(B) inflammation of the sternum
(C) inflammation of the vertebrae
(D) narrowing or stricture of a duct or canal
(E) stoppage of blood flow in a part of the body

133. Phlebitis is most closely associated with which type of injections?

(A) IV
(B) IM
(C) Intradermal
(D) Subcutaneous (SC)
(E) Both IM and IV

134. A 60-year-old patient with congestive heart failure who has been stabilized for 3 months on digoxin, hydrochlorothiazide, and potassium chloride is gradually placed on the following additional medicines. Which of these drugs is most likely to cause a problem?

(A) Nitroglycerin
(B) Temazepam (Restoril)
(C) Meperidine HCl (Demerol)
(D) Aspirin
(E) Quinidine

135. Which of the following diuretics would be LEAST likely to produce a hypokalemic effect in a patient?

(A) Amiloride (Midamor)
(B) Torsemide (Demadex)
(C) Chlorthalidone (Hygroton)
(D) Furosemide (Lasix)
(E) Ethacrynic acid (Edecrin)

136. Mannitol is used therapeutically primarily as a (an)

(A) cardiac stimulant
(B) sucrose substitute
(C) antianginal agent
(D) osmotic diuretic
(E) plasma expander

137. The tricyclic antidepressant imipramine (Tofranil) has been approved by the U.S. Food and Drug Administration (FDA) for use in the treatment of

(A) peptic ulcer disease
(B) manic–depressive illness
(C) hypertension
(D) enuresis
(E) supraventricular tachycardias

138. Which of the following agents is (are) classified as an HMG-CoA reductase inhibitors?

I. Lovastatin
II. Simvastatin
III. Nystatin

(A) I only
(B) III only
(C) I and II only
(D) II and III only
(E) I, II, and III

139. Cyclosporine (Sandimmune) is a (an)

    (A) aminoglycoside antibiotic
    (B) third-generation cephalosporin
    (C) antineoplastic agent
    (D) antifungal agent
    (E) immunosuppressant

140. A potential problem of using nalbuphine (Nubain) in a patient who is dependent on codeine is

    (A) additive respiratory depression
    (B) increased tolerance to codeine
    (C) precipitation of narcotic withdrawal symptoms
    (D) impaired renal excretion of codeine
    (E) excessive CNS stimulation

141. The advantage naltrexone (Trexan) has over naloxone (Narcan) is

    (A) its more rapid onset of action
    (B) it is not addictive
    (C) its availability as sublingual tablets
    (D) that it does not have to be reconstituted immediately before use
    (E) its longer duration of action

142. Which of the following would be appropriate for the treatment of candidal vulvovaginitis?

    I. Clotrimazole
    II. Nystatin
    III. Miconazole

    (A) I only
    (B) III only
    (C) I and II only
    (D) II and III only
    (E) I, II, and III

143. Polycythemia refers to an elevated number of

    (A) erythrocytes
    (B) leukocytes
    (C) thrombocytes
    (D) reticulocytes
    (E) granulocytes

144. In treating excessive heparin therapy with protamine sulfate, caution must be exercised to avoid using more protamine than is necessary because

    (A) protamine sulfate is toxic in small amounts
    (B) protamine sulfate is a cardiotoxic agent
    (C) the production of endogenous heparin will be stimulated
    (D) the strongly basic protamine will produce alkalosis
    (E) protamine sulfate is also an anticoagulant

145. If a patient on oral anticoagulant therapy experiences mild to moderate bleeding, the desirability of administering vitamin K should be weighed carefully against the underlying need for anticoagulant therapy because

    (A) rapid correction of vitamin K deficiency may precipitate thromboembolism
    (B) vitamin K will displace the oral anticoagulant from protein-binding sites and produce a transient increase in anticoagulant effect
    (C) it requires a minimum of 18 hours for vitamin K to become effective
    (D) the use of vitamin K will make it much more difficult to retitrate the patient on the oral anticoagulant
    (E) if anticoagulant therapy is to be resumed, an oral anticoagulant having a different mode of action will have to be used

146. Which of the following anticoagulants would be the best choice for use in a pregnant patient near the anticipated time of delivery?

    (A) Ticlopidine (Ticlid)
    (B) Warfarin (Coumadin, Panwarfin)
    (C) Aspirin
    (D) Heparin
    (E) Dipyridamole (Persantine)

147. Heparin Sodium USP should always be ordered by the physician in units rather than milligrams because

(A) heparin syringes are calibrated in units only

(B) the use of a standard units/mL of preparation gives a more reproducible dose

(C) a conversion table is difficult to use

(D) many different strengths are available

(E) it is difficult to measure milligrams accurately

148. The prothrombin time of patients on anticoagulant therapy with coumarin derivatives will be decreased by

(A) clofibrate (Atromid-S)

(B) metronidazole (Flagyl)

(C) heparin

(D) phenylbutazone (Butazolidin)

(E) phytonadione

149. The Schilling Test is useful for the detection of pernicious anemia. This test utilizes orally administered

(A) vitamin B_{12} labeled with $_{59}Fe$

(B) intrinsic factor labeled with $_{59}Fe$

(C) intrinsic factor labeled with $_{57}Co$

(D) red blood cells labeled with $_{59}Fe$

(E) vitamin B_{12} labeled with $_{57}Co$ or $_{58}Co$

150. Which one of the following drugs is a dopamine agonist used to treat hyperprolactinemia?

(A) Chlorpromazine (Thorazine)

(B) Selegiline (Eldepryl)

(C) Benztropine (Cogentin)

(D) Diphenhydramine (Benadryl)

(E) Bromocriptine (Parlodel)

151. The only insulin preparation that can be given IV is

(A) crystalline zinc (regular) insulin

(B) protamine zinc insulin (PZI)

(C) lente insulin

(D) isophane insulin

(E) prompt insulin zinc

152. Which of the following insulins would be expected to exert the longest duration of action?

(A) Semilente

(B) NPH

(C) Protamine zinc

(D) Lente

(E) Regular

153. The most common cause of diabetic ketoacidosis and coma in the diagnosed and treated diabetic is

(A) insulin tolerance

(B) excessive physical activity

(C) electrolyte depletion

(D) use of the wrong type of insulin

(E) failure of the patient to use insulin properly

154. A diabetic patient has been taking cefaclor (Ceclor) 500 mg orally (PO) every 8 hours for a UTI. To determine whether this drug is interfering with the patient's urine glucose testing, a sample of urine is tested by both the Clinitest and the Tes-Tape methods. The results are 1% with Clinitest and 0.25% with Tes-Tape. The most appropriate conclusion from these data is that there is

(A) a false-positive with Clinitest

(B) Clinitest generally reads four times higher than Tes-Tape

(C) a false-positive with Tes-Tape

(D) a false-negative with Clinitest

(E) a false-negative with Tes-Tape

155. A mixture of regular insulin and PZI in a ratio of less than 1:1 would be expected to have about the same duration of action as

(A) the individual components of the mixture because there is no interaction
(B) NPH insulin because some free regular insulin will be present
(C) PZI alone if neutral regular insulin is used
(D) lente insulin because lente insulin is made from these components in this specific ratio
(E) PZI alone because the excess protamine in PZI will bind essentially all of the regular insulin, thereby converting it to PZI

156. Which one of the following benzodiazepines would be preferred as an anxiolytic drug for an elderly patient with a history of cirrhosis?

(A) Chlordiazepoxide (Librium)
(B) Diazepam (Valium)
(C) Clorazepate (Tranxene)
(D) Oxazepam (Serax) — glucoronidation (Ativan)
(E) Prazepam (Centrax)

157. Which of the following drugs is particularly useful for the treatment of acute hypoglycemic reactions when oral or IV administration of glucose is not possible?

(A) Acarbose (Precose)
(B) Glucocorticoids
(C) Glucagon
(D) Pancreatin
(E) Glyburide (Micronase)

158. Doses of 6-mercaptopurine (Purinethol) should be reduced in patients taking allopurinol (Zyloprim) because allopurinol

(A) enhances the absorption of 6-mercaptopurine
(B) inhibits the renal excretion of 6-mercaptopurine
(C) releases 6-mercaptopurine from protein-binding sites
(D) inhibits tubular secretion of 6-mercaptopurine

(E) inhibits the metabolism of 6-mercaptopurine

159. A patient is admitted to the emergency room (ER) with marked hypotension and appears to be in shock. The drug of choice to treat the condition is probably

(A) dobutamine
(B) dopamine HCl (Intropin)
(C) epinephrine HCl
(D) diazoxide (Hyperstat)
(E) nitroprusside

160. Which of the following agents is/are progestin-only oral contraceptive products?

I. Modicon
II. Ovrette
III. Micronor

(A) I only
(B) III only
(C) I and II only
(D) II and III only
(E) I, II, and III

161. The erythrocytes of an iron-deficient patient would be described as

(A) microcytic and hyperchromic
(B) macrocytic and hypochromic
(C) microcytic and hypochromic
(D) macrocytic and hyperchromic
(E) normocytic and hyperchromic

162. Which one of the following is considered to be the drug of choice for treating trigeminal neuralgia (tic douloureux)?

(A) Procainamide (Pronestyl)
(B) Pentazocine (Talwin)
(C) Cyclandelate (Cyclospasmol)
(D) Zolpidem (Ambien)
(E) Carbamazepine (Tegretol)

163. Which of the following is (are) NOT typical of parkinsonism?

I. Rigidity
II. Posture disturbances

III. Mental deterioration

(A) I only
(B) III only
(C) I and II only
(D) II and III only
(E) I, II, and III

164. Lomotil should NOT be given to patients taking oral clindamycin because

(A) toxic effects of clindamycin may be enhanced
(B) aplastic anemia may be more likely to occur
(C) an insoluble complex will be formed
(D) the rate of hydrolytic destruction of clindamycin in the GI tract will increase
(E) the antimicrobial action of clindamycin will be imparied

165. An advantage of loperamide (Imodium) over diphenoxylate (Lomotil) as an antidiarrheal is the fact that loperamide

(A) has a relatively short biologic half-life and therefore is not as likely to be abused
(B) has a direct effect on the CNS and therefore works more rapidly than does diphenoxylate
(C) is not a controlled substance
(D) does not appear to have opiate-like effects
(E) can be given parenterally

166. Tricyclic antidepressants should NOT be used in patients also taking

(A) phenytoin (Dilantin)
(B) methyldopa (Aldomet)
(C) guanethidine (Ismelin)
(D) baclofen (Lioresal)
(E) furosemide (Lasix)

167. Side effects of cyclobenzaprine (Flexeril) would be expected to be most similar to the side effects of

(A) methocarbamol (Robaxin)
(B) dantrolene (Dantrium)

(C) diazepam (Valium)
(D) meprobamate (Equanil)
(E) amitriptyline (Elavil)

168. A patient under the influence of crack cocaine is brought to an acute-care facility. The symptoms of cocaine intoxication are most similar to

(A) morphine
(B) heroin
(C) ethanol
(D) tetrahydrocannabinol (THC)
(E) dextroamphetamine

169. The initiation of therapy with which one of the following agents would be LEAST likely to cause therapeutic problems in a patient already taking warfarin (Coumadin)?

(A) Metronidazole
(B) Aspirin
(C) Phenytoin
(D) Acetaminophen
(E) Cimetidine

170. When treating a patient with dopamine infusion, which one of the following procedures should be followed if the patient's blood pressure increases to 165/100?

(A) Discontinue the infusion.
(B) Increase the infusion rate.
(C) Administer a hypotensive agent.
(D) Discontinue dopamine and start dobutamine.
(E) Continue the infusion while monitoring the patient closely.

171. A nutritional product is said to contain 14 g of protein, 18 g of carbohydrate, and 10 g of fat in each 100-mL serving. The caloric content of a serving would be

(A) 238 kcal
(B) 198 kcal
(C) 218 kcal
(D) 168 kcal
(E) 378 kcal

172. Portagen is a dietary product used to treat patients with

    (A) milk allergy
    (B) diabetes mellitus
    (C) fat malabsorption
    (D) calcium deficiencies
    (E) kidney failure

173. An electrolyte supplement used to replenish electrolytes lost as a consequence of a diarrheal condition is

    (A) Lyphocin
    (B) K-Lyte
    (C) Isomil
    (D) Pedialyte
    (E) Kayexalate

174. Parenteral administration of 1 L of 5% dextrose in water provides the patient with approximately how many kilocalories of energy?

    (A) 100 to 125 kcal
    (B) 170 to 200 kcal
    (C) 450 to 500 kcal
    (D) 800 to 850 kcal
    (E) 1000 kcal

175. Lofenalac is a dietary product used in patients suffering from

    (A) celiac disease
    (B) pancreatic insufficiency
    (C) steatorrhea
    (D) hyperlipidemia
    (E) phenylketonuria (PKU)

176. Six weeks ago, a 32-year-old female patient with a history of recurrent UTIs was treated sucessfully with a 10-day course of ampicillin (250 mg q6h) for an *E coli* UTI. She now presents with signs and symptoms of another UTI. Pending culture and sensitivity results, this patient should be started on

    (A) ampicillin (Omnipen)
    (B) trimethoprim–sulfamethoxazole (Bactrim)

    (C) tetracycline (Achromycin)
    (D) gentamicin (Garamycin)
    (E) nitrofurantoin (Macrodantin)

177. Which of the following would be (a) good alternative(s) to penicillin V in a pregnant patient allergic to penicillins?

    I. Erythromycin (Ilotycin)
    II. Trimethoprim (Trimpex)
    III. Demeclocycline (Declomycin)

    (A) I only
    (B) III only
    (C) I and II only
    (D) II and III only
    (E) I, II, and III

178. Which one of the following sulfonamides is best suited for the topical prophylactic treatment of burns?

    (A) Sulfacetamide (Sulamyd)
    (B) Mafenide (Sulfamylon)
    (C) Sulfisoxazole (Gantrisin)
    (D) Sulfamethoxazole (Gantanol)
    (E) Sulfasalazine (Azulfidine)

179. Which of the following drugs would be most appropriate to use for the treatment of gonorrhea in a poorly compliant patient with a documented penicillin allergy?

    (A) Cefprozil (Cefzil)
    (B) Pipericillin (Pipracil)
    (C) Tetracycline (Achromycin V)
    (D) Clindamycin (Cleocin)
    (E) Spectinomycin (Spectrobid)

180. Which of the following drugs used in the treatment of gout does (do) NOT affect urate metabolism or excretion?

    I. Colchicine
    II. Probenecid (Benemid)
    III. Allopurinol (Zyloprim)

    (A) I only
    (B) III only
    (C) I and II only

(D) II and III only

(E) I, II, and III

181. A pharmacist wishes to dispense Opticrom 4% ophthalmic solution for use by a patient. Which one of the following statements is true of this drug product?

(A) It is administered at regular intervals to treat allergic ocular disorders.

(B) It is administered at regular intervals to treat herpes simplex keratitis.

(C) It is administered at regular intervals to treat cataracts.

(D) It is administered on a PRN basis to treat bacterial infections.

(E) It is used at regular intervals to control cytomegalovirus (CMV).

182. Thiazides may produce

(A) increased intraocular pressure

(B) hyperkalemia

(C) impaired glucose tolerance

(D) hypernatremia

(E) increased renal excretion of ammonia

183. An important advantage of using dopamine (Intropin) in cardiogenic shock is that dopamine

(A) will not cross the blood–brain barrier and cause CNS effects

(B) has no effects on alpha and beta receptors

(C) can be given orally

(D) will not increase blood pressure

(E) produces dose-dependent increases in cardiac output and renal perfusion

184. A male patient experiencing acute alcohol withdrawal is given 100 mg of chlordiazepoxide (Librium) IM. Because of an inadequate response, he is given another 100 mg IM dose 30 minutes later and a third 100 mg IM dose in 30 minutes after the second injection. Several hours later the patient becomes extremely ataxic and stuporous. These symptoms (ataxia and stupor) are most likely due to

(A) delayed absorption of relatively large amounts of drug

(B) the short duration of activity of the chlordiazepoxide

(C) the combined effects of alcohol and chlordiazepoxide

(D) the ineffectiveness of chlordiazepoxide in acute alcohol withdrawal

(E) toxicity of the "special" diluent in which the drug is reconstituted

185. A male patient who has been stabilized on 300 mg of Dilantin Kapseals once daily is having difficulty swallowing capsules. His physician writes a new prescription for Dilantin suspension 300 mg once daily. This change is likely to

(A) reduce the phenytoin level because of decreased bioavailability from the suspension

(B) increase the phenytoin level because of increased bioavailability from the suspension

(C) have no impact on the phenytoin level

(D) decrease the phenytoin level because the 300-mg dose of suspension contains less of the active form of the drug

(E) increase the phenytoin level because the 300-mg dose of suspension contains more of the active form of the drug

186. Dobutamine (Dobutrex) is a (an)

(A) local anesthetic

(B) antipsychotic drug

(C) beta-adrenergic agonist

(D) antihypertensive drug

(E) narcotic analgesic

187. A patient for whom you dispensed a new prescription for amitriptyline (Elavil) (25 mg TID) 4 days ago returns to your pharmacy and complains that the drug is causing drowsiness, dry mouth, and that the drug has not improved symptoms of depression. The pharmacist should

(A) inform the prescribing physician that the drug is not effective in this patient

(B) inform the prescribing physician that an anticholinergic agent must be prescribed for this patient

(C) explain to the patient that these are expected effects of early treatment of the drug

(D) contact the prescribing physician and report the adverse effects experienced by the patient

(E) should question the patient about apparent noncompliant behavior

188. A diabetic recovering from surgery receives insulin continuously by slow IV infusion in successive liter bottles of 5% dextrose in water. Urinary glucose tests indicate that blood glucose was markedly elevated after the first liter was administered. Similar testing after the second and third IVs were administered indicated noticeably improved control of blood glucose. Assuming that the insulin dose was adjusted initially for the stress of surgery, the hyperglycemia following the first IV was probably due to

(A) adsorption of insulin onto the walls of the infusion set

(B) the initial loading of the circulatory system with glucose from the IV dextrose

(C) error in quantity of insulin added to the first IV

(D) inadequate insulin dosing

(E) rapid diuresis in response to the initial fluid load followed by an apparent hyperglycemia

189. A male diabetic patient reports that he is planning a 4-week trip to Europe and will not have continued access to a refrigerator in which to store insulin. What information would you give him?

(A) Store the insulin in a small styrofoam box that can be kept cold with several ice cubes.

(B) Be sure that insulin is available wherever you travel and purchase a fresh vial at least every third day.

(C) Increase your insulin dose by 10% to compensate for any deterioration.

(D) The insulin will remain stable at room temperature during the time period in which a single vial will be used.

(E) See your doctor to prescribe a mixture of insulins that will be more stable.

190. Which of the following are true of isotretinoin (Accutane)?

I. Pregnancy category X
II. Likely to cause cheilitis
III. Vitamin A derivative

(A) I only
(B) III only
(C) I and II only
(D) II and III only
(E) I, II, and III

191. Peripheral veins are seldom used for the administration of total parenteral nutrition (TPN) fluids because

(A) TPN fluids tend to infiltrate surrounding tissue

(B) the hypotonic solution causes local hemolysis

(C) large-bore needles must be used

(D) the blood flow in peripheral vessels is not great enough to protect the peripheral vessels from irritation

(E) the vessels are easily occluded

192. An elderly insulin-dependent diabetic is about to be placed on a beta blocker for hypertension. Which of the following beta blockers would be most appropriate for this type of patient?

(A) Propranolol (Inderal)
(B) Pindolol (Visken)

(C) Atenolol (Tenormin)

(D) Nadolol (Corgard)

(E) Timolol (Blocadren)

193. When used to treat angina, nifedipine (Procardia) is much more likely than verapamil (Calan, Isoptin) and diltiazem (Cardizem) to cause

(A) hypokalemia

(B) tachycardia

(C) cardiac arrhythmias

(D) mental depression

(E) bronchospasm

194. Which of the following complications associated with the administration of TPN solutions is most likely to occur after the infusions have been discontinued?

(A) Alkalosis

(B) Hyperchloremic metabolic acidosis

(C) Hyperosmotic nonketotic hyperglycemia

(D) Hypoglycemia

(E) Pulmonary edema

195. Which one of the following provides the greatest number of calories per gram?

(A) Ethanol

(B) Proteins

(C) Anhydrous dextrose

(D) Hydrous dextrose

(E) Fats

196. A patient requires high-dose cisplatin (Platinol) therapy for the treatment of advanced bladder cancer. During the cisplatin therapy, the patient develops severe nausea and vomiting. Which of the following drugs would be appropriate to administer to control these symptoms?

(A) Methylphenidate (Ritalin)

(B) Granisetron (Kytril)

(C) Danazol (Danocrine)

(D) Amantadine (Symmetrel)

(E) Triazolam (Halcion)

197. The mechanism of action of amiloride (Midamor) is most similar to that of

(A) spironolactone (Aldactone)

(B) hydrochlorothiazide (HydroDIURIL)

(C) triamterene (Dyrenium)

(D) metolazone (Zaroxolyn)

(E) chlorthalidone (Hygroton)

198. A 50-year-old hypertensive patient has been maintained on spironolactone with hydrochlorothiazide (Aldactazide), methyldopa (Aldomet), and potassium (K-Tabs). The patient is admitted to the hospital for elective surgery and is found to be hyperkalemic (serum K of 6.4 mEq/L; normal range is 3.5–5.5 mEq/L) with no symptoms and a normal electrocardiogram. This patient should be treated with

(A) IV calcium

(B) IV sodium bicarbonate

(C) IV glucose plus insulin

(D) rectal sodium polystyrene sulfonate (Kayexalate)

(E) hemodialysis

199. A 55-year-old patient with a 5-year history of angina and a recent myocardial infarction is admitted to the hospital because of malignant hypertension. Diazoxide should NOT be used in this patient because

(A) of its hepatotoxicity

(B) of its slow onset of activity

(C) it tends to increase uric acid levels

(D) it is likely to cause orthostatic hypotension

(E) of its cardiostimulating effects

200. Which of the following antihypertensives would be preferred in the patient described in Question 199?

(A) Propranolol (Inderal)

(B) Trimethaphan (Arfonad)

(C) Nitroprusside (Nitropress)

(D) Hydralazine (Apresoline)

(E) Minoxidil (Loniten)

201. Which of the following agents is NOT employed in the treatment of depression?

    (A) Venlafaxine (Effexor)
    (B) Nefazodone (Serzone)
    (C) Paroxetine (Paxil)
    (D) Sertraline (Zoloft)
    (E) Zolpidem (Ambien)

202. The use of olsalazine (Dipentum) is contraindicated in patients with a history of hypersensitivity to

    (A) sulfonamides
    (B) salicylates
    (C) phenothiazines
    (D) imidazolines
    (E) beta-adrenergic blocking agents

203. A patient has been receiving 50 mg of hydrocortisone (Solu-Cortef) by IV every 6 hours for an acute exacerbation of ulcerative colitis. After several days of IV therapy, the physician wishes to switch the patient to an equivalent dose of oral prednisone. The equivalent total daily dose of prednisone would be

    (A) 10 mg
    (B) 25 mg
    (C) 50 mg
    (D) 100 mg
    (E) 200 mg

204. A 50-year-old patient with congestive heart failure is stabilized on digoxin 0.25 mg daily, hydrochlorothiazide 50 mg daily, and a low-sodium, high-potassium diet. The patient then develops polyarteritis, which requires corticosteroid therapy. Which of the following glucocorticoids would be most appropriate for this patient?

    (A) Hydrocortisone
    (B) Cortisone
    (C) Prednisolone
    (D) Dexamethasone
    (E) Prednisone

205. An asthmatic patient is stabilized to a therapeutic theophylline level on an IV aminophylline (dihydrate) infusion of 50 mg/h. The physician wishes to put the patient on an equivalent amount of sustained-release anhydrous theophylline (eg, Theo-Dur). An appropriate total daily dose of Theo-Dur would be

    (A) 1500 mg
    (B) 1200 mg
    (C) 900 mg
    (D) 600 mg
    (E) 300 mg

206. A 20-year-old asthmatic patient has been treated with Theo-Dur 500 mg twice daily. Despite a good therapeutic steady-state serum concentration of 16 μg/mL, the patient has brief episodes of bronchospasm several times a week. The physician would like to give the patient additional bronchodilator therapy with an oral beta-adrenergic agonist. Which of the following drugs would be LEAST desirable?

    (A) Albuterol (Ventolin)
    (B) Metaproterenol (Alupent)
    (C) Terbutaline (Brethine)
    (D) Ephedrine
    (E) Isoetherine (Bronkosol)

207. A patient with rheumatoid arthritis cannot swallow tablets. Which of the following salicylates is available in a liquid dosage form?

    (A) Sodium salicylate
    (B) Magnesium salicylate
    (C) Salsalate
    (D) Choline salicylate
    (E) Salicylic acid

208. A prescriber wishes to prescribe Lanoxicaps for a patient who has been receiving Lanoxin 0.25 mg tablets. Which strength of Lanoxicaps should be recommended by the pharmacist?

    (A) 0.05 mg
    (B) 0.1 mg

(C) 0.2 mg

(D) 0.3 mg

(E) 0.5 mg

209. A secondary means of contraception should be recommended to patients using oral contraceptives when which of the following drugs is (are) also to be taken?

   I. Rifampin
   II. Antihistamines
   III. B-complex vitamins

(A) I only

(B) III only

(C) I and II only

(D) II and III only

(E) I, II, and III

210. Sumatriptan succinate (Imitrex) is a useful agent employed in the treatment of

(A) prostatic hyperplasia

(B) migraine headaches

(C) muscle spasm

(D) ulcerative colitis

(E) endogenous depression

Answers and Explanations

1. **(C)** When administered intravenously, diazepam (Valium) is a rapidly acting anticonvulsant with less tendency to produce respiratory depression than the barbiturates. Diazepam is effective in grand mal, focal motor, and petit mal seizures and in status epilepticus. Because of its wide range of effectiveness, intravenous (IV) diazepam or a similar drug, lorazepam, are probably the drugs of choice for initial therapy of status epilepticus. Intravenous phenytoin is an important secondary drug but is likely to decrease heart rate and produce hypotension. Paraldehyde is also an effective drug but, like the barbiturates, is likely to cause respiratory depression. *(5:1217)*

2. **(E)** Chronic (longer than 6 months) high-dose administration of hydralazine can produce an acute rheumatoid state in approximately 10% of patients taking the drug. A syndrome clinically indistinguishable from disseminated lupus erythematosus develops in a smaller percentage of users. This lupus-like syndrome (fever, arthralgia, splenomegaly, edema, and the presence of lupus erythematosus cells in the peripheral blood) has also been associated with procainamide use. *(6:795)*

3. **(E)** Following slow uptake by the adrenergic nerve, guanethidine replaces norepinephrine in storage granules and accumulates in the nerve in place of norepinephrine. After several days of guanethidine administration, the sympathetic nerves no longer contain sufficient amounts of norepinephrine to maintain normal venomotor tone. Tricyclic antidepressants inhibit the uptake of guanethidine into the adrenergic neuron, thereby inhibiting the antihypertensive effect of guanethidine. *(8:481)*

4. **(E)** Metoprolol (Lopressor) blocks beta-adrenergic receptors. It differs from timolol (Blocadren) primarily in that it has some preferential effect on beta$_1$-adrenoreceptors, which are located chiefly in cardiac muscle. This preferential effect is not absolute and, at higher doses, metoprolol also inhibits beta$_2$-adrenoreceptors, which are located chiefly in bronchial and vascular musculature. Although the mechanism of its antihypertensive effect is not known, the drug is indicated in the management of hypertension either alone or in combination with other antihypertensives. *(3:1576)*

5. **(A)** Terazosin is believed to be a peripheral vasodilator. Side effects of therapy may include a precipitous fall in blood pressure, possibly with tachycardia and loss of consciousness following the first dose. The initial dose of terazosin is usually 1 mg at bedtime and can be increased slowly to 20 mg daily if required. *(3:163p)*

6. **(D)** CD4 cells are a type of T lymphocytes whose primary role is to stimulate other cells in the immune response. The lower the level of these cells in the patient's blood, the more susceptible the patient becomes to the development of opportunistic infections such as *Pneumocystis carinii* pneumonia. *(5:1651)*

7. **(C)** Diazoxide has marked antihypertensive activity when given by rapid IV injection. It appears to lower blood pressure by a direct

dilation of the arterioles, which minimizes the incidence of orthostatic hypotension. Both cardiac output and renal blood flow are increased. Initial doses of 1–3 mg/kg are used. Diazoxide is used orally in the treatment of hypoglycemia. (3:167d)

8. **(D)** Normal doses of doxycycline are not eliminated by the same pathways as the other listed tetracyclines. Because it does not appear to accumulate in the blood, it is one of the safest tetracyclines for treating extrarenal infections in patients with renal failure. (6:1127)

9. **(E)** Ramipril (Altace), an angiotensin converting enzyme (ACE) inhibitor, would be the best choice because depression is a major side effect of reserpine, guanethidine, methyldopa, and clonidine. The principal serious side effects of ramipril are headache, dizziness, rash, and fever. (3:195e)

10. **(A)** All of the agents listed, except ketoconazole, are employed in the treatment of *Helicobacter pylori*–related peptic ulcer disease. Ketoconazole is an antifungal agent. (5:711)

11. **(E)** Cholestyramine is a basic anion exchange resin. This quaternary ammonium chloride compound exchanges the chloride ion for the negatively charged bile acids, thereby preventing their reabsorption. Cholestyramine binds many organic acids, including all of the drugs listed in this question. (6:888)

12. **(C)** If drug B has a greater affinity (ie, higher association constant) for specific proteinbinding sites than does drug A, it will have a tendency to displace drug A from these sites. Further, if drug B is given in large doses, the degree of this displacement will increase because there will be a greater amount of drug B competing with drug A for the binding sites. (6:1708)

13. **(D)** Each of the three major drugs used to treat convulsive disorders (phenobarbital, phenytoin, and primidone) can disturb folic acid metabolism. The hematologic problems associated with folic acid deficiency are rela-

tively easy to detect. However, the abnormal mental states that may develop are considerably more difficult to diagnose. These symptoms may range from mild confusion to psychoses resembling schizophrenia. (5:1868)

14. **(D)** Acetylsalicylic acid (aspirin) and the NSAID, naproxen sodium, exhibit antiplatelet action. Acetaminophen (NAPAP) does not. (6:1353)

15. **(E)** Penetration of the cornea by *Pseudomonas aeruginosa* will often lead to destruction of the cornea and interior portions of the eye. Blindness may result. This organism is a common contaminant in water. The need for sterility of ophthalmic products is well recognized. (1:1588)

16. **(A)** Boils caused by *Staphylococcus* organisms form in the anterior portion of the external auditory meatus. They are usually self-limiting, and treatment with antibiotic ointments prevents spreading. (2a:597)

17. **(D)** Idoxuridine is an antimetabolite that inhibits the replication of viral DNA with greater selectivity than does that of the host cell. It is used primarily in the treatment of herpes simplex keratitis, a disease of viral origin that can cause blindness. (5:2049)

18. **(C)** Although tolnaftate is effective against several types of fungi, it is ineffective against *Candida* organisms. Miconazole, clotrimazole, and ciclopirox olamine (Loprox) are relatively broad-spectrum antifungal agents with activity against some species of *Candida*. (3:577)

19. **(E)** Although methotrexate is not curative, it suppresses psoriatic lesions and induces prolonged remissions. Baseline and regular liver function and hematologic testing should be performed before initiating therapy. (5:1828)

20. **(E)** Complications of corticosteroid therapy are usually related to the length of time that they have been administered and the dosage used. Corticosteroids suppress normal tissue responses to infection (increasing susceptibil-

ity to infection) and allow further dissemination of existing infections. Because tissue responses to infection are suppressed, the subjective, objective, and laboratory manifestations of infection may be masked. *(6:1475)*

21. **(C)** Although the NSAIDs are structurally different, they all possess similar pharmacologic properties and all inhibit prostaglandin synthesis. Furthermore, these drugs produce similar adverse effects, including gastrointestinal (GI) intolerance. Piroxicam has the longest half-life of the group (approximately 38 hours) and is recommended to be given on a once-a-day basis. *(6:618)*

22. **(D)** Perhaps the most significant difference among these drugs is the prolonged biologic half-life of oxaprozin (42 hours). The other drugs have half-lives ranging from 1 to 3 hours. Because of this long biologic half-life, oxaprozin can be administered on a once-daily regimen. This may be of value to patients who have difficulty complying with dosing schedules that require more frequent dosing. *(3:251)*

23. **(C)** Fluorouracil is used topically for the treatment of multiple premalignant actinic keratoses. It prevents further development of existing lesions and results in cosmetic improvement. If an occlusive dressing is applied, there may be an increased incidence of inflammatory reaction in the adjacent normal skin. However, even without an occlusive dressing, such responses occasionally occur in skin that appears clinically normal. This is due to the presence of subclinical actinic keratoses. *(10)*

24. **(D)** In the condition known as hypoprothrombinemia, there is a reduction in the levels of prothrombin in the blood. This substance is essential in the blood-clotting mechanism. *(27:753)*

25. **(B)** Rapid reversal of drug-induced hypoprothrombinemia requires the use of a source of prothrombin such as fresh blood or plasma. The various vitamin K derivatives can be used if the situation is not urgent or as a sup-

plement to one of the immediate sources of prothrombin (ie, blood or plasma). *(19:12.16)*

26. **(E)** Phenazopyridine (Pyridium) is a red dye that commonly causes discoloration of the urine. It is used primarily as a urinary tract analgesic. *(3:731)*

27. **(D)** Menotropins (Pergonal, Humegon) is an agent that has moderate follicle stimulating hormone (FSH) and luteinizing hormone (LH) activity. It has been used successfully to induce ovulation in many patients with amenorrhea and other conditions that cause anovulatory cycles. *(3:115e)*

28. **(E)** Once conception has taken place, the body starts to produce chorionic gonadotropin. The e.p.t. Quick Stick Test assays for the presence of this hormone in the urine. *(3:246a)*

29. **(A)** Animal testing of a new drug is completed before the investigational new drug (IND) status is obtained for clinical testing. In Phase I of the study, healthy volunteers are tested to determine drug tolerance, dosing schedules, side effects, and pharmacokinetic data. This is followed by Phase II, in which actual patients suffering from the disease are tested with the drug. Drug efficacy is observed, and side effects not evident in healthy volunteers may occur. Phase III involves administration of the drug to large numbers of patients by private practitioners. Phase IV is the continuous investigation or monitoring of the drug after marketing. *(6:56)*

30. **(A)** Hypoparathyroidism usually presents itself as a disorder of calcium metabolism in which serum calcium levels of the patient decrease while levels of phosphate increase in an inversely proportional manner. Low serum calcium levels may precipitate a potentially serious condition known as tetany. To prevent the development of this disorder and to treat the hypoparathyroidism, calcium supplements such as calcium gluconate, calcium carbonate, calcium lactate, or calcium gluceptate are often prescribed. *(6:1528)*

31. **(C)** Amikacin and other aminoglycoside antibiotics (gentamicin, tobramycin, etc) may produce neuromuscular blockade; this can enhance the blockade produced by skeletal muscle relaxants such as tubocurarine. *(8:204)*

32. **(C)** The hypothyroid state is characterized by marked retardation of mental and physical activity; hoarseness; dry sparse hair; thickening of the skin and subcutaneous tissues; constipation; cold intolerance; anemia; and dry, pale, coarse skin. However, because of the nature of the general symptoms, hypothyroidism is usually recognized and treated before all of the previously mentioned symptoms develop. *(5:1536)*

33. **(E)** *(5:1304)*

34. **(D)** Fiorinal is the only agent listed that contains aspirin. *(3:250e)*

35. **(D)** Hemochromatosis is an iron storage disorder characterized by excessive amounts of iron in parenchymal tissues with resultant tissue damage. Such a condition may be caused by a number of factors, one of which is the prolonged use of excessive doses of iron preparations. *(5:1863)*

36. **(A)** This syndrome generally occurs when erythromycin estolate is given to susceptible individuals for more than 10–14 days. It is more common after multiple exposures to the drug, although full recovery usually follows discontinuation of the medication. The reaction is unpredictable and is apparently due to individual hypersensitivity. It has not been observed with the use of erythromycin free base or with other derivatives of erythromycin. Because there is no established clinical superiority of the estolate salt, there is little justification for using it in light of the possibility of this potential toxicity. *(6:1140)*

37. **(C)** Vancomycin is bactericidal for gram-positive bacteria. Most pathogenic staphylococci are killed by a plasma concentration of 10 mg/mL or less. However, because vancomycin is highly irritating to tissue, thrombophlebitis following IV injection is common. The drug is also ototoxic and nephrotoxic. Consequently, it is used only for serious staphylococcal or enterococcal infections in patients who fail to respond to other drugs. *(6:1146)*

38. **(A)** Conventional antihistamines, or H_1-receptor antagonists, inhibit histamine-mediated contraction of the bronchi and gut. They do not, however, block the stimulatory effect of histamine on gastric acid secretion. Famotidine (Pepcid), a selective H_2-receptor antagonist, blocks gastric acid and pepsin secretion in response to histamine, gastrin, food, distention, and caffeine. *(6:904)*

39. **(E)** In questionable cases of penicillin allergy, skin tests may be performed using benzyl-penicilloyl–polylysine (Pre-Pen). Although a negative reaction to the test does not rule out the possibility of a hypersensitivity reaction, it does indicate that anaphylaxis is not likely to occur on administration of the drug. *(3:750a)*

40. **(B)** Amantadine (Symmetrel) inhibits the replication of certain myxoviruses (eg, influenza A, rubella, some tumor viruses) in humans. A daily oral dose of 200 mg for 2–3 days before and 6–7 days after influenza A infection reduces the incidence and severity of symptoms and the magnitude of the serologic response to the infection. *(6:1210)*

41. **(B)** Didanosine is a retroviral inhibitor approved for the treatment of HIV infection. Its major adverse reactions include peripheral neuropathy and pancreatitis. Ifosfamide is an antineoplastic alkylating agent and cytarabine is an antineoplastic antimetabolite. *(5:2363)*

42. **(A)** Patients with sinus headaches generally experience pain in the periorbital area. Pain is usually greatest on awakening because of the accumulation of fluid in the sinus cavities. *(2a:49)*

43. **(C)** Combined drug treatment is usually required because of the rapid development of resistant organisms when a single agent is

used. It has also been demonstrated that combined drug therapy enhances the tuberculostatic effects of the individual drugs. For example, a combination of streptomycin and isoniazid is significantly more tuberculostatic than is either agent used alone. (5:2112)

44. **(D)** The color change imparted to urine and sweat is a predictable and harmless side effect. Patients should be told to expect this effect so that they are not alarmed by it. (3:388)

45. **(E)** Ticlopidine (Ticlid) is a platelet aggregation inhibitor used to reduce the risk of thrombotic stroke. While using this drug the patient may be at higher risk for abnormal bleeding. (10)

46. **(B)** (6:1077)

47. **(C)** Pseudomembranous colitis is a severe and occasionally fatal complication of antibiotic therapy. One etiology appears to be the presence of an exotoxin produced by overgrowth of Clostridium difficile in the bowel. Clindamycin, lincomycin, and ampicillin have been the most commonly implicated antibiotics, although other antibiotics have also been implicated. Treatment is directed against the offending organism and its exotoxin. Oral vancomycin in doses of 125–500 mg three to four times daily for 7–14 days is most commonly used. Cholestyramine resin may also be used to bind the bacterial exotoxin. (5:2130)

48. **(B)** Cushing syndrome is a condition characterized by adrenal hyperplasia caused by overproduction of ACTH by the pituitary gland. Patients with this disease will often have obesity, hypertension, and gonadal dysfunction. (5:1550)

49. **(B)** The aminoglycosides have activity against a wide range of microorganisms. After parenteral administration, they are excreted unchanged in the urine. Because of their well-established nephrotoxicity and ototoxicity, they are not suitable for long-term treatment of chronic tract infections. (6:1110)

50. **(D)** Loracarbef, cefazolin, and cefotaxime are not adequately absorbed from the GI tract and therefore must be administered parenterally for systemic therapy. Although both cefaclor and cephradine are adequately absorbed, only cephradine is commercially available in both oral and parenteral dosage forms. (3:335g)

51. **(D)** For the prophylactic treatment of asthma, cromolyn sodium is available in several forms: powder-filled capsules for inhalation; a solution for use with a nebulizer; and an aerosol spray. Cromolyn is used to prevent asthma attacks, not to treat acute attacks. (3:182g)

52. **(B)** A major advance in steroid therapy for asthma has been the development of corticosteroid aerosols such as beclomethasone (Vanceril). Like cromolyn (Intal), beclomethasone is a prophylactic agent that must be used regularly. It is not suitable for an acute asthmatic attack. The primary value of steroid therapy by inhalation is to avoid systemic side effects in patients who require steroids for the first time or to permit significant dosage reductions of oral steroids in patients on maintenance therapy. (5:579)

53. **(B)** Vasopressin, which is a purified preparation of antidiuretic hormone, is used therapeutically in the treatment of diabetes insipidus, a disease of pituitary origin. When administered in any one of a number of available dosage forms (IM, IV, subcutaneous [SC], and nasal insufflation or spray), vasopressin usually reverses the symptom of excessive urination (polyuria), which is the primary symptom of patients suffering from this disease. The initially observed action of the hormone was vasoconstriction, which led to the name vasopressin; this is still the official USP designation. (6:726)

54. **(E)** Lithium carbonate (Lithane, Eskalith) is primarily indicated for treating manic episodes in patients with manic–depressive illness. It is administered orally in daily divided doses of 600 mg to 1.8 g and generally should not be administered with diuretics,

because retention of lithium may occur. (5:1427)

55. **(A)** The rate of excretion of lithium carbonate is generally independent of urine flow and dietary sodium. However, in the presence of sodium deficiency, the excretion of lithium is markedly decreased and toxic levels can accumulate rapidly. Conversely, high sodium intake enhances lithium excretion. (5:1434)

56. **(D)** Glucose-6-phosphate (G6PD) dehydrogenase controls the initial step in the pentose–phosphate pathway, bringing about the oxidation of glucose-6-phosphate to 6-phosphogluconate, which reduces NADP to NADPH. Many oxidant drugs (eg, primaquine, sulfisoxazole, probenecid) increase the rate of oxidation of glutathione. This increases the intracellular demand for NADPH to maintain glutathione in the reduced form. In patients with a deficiency in erythrocyte G6PD, oxidized glutathione accumulates and, by some unknown mechanism, disrupts erythrocyte membrane integrity with subsequent hemolysis. (6:972, 978)

57. **(D)** The anticoagulant effect of heparin is quantitated by the activated partial thromboplastin time (APTT). The usual therapeutic goal is to prolong the APTT to 2–2.5 times that of the laboratory control. (5:407)

58. **(E)** Because of heparin's brief duration of action, mild hemorrhaging is usually treated by simply withdrawing the drug. In the presence of severe hemorrhage, the use of a specific heparin antagonist (eg, protamine sulfate) is imperative. Usually, 1 mg of protamine sulfate will neutralize 100 units of heparin. However, after the IV administration of heparin, the quantity of protamine required decreases rapidly with time. Only 0.5 mg of protamine is required to neutralize 100 units of heparin 30 minutes after IV administration of heparin. (5:411)

59. **(E)** Cimetidine potentiates the effects of oral anticoagulants by decreasing the rate of hepatic metabolism of warfarin. Cimetidine causes a reversible but significant increase in plasma warfarin concentration and, consequently, in the prothrombin time. In this case, it is necessary to recognize this interaction and decrease the dose of warfarin or use a safer alternative to cimetidine. (8:308)

60. **(A)** Normal fasting blood sugar values for adults range from 80 to 120 mg/dL (or 80 to 120 mg%). When the fasting blood sugar levels exceed 120 mg/dL, diabetes mellitus should be suspected. Levels below 60 mg/dL may suggest insulin overdosage, glucagon deficiencies, and/or hypoactivity of various endocrine glands. (19:48.5)

61. **(B)** The administration of pharmacologic doses (0.4 mg/day or more) of folic acid can stimulate reticulocytosis and improve the anemia associated with vitamin B_{12} deficiency. However, folic acid administration does not prevent the development or progression of the neurologic manifestations of pernicious anemia. (2a:373)

62. **(C)** Calcium-containing products tend to increase the release of gastrin in the stomach. Gastrin release promotes more HCl production. (2a:207)

63. **(A)** By revealing the relative proportions of the various white blood cells, the white cell differential count may direct the physician's attention toward a particular disease or group of diseases. For example, eosinophils are increased in parasitic infections and allergic conditions; neutrophils are increased in most bacterial infections; basophils may be increased in certain blood dyscrasias; and monocytes are often greatly increased in chronic infections such as tuberculosis. (5:1931)

64. **(E)** Creatine kinase (CK) is an enzyme that is found primarily in muscle tissue. It is released into the blood in response to muscle injury. Serum concentrations of CK are elevated in disorders involving muscle damage such as myocardial infarction, muscular dystrophy, muscle trauma, and muscular inflammation. (19:4.10)

65. **(B)** Whole blood treated with anticoagulant is centrifuged in a calibrated hematocrit tube. The volume ratio of the packed red blood cells to total blood volume is determined. The hematocrit is normally 39–49 for men and 33–43 for women. It gives some indication of both the number and size of the red blood cells present in an individual. *(19:4.14)*

66. **(E)** A reticulocyte is an immature erythrocyte. *(19:4.14)*

67. **(D)** *(1:1753)*

68. **(E)** Aspirin, the NSAID, and acetaminophen are capable of reducing elevated body temperature by altering the hypothalamic set-point. *(2a:56)*

69. **(D)** Clinistix contains glucose oxidase and is therefore specific for glucose. Tes-Tape and Diastix also use the glucose oxidase method. Ascorbic acid, levodopa, salicylates, and phenazopyridine (Pyridium) may produce false-negative results with these agents. *(1:519)*
(A–incorrect; C–incorrect) Benedict's qualitative test and Clinitest tablets are based on the copper reduction method. *(1:519)*
(B–incorrect; E–incorrect) Acetest tablets and Ketostix are used to detect the presence of ketones in the urine. Levodopa and phenazopyridine may interfere. *(1:519)*

70. **(A)** Zollinger-Ellison syndrome is a condition characterized by gastric acid hypersecretion and recurrent peptic ulceration. It is generally the result of a gastrin-producing tumor. The proton pump inhibitors such as omeprazole are effective in managing the acid secretion in this condition. *(5:718)*

71. **(E)** The administration of a drug by intermittent (rather than continuous) IV injection is accomplished over a period of minutes (rather than hours). Stability and/or compatibility problems are less likely to occur because the drug does not remain in contact with a large-volume IV fluid for long periods of time. The potential for thrombophlebitis is reduced because the drug is not in constant contact with the blood vessel tissue at the site of the injection. Finally, the greater concentration gradient produced by a more rapid injection may promote better diffusion of some drugs into tissues. *(1:1545)*

72. **(B)** The use of the milliequivalent unit takes into consideration the chemical-combining capacity of various ionic species. *(1:101)*

73. **(E)** Aspirin should be avoided during the last trimester of pregnancy. Aspirin exerts a dose-dependent action on uric acid excretion. *(2a:60)*

74. **(E)** *Martindale's Extra Pharmacopoeia* is probably one of the most comprehensive, international, single-volume references on drugs and drug products. *Martindale's* is divided into three parts: The first part consists of monographs on drugs and ancillary substances. (Although drugs that are manufactured in the United Kingdom are stressed, generic and proprietary products from many other countries are included.) The monographs includes physiochemical data, storage, incompatibilities, uses, doses, and toxic effects. The second part contains a supplementary discussion of new drugs, obsolete drugs, and miscellaneous substances. The third part lists formulas of OTC products sold in the United Kingdom. There is also a directory of worldwide pharmaceutical manufacturers. *(1:54)*

75. **(E)** Although drug literature abstracts often appear to provide sufficient detail to answer certain questions, it must be recognized that an abstract may contain statements taken out of context and that supporting detail and/or qualifications for such statements have been excluded. It is the obligation of the individual providing the information to retrieve the entire article to ascertain whether the information provided is accurate and complete. *(1:55)*

76. **(A)** Kernicterus is a neurologic syndrome in which damaging bile pigments are deposited in the basal ganglia in the CNS. It may develop in the neonate following therapy with the sulfonamides. Bilirubin is a normal

breakdown product of hemoglobin; it is generally conjugated in the liver to a water-soluble glucuronide that is excreted in the bile. Because of a deficiency in the enzyme glucuronyl transferase, neonates have a limited capacity to metabolize bilirubin. Sulfonamides are implicated in this disorder because of their ability to displace unconjugated bilirubin from protein-binding sites. Sulfonamides should be avoided in pregnant women near term because these drugs cross the placenta, and also by nursing mothers because they are excreted in breast milk. *(6:1046)*

77. **(A)** Although the presence of impaired renal function or renal failure does not contraindicate the use of drugs that are directly excreted or the active metabolites of which are excreted by the kidney, it does modify the dose required to produce a given therapeutic effect. Renal impairment or renal failure allows these drugs or their metabolites to accumulate in the blood. Drug accumulation in these situations can be avoided by reducing the dose and/or the dosage schedule of the drug. Careful monitoring of drug concentrations in the blood and of remaining renal function should also be done. *(6:17)*

78. **(E)** No significant difference in clinical response can be identified between patients who acetylate isoniazid slowly and those who do so rapidly. *(6:1158)*
(B–incorrect) Although slow acetylators of isoniazid are more likely to develop peripheral neuropathy from the drug, they respond equally well to pyridoxine therapy as rapid acetylators. *(6:1158)*

79. **(C)** Cold sores or fever blisters are generally caused by herpes simplex type 1 virus. They usually occur on the lip or on areas surrounding the lips. Cold sores tend to be self-limiting and disappear within 10–14 days. *(2a:525)*

80. **(E)** Plantago (psyllium) is a bulk-forming laxative agent. Patients using it should mix the dose with a glass of water or other fluid and drink it down quickly. This should be followed with more fluids. *(2a:229)*

81. **(C)** The relative concentration of different anions and cations varies considerably between intracellular and extracellular fluids of the body. Intracellular body fluids contain high concentrations of potassium (a cation) and phosphate (an anion), whereas extracellular fluid contains high concentrations of sodium (a cation) and chloride (an anion). *(19:4.3)*

82. **(B)** Acute fluoride ingestion is generally treated with dilute calcium hydroxide solution or with another calcium source. The calcium reacts with the unabsorbed fluoride and prevents its absorption. It also prevents the development of hypocalcemia in the patient. *(2a:386)*

83. **(C)** There is a reciprocal relationship between the concentration of calcium and phosphorus in the blood. For example, hypoparathyroidism is characterized by low serum calcium and high serum phosphorus, whereas hyperparathyroidism is characterized by low serum phosphorus and high serum calcium. *(19:4.8)*

84. **(A)** Pyrantel pamoate is used in the treatment of pinworms. It is available as an oral suspension. A single dose of 11 mg/kg generally is administered. The drug is well tolerated but may cause nausea, vomiting, diarrhea, or dizziness in some individuals. *(3:418)*

85. **(E)** Acetaminophen is metabolized in the liver primarily by conjugation to glucuronide or sulfate metabolites. A small percentage is metabolized by the hepatic cytochrome P-450 mixed-function oxidase system to a toxic intermediate metabolite. Normally, this metabolite is preferentially conjugated to glutathione and excreted in the urine. When large doses of acetaminophen are ingested, the glucuronide and sulfate pathways become saturated, and stores of glutathione become inadequate to conjugate the amount of toxic metabolite that is produced. The metabolite binds covalently to hepatocytes and produces hepatic necrosis. *(6:73)*

86. **(B)** Because the drug was ingested 6 hours ago, the likelihood of removing a large amount of drug from this patient's stomach with ipecac syrup is small. Activated charcoal effectively binds acetaminophen if given soon after ingestion, but its use here is also unlikely to be of value because of the elapsed time. Glutathione would seem a logical antidote (see commentary for Question 85), but it does not enter cells readily and therefore will not prevent hepatic necrosis. *N*-acetylcysteine serves as a glutathione substitute that effectively binds the toxin and permits it to be excreted in the urine. *N*-acetylcysteine is given orally or by lavage tube. Cysteamine, a glutathione precursor, has also been used successfully. It is given by IV. *(19:104.20)*

87. **(C)** Because of sulfasalazine's poor absorption from the GI tract, its localized activity is valuable as one of the first-line treatments for various forms of colitis and enteritis. The drug is available as oral tablets and as a suspension. *(3:365)*

88. **(E)** Aspirin allergy in association with asthma is cause for serious concern. Asthma, rhinorrhea, and nasal polyps usually accompany this type of aspirin intolerance, which occurs in about 4% to 20% of asthmatic patients. These patients appear to exhibit a high degree of cross-reactivity to other NSAIDs, such as ibuprofen. *(5:637)*

89. **(D)** Because of the structural similarity between the penicillins and the cephalosporins, cross-sensitivity may be a problem in these patients. Although the possibility exists, the incidence of cross-sensitivity is probably less than 5%. However, patients allergic to penicillin should be watched carefully when initiating cephalosporin therapy. *(6:1086)*

90. **(B)** Torsemide (Demadex) is a loop diuretic that is capable of producing ototoxicity, which would enhance the similar toxicity produced by gentamicin. *(3:138c)*

91. **(E)** Nitroprusside sodium (Nitropress) is a drug administered by IV infusion in the emergency treatment of acute hypertensive crisis. It causes a rapid fall in blood pressure that can be controlled by adjusting the infusion rate of the drug. *(3:166e)*

92. **(E)** An infant nasal aspirator is a bulb device that can be used to remove nasal mucus by suction. It is a safe nondrug approach to relieving symptoms of congestion in infants. *(1:1879)*

93. **(E)** Sodium nitroprusside is a powerful vasodilator that acts directly on the smooth muscle of blood vessels. Because of its rapid conversion to thiocyanate in the body, the effects of nitroprusside are quite transient. Following termination of the drug infusion, blood pressure begins to rise immediately and reaches the pretreatment level in 1–10 minutes. It is extremely important that the blood pressure and the flow rate of the solution be monitored carefully. Although the dose range is quite large, the average adult dose is 0.25–1.5 μg/kg/min. Nitroprusside is used when short-term rapid reduction in blood pressure is necessary. *(6:798)*

94. **(C)** Phenelzine (Nardil) is a monamine oxidase (MAO) inhibitor that may interact with pressor amines such as tyramine in some cheeses, wines, beers, etc, to produce a hypertensive crisis that may be life threatening. *(8:580)*

95. **(D)** Frequent urination (polyuria) is a common symptom of diabetes mellitus. *(5:1490)*

96. **(E)** Ergocalciferol is one of a number of active compounds collectively called vitamin D. Administration of vitamin D to a patient suffering from hypoparathyroidism is indicated because it will tend to elevate serum calcium levels and lower serum phosphate levels to acceptable ranges. *(6:1529)*

97. **(A)** Sotalol (Betapace) is used primarily for its ability to block beta-adrenergic activity, and is therefore useful in treating patients suffering from ventricular arrhythmias. However, because beta-adrenergic blockade also tends to increase airway resistance, the drug is usually contraindicated for use in patients

suffering from asthma or severe allergies. (6:855)

98. **(B)** The phenothiazine group of drugs can be subdivided into three groups according to chemical structure: dimethylaminopropyl derivatives (eg, chlorpromazine); piperazine derivatives (eg, perphenazine, prochlorperazine, trifluoperazine); and the piperidyl derivatives (eg, thioridazine). Generally, the piperidyl group is the least likely to produce extrapyramidal symptoms and the piperazine group is the most likely to do so. (6:403)

99. **(C)** Tardive (late-occurring) dyskinesia (involuntary muscular movements) is a drug-induced neurologic disorder that appears to be irreversible and unresponsive to drug treatment. It is characterized by involuntary movement of the lips, tongue, or jaw and is commonly observed as a smacking of the lips, rhythmical movement of the tongue, or facial grimaces. This disorder may be due to hypersensitivity of dopaminergic receptors to endogenous dopamine after long-term blockade by antipsychotic drugs.
(A–incorrect) Akathisia is a feeling of restlessness or a compelling need for movement. (5:1383)

100. **(B)** Losartan (Cozaar) is the first angiotensin II receptor antagonist. It is employed in the treatment of hypertension. (3:165q)

101. **(E)** Metoclopramide exerts a potent antiemetic effect by inhibiting the chemoreceptor trigger zone (CTZ). It also stimulates GI motility and increases the rate of gastric emptying. This enhances the antiemetic activity by eliminating stasis that precedes vomiting. All of the other drugs listed decrease the rate of gastric emptying. (19:105.7)

102. **(E)** Most antiparkinson agents act by increasing dopaminergic activity. (6:511)

103. **(B)** Tacrine (Cognex) is a centrally acting cholinesterase inhibitor that increases acetylcholine levels in cortical neurons and may, therefore, slow progression of Alzheimer's disease symptoms. (6:172)

104. **(C)** Metformin is a biguanide that, in rare cases, may cause lactic acidosis. This is a condition that may be fatal in 50% of cases. (3:130n)

105. **(C)** A satisfactory approximation of the temperature of the internal organs can be made by inserting a clinical thermometer into either the mouth or rectum. These are both closed cavities with good blood supply. The accepted average oral temperature is 98.6° F, with recognition that both individual and diurnal variations occur regularly. The rectum is about 1° F warmer. Rectal and oral thermometers have the same temperature scales and markings, differing only in the shape of the bulb. To avoid the potential confusion and errors in subtracting or adding degrees from readings, physicians prefer that the actual temperature and the method be reported; for instance, 102.5° F taken rectally. (2a:55)

106. **(B)** Immediate counteraction to the burn is recommended. Application of cold water will often reduce the severity of the burn. The burn area should be kept in cold water until no further pain is experienced whether in or out of the water. If necessary, a physician may then be contacted. (2a:639)

107. **(A)** (5:1795)

108. **(D)** Pilocarpine is a cholinergic drug that produces a miotic effect (pupillary constriction). (3:479a)

109. **(A)** The Ocusert pilocarpine unit is a drug delivery system that has a centrally located reservoir of pilocarpine. The Ocusert is placed in the upper or lower cul-de-sac of the eye. Pilocarpine then diffuses across two outer polymeric layers that serve as rate-controlling membranes. The Ocusert is a clear oval device with a visible rigid white margin to aid in placement and removal. The unit is available in two strengths, Pilo-20 and Pilo-40, for use in chronic open-angle glaucoma. The numbers designate the rate of release of

drug: 20 mg/h and 40 mg/h respectively. Each Ocusert unit contains sufficient drug for 1 week. *(3:481)*

110. **(C)** Although each of the other choices will produce a constriction of the iris (miosis) and will most likely aid in reducing the patient's intraocular pressure, homatropine will produce mydriasis, which will further aggravate the patient's condition and possibly lead to blindness. *(5:1790)*

111. **(E)** The usual categories of drugs used to treat glaucoma include cholinomimetics (eg, pilocarpine), sympathomimetics (eg, epinephrine), and carbonic anhydrase inhibitors (eg, acetazolamide). The most widely used cholinomimetic, pilocarpine, is relatively short-acting, causing accommodative spasm and miosis. Levobunolol (Betagan), a beta-receptor antagonist, is believed to reduce elevated intraocular pressure by decreasing the production of aqueous humor. Levobunolol exerts its maximal effect within 1–2 hours and maintains significant effects for as long as 24 hours following a single topical dose. There seems to be little or no effect on pupil size, visual acuity, or accommodation. *(3:478l)*

112. **(B)** Atropine is a mydriatic used for retraction work and ophthalmoscopy. In a few instances, it has precipitated acute attacks of angle-closure glaucoma. *(6:151)*
(A–incorrect) Carbachol is used as a replacement when resistance or intolerance to pilocarpine occurs. *(6:1634)*
(C–incorrect) Demecarium is a long-acting anticholinesterase used to treat primary open-angle glaucoma, glaucoma in aphakia, and accommodative esotropia. *(6:1634)*
(D–incorrect) Physostigmine is a short-acting anticholinesterase used in the treatment of primary open-angle glaucoma and for emergency treatment of angle-closure glaucoma. *(6:1634)*
(E–incorrect) Betaxolol (Betoptic) is a beta-blocking drug similar to timolol. *(6:1636)*

113. **(A)** Epinephrine effectively reduces intraocular pressure in open-angle (chronic) glaucoma by both increasing the outflow of aqueous humor from the anterior chamber of the eye and inhibiting the formation of aqueous humor. Because of its mydriatic action (pupillary dilation), epinephrine is contraindicated in narrow-angle glaucoma. Dilation of the pupils may precipitate acute-angle closure. *(5:1793)*

114. **(A)** *(2a:659)*

115. **(E)** The distinctive lesion is a vivid red macule, papule, or plaque covered by silvery lamellated scales. Usually the scalp, elbows, knees, and shins are affected first. *(5:1824)*

116. **(B)** If morphine allergy is present, codeine should also be avoided because both codeine and morphine are structurally similar phenanthrene derivatives. Also, codeine is partially (10%) demethylated to morphine. *(6:536)*

117. **(C)** Nitrol is a nitroglycerin topical ointment applied onto the chest or back using an applicator or a dose-measuring paper over at least a $2\,^1/_4 \times 3\,^1/_2$-inch area. *(3:144a)*

118. **(B)** Ascorbic acid is added to a number of iron preparations with the claim that it will enhance iron absorption. Ascorbic acid maintains iron in the ferrous state and forms a soluble and absorbable chelate with iron that is present in the ferric state. Doses of 200 mg of ascorbic acid are given for each 30 mg of elemental iron. *(2a:382)*

119. **(E)** Clonidine is a central alpha-adrenergic stimulant that reduces peripheral vascular resistance and heart rate. Patients who use oral clonidine are susceptible to rebound hypertension if they discontinue their use of the tablets. The transdermal dosage form (Catapres TTS) releases clonidine at a constant rate for about 7 days, thereby improving compliance and reducing the likelihood of rebound hypertension. *(3:161g)*

120. **(A)** Raising the intragastric pH from 1.5 to 3.5 neutralizes 99% of the acid and greatly reduces the proteolytic activity of pepsin, thus attenuating the two primary factors known

to overwhelm gastric mucosal resistance. Buffering to a higher pH serves no useful puprose. *(2a:196)*

121. **(A)** Carbidopa inhibits dopa decarboxylase peripherally but does not cross the blood–brain barrier. Inhibiting the peripheral metabolism of levodopa leaves a greater fraction of intact levodopa available to cross the blood–brain barrier where metabolism to dopamine is desired. If a larger fraction of a given dose of levodopa reaches the brain, then a smaller original dose can be used with a reduction in side effects of therapy. This combination of carbidopa and levodopa is commercially available as Sinemet tablets. *(3:290e)*

122. **(D)** Sinemet is a combination product containing carbidopa and levodopa in a ratio of 1:4 or 1:10. Because carbidopa inhibits the peripheral decarboxylation of levodopa, much smaller doses of levodopa can be used. This in turn generally reduces the peripheral side effects associated with high doses of levodopa. Dosage levels of levodopa can be decreased by approximately 75%. *(3:290e)*

123. **(B)** The administraton of pyridoxine, even in the small doses (5 mg or more) contained in ordinary vitamin preparations, is equivalent to a reduction in dosage of levodopa. Pyridoxine is believed to be a cofactor for the enzyme dopa decarboxylase, which is responsible for the peripheral metabolism of levodopa. The decarboxylated metabolic product cannot enter the brain, which is the desired site of action. *(8:666)*

124. **(D)** Pergolide mesylate (Permax) is a dopamine receptor agonist that exhibits little, if any, anticholinergic action. *(5:1254)*

125. **(A)** The gray-baby syndrome occurs in premature and term newborn infants when chloramphenicol is administered during the first few days of life. The syndrome results from the inability of the infant to metabolize the drug because of a deficient enzyme, glucuronyl transferase, which is required to detoxify the drug by changing it to the glu-

curonide. Symptoms consist of cyanosis, vascular collapse, and elevated chloramphenicol levels in the blood. *(6:1134)*

126. **(B)** *(27:1481)*
(A–incorrect) Inflammation of the eyelid is blepharitis.
(D–incorrect) Gastritis is an inflammation of the stomach wall.
(E–incorrect) Inflammation of the tongue would be known as glossitis.

127. **(C)** Polyphagia is defined as an excessive craving for food. *(27:1237)*

128. **(B)** *(27:746)*
(A–incorrect) An abnormal increase in cell number in a tissue is hyperplasia.
(C–incorrect) Excessive sweating is hyperhidrosis.
(D–incorrect) Increased motor activity (excessive movement) is called hyperkinesia.
(E–incorrect) Excessive sensitivity to stimulation is hyperesthesia.

129. **(E)** *(27:480)*
(A–incorrect) Restlessness is dysphoria.
(B–incorrect) Difficulty in swallowing is dysphagia.
(C–incorrect) Impairment of digestive functioning is dyspepsia.
(D–incorrect) Painful or difficult urination is dysuria.

130. **(D)** Myopia is the condition of nearsightedness. *(27:1018)*
(A–incorrect) Myalgia is pain in a muscle.
(B–incorrect) Myocardia pertains to the heart muscle.
(C–incorrect) Myoclonus is muscular twitching or contraction.
(E–incorrect) Myositis is inflammation of a voluntary muscle.

131. **(E)** The deficiency is usually due to a constriction or actual obstruction of a blood vessel. For example, myocardial ischemia is a deficiency of the blood supply to the heart muscle. *(27:803)*
(C–incorrect) Icterus is a synonym for jaundice.

132. **(D)** Aortic stenosis, for example, is the narrowing of the aortic orifice of the heart. Pyloric stenosis is obstruction of the pyloric orifice of the stomach, caused by hypertrophy of the pyloric muscle. *(27:1473)*
(A–incorrect) Sclerosis is generally caused by overgrowth of fibrous tissue.
(C–incorrect) Refers to spondylitis.
(E–incorrect) Refers to stasis.

133. **(A)** Phlebitis indicates vein inflammation. It results from injury to the endothelial cells of a blood vessel, usually the vein at an IV injection site. The earliest sign is tenderness at the site. The area around the vein then becomes red, warm, and painful, often with edema and stiffness. In some instances thrombophlebitis occurs. This term implies that a clot (thrombus) has formed in the blood vessel at the site of the inflammation. Breakage of the thrombus from the site of formation may lead to an embolism (ie, obstruction or occlusion of a blood vessel at some site removed from the site of clot formation). *(27:1186)*

134. **(E)** Although digoxin and quinidine are frequently used together, it is well documented that administering quinidine to a patient previously stabilized on digoxin will cause serum digoxin levels to rise an average 2- to 2.5-fold. The mechanism of this interaction may involve both a displacement of digoxin from tissue-binding sites and a reduction in renal clearance of digoxin. Even though the significance of this interaction remains controversial, many clinicians suggest reducing the dose of digoxin by 50% when adding quinidine. In any case, the patient should be monitored carefully for signs of digoxin toxicity. *(8:191)*

135. **(A)** Under normal circumstances, diuresis induced by amiloride is accompanied by either no appreciable difference or only a slight increase in potassium excretion. However, a sharp reduction in potassium output is observed when either amiloride (Midamor) or triamterene (Dyrenium) is given with other natriuretic drugs. This potassium-sparing action is the rationale for concomitant drug therapy with amiloride. Because of the possibility of inducing serious hyperkalemia, potassium supplements should not be given to patients being treated with amiloride or triamterene. Spironolactone (Aldactone) is an aldosterone antagonist also used to decrease the potassium loss that occurs secondary to the use of other diuretics. *(6:704)*

136. **(D)** Mannitol is usually administered by IV as a hypertonic 10% to 25% solution (an isotonic solution is about 5.5%). The introduction of a hypertonic solution provokes urine flow. Mannitol solutions are used in prophylaxis of acute renal failure, in the evaluation of acute oliguria, and for the reduction of the pressure and volume of the intraocular and cerebrospinal fluids. *(6:694)*

137. **(D)** Because many patients who took imipramine for depression reported difficulty in urination, it was reasoned that the drug might be of value in treating enuresis. Now the drug is used routinely to treat nocturnal enuresis, especially in children. It is not recommended for children younger than 6 years of age. Doses of imipramine range from 25 to 75 mg, lower than those used for treatment of depression. Other brands besides Tofranil are Janimine and SK-Pramine. *(5:1305)*

138. **(C)** Nystatin is an antifungal agent employed in the treatment of candidiasis (yeast) infections. *(3:520b)*

139. **(E)** Cyclosporine (Sandimmune, Neoral) is a cyclic polypeptide immunosuppressive agent that prolongs survival of allogenic transplants (heart, kidney, liver, and other organs) in humans and other animals. Nephrotoxicity has been noted in 25% to 38% of organ transplant recipients using cyclosporine. Synergism with nephrotoxic drugs may occur. Hypertension, hirsutism, and gum hyperplasia are other adverse reactions. The oral solution (100 mg/mL) is taken immediately after mixing with milk, chocolate milk, or orange juice. Soft gelatin capsules and an IV dosage form are also marketed. Cyclosporine may be administered concurrently with adrenal cor-

ticosteroids but not with other immunosuppressants. *(3:738k)*

140. (C) Nalbuphine (Nubain) is a mixed narcotic agonist–antagonist capable of relieving moderate to severe pain. In subjects dependent on such narcotics as morphine and codeine, nalbuphine precipitates a withdrawal syndrome. Although it is capable of producing euphoriant effects similar to morphine, its effect on respiration seems to exhibit a ceiling effect, such that doses higher than 30 mg produce no further respiratory depression. *(6:547)*

141. (E) Naltrexone (ReVia) is a pure opioid antagonist that is used in managing opioid addiction. A single dose of 50 mg once daily is adequate for most patients. *(3:709b)*

142. (E) Each of these agents exerts an antifungal action against *Candida* (yeast) organisms. *(2a:95)*

143. (A) Mild polycythemia is normal in persons who exercise excessively and in persons who live at high altitudes. Polycythemia vera is a state in which the rate of red cell production is far greater than normal, even though there is no apparent physiologic need for the increased production. It is believed that this disease may result from some sort of tumor of the bone marrow. Phlebotomy whenever the hematocrit rises higher than 55% may suffice as the only treatment for patients who do not have severe thrombocytosis. Drugs used to treat polycythemia include busulfan (Myleran) and radioactive phosphorus ($_{32}$P). *(5:608)*

144. (E) Protamine is a strongly basic substance that combines with the strongly acidic heparin to produce a stable salt and a loss of anticoagulant activity. Because protamine itself possesses anticoagulant properties, it is unwise to administer more than 100 mg of protamine over a short period of time unless it is known that there is a definite need for a larger amount. *(6:1346)*

145. (D) Administration of vitamin K_1 (phytonadione) will correct oral anticoagulant–induced bleeding within a few hours. This form of treatment, however, should only be used in severe cases of hemorrhage because the patient may become temporarily refractory to renewed oral anticoagulant therapy. *(5:416)*

146. (D) Althogh the risk of hemorrhage in the fetus can be minimized by monitoring the prothrombin time of the mother closely, it is probably best to use heparin if anticoagulant therapy is necessary under these circumstances. Because heparin is a high molecular weight mucopolysaccharide, it does not cross the placenta. *(5:416)*

147. (B) Heparin is not a uniform molecular species, and therefore should be prescribed in units rather than milligrams. The old equivalent of 100 mg = 10,000 units is a poor approximation because the USP specifies that the potency must be not less than 120 U/mg when derived from lung tissues and not less than 140 U/mg when derived from other tissues. Potency must be within 90% to 110% of what is stated on the label. If a physician orders 100 mg of heparin, it is not clear whether 10,000 units, 12,000 units, or some other quantity is meant. Other nations use an international unit that is not identical to the USP heparin unit. *(3:88c)*

148. (E) Prothrombin time (PT) is a measure of the time it takes for fibrin to gel in plasma after addition of calcium and thromboplastin. The PT of patients on coumarin drugs is prolonged because of the reduced activity of several blood factors. Phytonadione (vitamin K_1) antagonizes the action of these anticoagulants and therefore shortens PT. The other drugs listed will increase PT. *(19:12.4)*

149. (E) In normal individuals, more than 50% of an oral dose of vitamin B_{12} is absorbed from the GI tract. This absorption occurs only in the presence of the intrinsic factor of Castle, with which the vitamin must presumably combine in order to pass through the intestinal walls. By means of radioactive cobalt–labeled cyanocobalamin, it has been shown that more than one-half of an oral dose soon appears in the blood. Normally, only a small amount of radioactivity appears in the urine. However, if a large "flushing" dose (1000 mg) of vitamin B$_{12}$ is given parenterally within an hour of the tagged oral dose, the renal threshold for B$_{12}$ is exceeded and radioactivity is observed in the urine. In patients with pernicious anemia, there is a deficiency in intrinsic factor that results in poor absorption of the radioactive B$_{12}$. Most of the radioactivity in these patients will be detected in the feces. (6:1329)

150. (E) Bromocriptine is an ergot alkaloid derivative that acts on the anterior pituitary gland to suppress prolactin secretion. The drug may be indicated in the treatment of amenorrhea and galactorrhea associated with hyperprolactinemia. It is available as 2.5 mg tablets, and the usual therapeutic dose is one tablet, two or three times daily. (6:1371)
(A–incorrect) Chlorpromazine is a dopamine antagonist.   (6:402)
(C–incorrect) Benztropine is an anticholinergic drug.   (6:156)
(D–incorrect) Diphenhydramine is an antihistaminic drug.   (6:552)

151. (A) Insulin injection (regular or crystalline zinc) is used in situations in which rapid onset and brief duration of action are desired. It is the only preparation that can be given by IV; it is so used in the treatment of diabetic ketoacidosis. In this emergency situation, the drug is often used in conjunction with subcutaneously administered and longer-acting insulin preparations. (3:129f)

152. (C) Protamine zinc insulin exerts an action for as long as 24–36 hours. The shortest duration is exhibited by regular insulin, which may act for only 6–8 hours. (3:129f)

153. (E) Diabetic ketoacidosis is a direct result of the lack of insulin. The omission of insulin doses or errors in adjusting the insulin dosage in response to changes in food intake or physical activity is probably the most common cause of diabetic ketoacidosis. Other

common causes include infections and myocardial infarctions. (5:1512)

154. (A) Although copper reduction tests (eg, Clinitest) are more quantitative measures of glucosuria than are the glucose oxidase tests (eg, Tes-Tape), they are less specific for glucose. It is well documented that the cephalosporin antibiotics may cause false-positive readings with copper reduction tests. To enable a patient to use the copper reduction method of urine testing while taking cefaclor, it is desirable to determine whether the drug is interfering with the test. In this example, the fact that the tests yielded different results indicates that there is an interference. The fact that cephalosporins do not interfere with Tes-Tape indicates that the interference is a false-positive with Clinitest. (5:1505)

155. (E) (5:1500)

156. (D) Chlordiazepoxide, diazepam, clorazepate, and prazepam are all metabolized by oxidation in the liver to desmethyldiazepam, an active metabolite with a very long half-life. This process is impaired in the elderly and in the presence of liver disease (eg, cirrhosis), resulting in drug accumulation and the risk of oversedation. Oxazepam (Serax) and lorazepam are metabolized by glucuronidation, a process that is much less dependent on liver function than on oxidation. Furthermore, the metabolites of oxazepam and lorazepam are inactive. (6:368, 423)

157. (C) The usual method of treating an acute hypoglycemic reaction is to give glucose orally or, in unconscious patients, by IV in concentrated solutions. However, if these routes cannot be used, 0.5 to 1 mg of glucagon may be given SC or IM as well as by IV. Glucagon is an endogenous hormone produced by the alpha cells of the pancreatic islets of Langerhans. Glucagon increases blood glucose by stimulating hepatic gluconeogenesis and glycogenolysis. (5:1506)

158. (E) Because 6-mercaptopurine is metabolized by the enzyme xanthine oxidase, con-

comitant administration of allopurinol, which is a xanthine oxidase inhibitor, will decrease the rate of metabolism of 6-mercaptopurine. This will potentiate the effects and toxicity of 6-MP unless the dose of 6-MP is reduced to 25% to 30% of its usual therapeutic level. *(8:412)*

159. **(B)** Dopamine exerts a positive inotropic effect by direct action on beta-adrenergic receptors and causes a release of norepinephrine from storage sites. A major advantage of the drug is that its hemodynamic effects can be varied by controlling the infusion rate. *(6:211)*

160. **(D)** Modicon is a monophasic oral contraceptive containing estrogen and progestin. *(3:108f)*

161. **(C)** In the iron-deficient state, the iron storage compartment becomes depleted. This is followed by a reduction in plasma transferrin saturation. Subsequently, the number and size of the erythrocytes as well as their hemoglobin content will be decreased. *(6:1317)*

162. **(E)** Trigeminal neuralgia is a disorder characterized by sudden attacks of severe pain along the distribution of the fifth cranial nerve. Attacks are often precipitated by stimulation of a "trigger zone" in the area of the pain. Carbamazepine (Tegretol) is remarkably effective in both relieving and preventing the pain of trigeminal neuralgia. Anticonvulsants such as phenytoin (Dilantin) may also be beneficial in some cases. Other drugs that have been effective are vitamin B_{12} in massive doses (1 mg) and injection of alcohol into the ganglion or the branches of the trigeminal nerve. *(6:475)*

163. **(B)** Although aged people with parkinsonism may have impairment of memory and judgment or mental disturbances due to other disease states or social isolation, these effects are not caused by the disease per se. *(5:1243)*

164. **(A)** The development of inflammatory conditions of the colon (eg, nonspecific colitis, or

a more severe pseudomembranous colitis) has been associated with antibiotic therapy. Although many antibiotics have been implicated, there have been a disproportionate number of reports specifically involving clindamycin and lincomycin. Colitis has been associated with both oral and parenteral administration of these drugs, and no clear predisposing conditions have been identified. Because antimotility drugs (eg, diphenoxalate) used to treat the resulting diarrhea seem to prolong the disease, they should not be used. *(5:2131)*

165. **(D)** Loperamide (Imodium) inhibits peristaltic activity by a direct effect on the musculature of the intestinal wall. Loperamide appears to be devoid of opium-like effects. Even after chronic administration of loperamide, the injection of the narcotic antagonist naloxone does not produce pupillary dilation. *(6:926)*

166. **(C)** Tricyclic antidepressants such as imipramine (Tofranil) and amitriptyline (Elavil) may block the uptake of guanethidine by adrenergic nerves, thereby inhibiting its antihypertensive action. *(8:481)*

167. **(E)** Cyclobenzaprine (Flexeril), an analogue of amitriptyline, is available for the treatment of acute voluntary muscle spasm. Because they are so alike in chemical structure, cyclobenzaprine and amitriptyline have essentially the same side effects and toxicity. *(3:2871)*

168. **(E)** Cocaine, like the amphetamines, is a potent CNS stimulant. The other agents listed are CNS depressants. *(5:1350)*

169. **(D)** Acetaminophen will not displace warfarin from its protein-binding sites or interfere with warfarin metabolism. It is less likely, therefore to cause a therapeutic problem in this patient. All of the other choices either have a high affinity for plasma proteins or may alter warfarin metabolism. *(2a:66)*

170. **(E)** Significant increases in blood pressure can be controlled by either reducing the infu-

sion rate or discontinuing the infusion until the blood pressure has been stabilized. Among the major drug interactions of dopamine is concurrent use of the MAO inhibitors. Because dopamine is metabolized by monamine oxidase enzymes, doses of dopamine may have to be reduced to 10% of normal when the patient has been medicated with an MAO inhibitor drug. *(6:211)*

171. **(C)** Each gram of protein supplies about 4 kcal, each gram of carbohydrate supplies about 4 kcal, and each gram of fat supplies about 9 kcal. It is obvious, therefore, that strictly on a weight basis, fats are better caloric sources than are other nutrients. *(19:35.5)*

172. **(C)** Portagen is a product used when conventional dietary fats may not be well absorbed, digested, or used. Its fat content consists of more than 95% medium-chain triglycerides, which are more rapidly absorbed than are the triglycerides of long-chain fatty acids present in conventional food fats. Patients suffering from steatorrhea (excessive loss of fats in the feces) are ideal candidates for dietary supplementation with Portagen. *(2a:412)*

173. **(D)** Pedialyte is an orally administered electrolyte solution containing dextrose; potassium chloride; and sodium, calcium, and magnesium salts. It is used to supply water and electrolytes in a balanced proportion in order to prevent serious deficits from occurring in patients suffering from mild to moderate fluid loss. The product does not contain protein or fat. *(2a:414)*

174. **(B)** Each gram of carbohydrate supplies 4 kcal of energy to a patient. Because a liter of dextrose 5% solution contains 50 g of dextrose, the administration of the liter will supply the patient with approximately 200 kcal. *(19:35.5)*

175. **(E)** Phenylketonuria (PKU) is an inherited metabolic disorder characterized by high plasma phenylalanine hydroxylase, which converts phenylalanine to tyrosine. Routine

testing of newborns for PKU is common in the United States. Treatment consists of following a low-phenylalanine diet that is started early in life and continued perhaps indefinitely. Lofenalac, a complete nutritional product except for its low phenylalanine content, is used in place of the usual milk in the diet of children with PKU. Untreated PKU results in mental retardation. Foods and beverages containing aspartame (NutraSweet) must bear label warnings for people with PKU, because aspartame is metabolized to phenylalanine (and aspartic acid and methanol). *(19:99.6)*

176. **(A)** Because this patient has a history of recurrent infections, the present symptoms probably indicate a reinfection. Therefore, ampicillin would be the most reasonable choice pending culture and sensitivity results. If this patient had been treated initially with a sulfonamide or a tetracycline, it would be desirable to switch to a different drug because bacteria frequently develop resistance to these drugs. *(19:63.8)*

177. **(A)** Of the drugs listed, erythromycin has the lowest degree of toxicity and the spectrum of action most similar to penicillin. Demeclocycline may inhibit skeletal growth in the fetus. Deposition of tetracyclines in the teeth of the fetus has been associated with enamel defects and staining of the teeth. Trimethoprim is a teratogenic drug. *(3:343)*

178. **(B)** Sulfamylon cream applied topically to burns has been found to be quite effective in inhibiting the invasion of the affected site by both gram-positive and gram-negative bacteria. The cream is usually applied to a thickness of about $1/16$ inch twice daily over the entire burned surface. Silver sulfadiazine is also used topically for the same purpose. *(3:559)*

179. **(E)** Spectinomycin (Trobicin) is an aminocyclitol antibiotic related to the aminoglycosides. Although it is active against many gram-positive and gram-negative organisms, it is generally reserved for the treatment of gonorrhea in patients who do not respond to

or tolerate the use of ceftriaxone. In the treatment of gonorrhea, spectinomycin is generally given in a dose of 2 g IM as a single dose, followed by 100 mg of doxycycline twice daily for 7 days. *(3:344c)*

180. **(A)** Colchicine is one of the most valuable drugs available for the treatment of an acute attack of gout. The mechanism of action is not known but is believed to be interference with the inflammatory response of gout. Colchicine may alter other inflammatory states, but the effects are less dramatic. The uricosuric drugs used for gout act by either increasing the rate of uric acid excretion by the kidney (ie, probenecid and sulfinpyrazone) or by decreasing the rate of synthesis of uric acid (ie, allopurinol). *(6:647)*

181. **(A)** Opticrom ophthalmic solution contains cromolyn sodium 4%. It is used to treat ocular allergic disorders such as vernal conjunctivitis. It is effective only if it is used at regular intervals. *(3:760)*

182. **(C)** Glucose tolerance is impaired by the thiazides, even though certain other sulfonamide derivatives are hypoglycemic agents. The degree of hyperglycemia induced by the thiazides is unimportant in patients with normal carbohydrate tolerance but may intensify the hyperglycemia of diabetes or precipitate glycosuria in persons predisposed to diabetes. *(5:1491)*

183. **(E)** Dopamine (Intropin) is a sympathomimetic drug that acts directly on alpha and beta receptors and produces indirect effects due to release of norepinephrine. Dopamine also dilates renal and mesenteric vessels through a dopamine receptor effect. The hemodynamic effects of dopamine are dose related. At low infusion rates (1–5 mg/kg/min), dopamine increases renal blood flow without much change in cardiac output or total peripheral resistance. In higher doses (5–20 mg/kg/min), cardiac output and heart rate increase, the increase in renal perfusion persists, and total peripheral resistance is variable. At higher infusion rates, renal vasoconstriction occurs, total peripheral resistance rises, and blood pressure increases. Consequently, the infusion rate must be adjusted and monitored carefully to achieve the desired response. *(6:211)*

184. **(A)** Because of the relatively poor aqueous solubility of chlordiazepoxide, the drug is reconstituted in a "special" diluent that consists primarily of propylene glycol. When injected IM, the drug is believed to precipitate at the injection site, forming a depot from which it slowly redissolves and becomes available for absorption. Compared to equal oral doses, IM chlordiazepoxide is absorbed more slowly and produces lower blood levels. If large IM doses of the drug are given repeatedly over a short period of time, it is quite likely that the patient will demonstrate symptoms of overdose several hours later, when large amounts of the drug are absorbed from the multiple injections. Also, the drug and its metabolites have long half-lives. *(3:261h)*

185. **(E)** Although there are no reported differences in bioavailability between phenytoin capsules and suspension, this patient's phenytoin level is most likely going to increase because the milligram-for-milligram conversion is equivalent to an increase in dose. The capsule form of Dilantin is the sodium salt and as such contains only 92% phenytoin. The suspension is the free acid and contains 100% phenytoin. In this situation, the patient would be going from a daily dose of 276 mg phenytoin (as 300-mg phenytoin sodium) to 300 mg phenytoin. *(3:283g)*

186. **(C)** Dobutamine (Dobutrex) is a beta-adrenergic agonist that is available for IV use as an inotropic drug. Although dobutamine is similar to isoproterenol (Isuprel) in terms of its inotropic effect, dobutamine is relatively less potent than isoproterenol as a stimulator of peripheral beta receptors that mediate vasodilation. Consequently, dobutamine produces an inotropic effect with comparatively little effect on preload, afterload, or heart rate. *(6:213)*

187. **(C)** The full therapeutic effect of the tricyclic antidepressants often takes several weeks to develop. During this period, many patients subjectively feel that their depression has worsened. However, the side effects of these drugs, sedation and anticholinergic effects, usually begin shortly after therapy is initiated. The pharmacist should discuss these anticipated effects with the patient. The pharmacist should also consult with the prescribing physician if it is apparent that an intensified depression may be serious enough to lead to suicide. *(19:78.4)*

188. **(A)** The theoretical advantage of administering insulin in IV glucose is that both insulin and glucose are delivered in constant proportions. Administration of insulin in this manner, however, can result in undesirable fluctuations in blood glucose levels. As much as 20% of the insulin added to an IV is bound to the container and tubing. Proportionally greater binding occurs with lower doses of insulin. If the same administration set is used for subsequent infusions, the binding sites on the set may be saturated with insulin. This would be observed clinically as some improvement in control of blood glucose, because subsequent binding would be to the IV container alone. Furthermore, even if the insulin dose is adjusted for binding by the container, hyperglycemia may still occur after the administration set is changed. This, of course, does not mean that insulin should not be administered by IV infusion, but that the adsorption of insulin by IV bottles and tubing should be considered in accounting for unusual changes in blood glucose levels and in determining insulin doses, especially when low doses are contemplated. *(19:48.35)*

189. **(D)** In general, all insulins are reasonably stable at room temperature (ie, 59° to 85° F). Traveling diabetics should be advised to avoid prolonged exposure of their insulin to very high temperatures, and told that it is not necessary to refrigerate the vial in use. Insulin vials stored in pharmacies are required to be refrigerated because they may be kept in stock for a long period of time. *(5:1504)*

190. **(E)** Isotretinoin (Accutane) is a vitamin A derivative indicated for the treatment of recalcitrant cystic acne in patients who do not respond to more conservative therapy. Approximately 90% of patients using this product experience cheilitis. *(3:543a)*

191. **(D)** Fluids employed in TPN are generally very hypertonic and hyperosmotic. Until the technique of subclavian vein catheterization was perfected, it was too irritating and inflammatory to use the usual sites of IV administration. Peripheral veins are seldom used in the administration of hypertonic nutrient solutions because blood flow is insufficient to provide the necessary dilution of the fluid to protect the intima of the vessel. The exception occurs when the slightly hypertonic amino acid solutions containing limited amounts of dextrose are administered. *(19:35.5)*

192. **(C)** Although all beta blockers are likely to mask the symptoms of acute hypoglycemia (eg, rapid pulse, tachycardia, tremor), the cardioselective beta blockers atenolol (Tenormin) and metoprolol (Lopressor) are more appropriate in diabetics; these drugs have much less of an effect on the metabolic and cardiovascular responses to hypoglycemia than do the nonselective beta blockers. They are therefore less likely to intensify hypoglycemia, precipitate hypertensive crises during hypoglycemia, and compromise peripheral circulation. Atenolol does not potentiate insulin-induced hypoglycemia and, unlike the nonselective beta blockers, does not delay recovery of glucose to normal levels. *(6:238)*

Cardio selective Atenolol, Lopressor

193. **(B)** Inhibition of calcium entry into arterial smooth muscle is associated with decreased arteriolar tone and systemic vascular resistance, resulting in decreased arterial pressure. This reduction in arterial pressure, in turn, causes a significant reflex tachycardia. Because other calcium channel blockers such as verapamil (Calan, Isoptin) and diltiazem (Cardizem) also decrease intracardiac conduction significantly, they are much less likely to cause tachycardia. *(6:771)*

194. **(D)** Suddenly discontinuing dextrose solution may cause a rebound hypoglycemia in response to the sudden elimination of the sustained glucose load of the TPN solution. It is best to maintain the patient on a nominal amount of dextrose such as D5W or to wean the patient slowly from the TPN solution. *(19:35.7)*
(B–incorrect) Hyperchloremic metabolic acidosis may occur during TPN therapy when the total chloride ion content is high. The amino acids in the protein salts are usually chloride or hydrochloride salts. Additional amounts of chloride are obtained when sodium or potassium chlorides are added to the TPN solutions. It may be useful to supply either sodium or potassium as acetate salts. (C–incorrect) Hyperosmotic nonketotic hyperglycemia is a result of infusing an overload of glucose. Causes include an overly rapid infusion rate, dextrose solutions that are too concentrated, and malfunction of pancreatic secretion of insulin.

195. **(E)** Fats provide approximately 9 kcal/g. Because of their isotonicity, fat emulsions can be administered safely through peripheral veins. A commercial example of a fat emulsion is Intralipid, a 10% soybean emulsion. *(19:35.5)*
(A–incorrect) Ethanol provides 7 kcal/g. Disadvantages associated with ethanol are the fact that excessively rapid infusion can cause heartburn and/or intoxication, and the fact that it cannot be used in patients with GI disease such as pancreatitis.
(D–incorrect) Hydrous dextrose provides 3.4 kcal/g. It is the usual source of calories in TPN formulations because of its safety, economy, and availability to the body.
(E–incorrect) Proteins provide 3 to 4 kcal/g.

196. **(B)** Granisetron (Kytril) is a selective 5-HT$_3$ receptor antagonist used to prevent nausea and vomiting associated with cancer chemotherapy. It is particularly useful in treating nausea and vomiting accompanying cisplatin therapy. Granisetron is administered orally or by IV infusion beginning 30 minutes prior to initiating emetogenic chemotherapy. An additional dose of the oral form may be given 12 hours after the first dose on the day of chemotherapy treatment. *(3:259r)*

197. **(C)** Amiloride is a potassium-sparing diuretic with a mechanism of action similar to that of triamterene. Both drugs exert a diuretic effect by promoting the exchange of sodium for potassium in the distal portion of the renal tubule. In contrast to spironolactone, neither of these drugs inhibits aldosterone. Metolazone and chlorthalidone are thiazide-like diuretics. *(6:704)*

198. **(D)** Treatment of hyperkalemia can be approached by three methods. First, in the presence of ECG changes, calcium should be given to counteract the effects of excess potassium on the heart. Secondly, bicarbonate or glucose plus insulin can be used to shift potassium rapidly from extracellular to intracellular fluid compartments. Thirdly, exchange resins (eg, Kayexalate) or dialysis can be used to remove potassium from the body. In this case, because there are no symptoms of ECG changes, the rectal administration of Kayexalate (enemas containing 50 g in 70% sorbitol solution) is the most appropriate option. *(5:1119)*

199. **(E)** The hypotensive activity of diazoxide is caused by a reduction in peripheral vascular resistance via direct arteriolar relaxation. As arterial pressure is lowered, baroreceptor reflexes are activated; this leads to cardiac stimulation with increased heart rate, stroke volume, and cardiac output. This, in turn, will increase myocardial oxygen demand, a potentially dangerous situation in a patient with ischemic heart disease. *(6:799)*

200. **(C)** Nitroprusside and trimethaphan both decrease total peripheral resistance rapidly, with minimal effects on myocardial oxygen consumption. Nitroprusside dilates both venous (capacitance) and arterial (resistance) vessels, therefore reducing preload and afterload on the heart. Nitroprusside is preferred over trimethaphan because tolerance develops rapidly to trimethaphan's hypotensive activity. Propranolol is not effective in hypertensive emergencies. Hydralazine and minoxidil are both likely to cause cardiac stimu-lation. (6:790, 797)

201. **(E)** Zolpidem (Ambien) is a nonbarbiturate, nonbenzodiazepine hypnotic. *(3:269h)*

202. **(B)** Olsalazine is a salicylate compound that is converted to 5-aminosalicylic acid in the gut. This agent produces an anti-inflamma-tory effect in the gut. *(3:326c)*

203. **(C)** Prednisone is approximately four times more potent than hydrocortisone. Because this patient was receiving a total daily dose of 200 mg of hydrocortisone, an equivalent anti-inflammatory dose of prednisone would be 50 mg/day. *(6:1474)* P = 4×H

204. **(D)** Glucocorticoids associated with a lesser degree of mineralocorticoid activity should be used in patients with conditions such as congestive heart failure in which sodium re-tention can be an aggravating factor. Because all glucocorticoids induce potassium loss re-gardless of their mineralocorticoid activity, even dexamethasone should be used with caution in this patient. *(6:1475)*

205. **(C)** At the infusion rate of 50 mg/hr, the pa-tient is receiving a total daily dose of 1200 mg (50 mg/hr × 24 hr) of aminophylline dihy-drate. Because aminophylline dihydrate con-tains the equivalent of 79% anhydrous theo-phylline, this patient is receiving a total daily dose of 948 mg anhydrous theophylline (0.79 × 1200 mg/day). The most practical dose of Theo-Dur would be 900 mg/day given in doses of 300 mg every 8 hours. *(3:179a)*

206. **(D)** Although a number of beta-adrenergic agonists are available for clinical use, only ephedrine, metaproterenol, terbutaline, and albuterol are available in oral dosage forms. Metaproterenol, terbutaline, and albuterol se-lectively stimulate beta$_2$-adrenergic receptors to a greater degree than beta$_1$-adrenergic re-ceptors. Therefore, they are somewhat less likely to cause cardiac stimulation. Ephedrine has both weak alpha as well as beta$_1$ and beta$_2$ activity. When compared to these other agents, ephedrine has a shorter duration of action, a lower peak effect, and more adverse effects. Ephedrine also adds little to the bron-chodilation produced by therapeutic doses of theophylline. Such a combination is, how-ever, likely to produce synergistic toxicity. *(6:664)*

207. **(D)** Choline salicylate (Arthropan) is a liquid salicylate dosage form that has a fishy odor. *(3:249)*

208. **(C)** Lanoxicaps contain digoxin in a more bioavailable form than in digoxin tablets. A 20% reduction in dosage is generally re-quired to achieve a comparable therapeutic response with Lanoxin tablets. *(3:142b)*

209. **(A)** Rifampin is a potent microsomal enzyme inducer and may reduce effectiveness of hor-mones supplied by oral contraceptive prod-ucts. *(3:107i)*

210. **(B)** Sumatriptan succinate (Imitrex) is a vaso-constrictor that is effective in controlling mi-graine headaches. When used parenterally, it is contraindicated in patients with ischemic heart disease or uncontrolled hypertension. The oral form of the drug tends to be better tolerated by most patients. *(3:256h)*

CHAPTER 7

Patient Profiles

The pharmacist, whether practicing in a community or an institutional setting, must constantly refer to patient profiles for information regarding the medical history of a specific patient. Analysis of profile data requires a strong knowledge base in the pharmacy disciplines already reviewed in this book.

In this section, there are 30 patient medication profiles. Some are related to community pharmacy practice and some to institutional practice.

Questions

Community Pharmacy Medication Record

Patient Name: David Harris
Address: 7 North Way
Age: 25
Sex: M
Allergies: penicillin, ragweed

Height: 6'2"
Weight: 180 lb

DIAGNOSIS

Primary	Secondary
1. tinea cruris	1.
2.	2.
3.	3.

MEDICATION RECORD

Date	Rx No.	Physician	Drug & Strength	Quantity	Sig	Refills
1. 7/21	34325	Jimes	Dimetapp Elixir	4 oz	5 mL p.r.n.	2
2. 7/21	34326	Jimes	E.E.S. 400	#40	1 q.i.d.	
3. 7/21	34327	Jimes	Afrin Spray	#1	spray b.i.d.	
4. 9/4	39856	Hunat	Fulvicin P/G 165 mg	#C	b.i.d.	2

PHARMACIST'S NOTES AND OTHER PATIENT INFORMATION

Date	Comment
1. 9/4	Hydrocortisone 0.25% 1 oz OTC

DIRECTIONS (Questions 1a through 1k): Each of the numbered items or incomplete statements in this section is followed by answers or by completions of the statement. Select the ONE lettered answer or completion that is BEST in each case.

1a. Tinea cruris is also known as

(A) jock itch
(B) athlete's foot
(C) candidiasis
(D) thrush
(E) atopic dermatitis

1b. Tinea cruris is caused by a

(A) virus
(B) protozoan
(C) gram-negative bacterium
(D) fungus
(E) gram-positive bacterium

1c. The active ingredient in Fulvicin P/G is

(A) desiccated
(B) macrocrystalline
(C) deliquescent
(D) efflorescent
(E) ultramicrosized

1d. Fulvicin P/G contains

(A) phenolated glycerin
(B) propylene glycol
(C) polyoxyethylene guaiacolate
(D) polyethylene glycol
(E) glycolated protein

1e. Patients receiving Fulvicin P/G should be advised to

I. avoid dairy products when using the medication
II. continue medication for the entire course of therapy
III. prevent excessive exposure to ultraviolet light

(A) I only
(B) III only
(C) I and II only
(D) II and III only
(E) I, II, and III

1f. The pharmacist should advise Dr. Hunat of

(A) Mr. Harris' penicillin allergy
(B) Mr. Harris' age
(C) Mr. Harris' ragweed allergy
(D) the dosage error made in prescribing Fulvicin P/G
(E) all of the above

1g. Which of the following products is most similar to Fulvicin P/G?

(A) Grifulvin V
(B) Grisactin Ultra
(C) Mycostatin
(D) Diflucan
(E) Nizoral

1h. A topical product that would be appropriate for this patient to use is

(A) bacitracin ointment
(B) metronidazole
(C) nystatin cream
(D) gentian violet
(E) clotrimazole

1i. The use of fluorinated steroids on areas affected by tinea is likely to result in

(A) local ulceration
(B) loss of hair in the area to which the steroid is applied
(C) spread of the organism
(D) increased blood glucose levels
(E) yellowish skin discoloration

1j. The patient's ragweed allergy could be a serious problem if he attempted to use a product containing

(A) malathion
(B) lindane
(C) pyrethrins
(D) menthol
(E) hydrocortisone

1k. If the patient complained of dry skin lesions, the appropriate dosage form of hydrocortisone would be

(A) cream
(B) gel
(C) suppository
(D) ointment
(E) aerosol spray

■ PROFILE NO. 2

Community Pharmacy Medication Record

Patient Name: Hattie Wilson
Address: 7 Wilson Dr.
Age: 78   Height: 5'4"
Sex: F   Weight: 120 lb
Allergies: codeine

DIAGNOSIS

Primary	Secondary
1. rheumatoid arthritis	1.
2. hypertension	2.
3.	3.

MEDICATION RECORD

Date	Rx No.	Physician	Drug & Strength	Quantity	Sig	Refills
1. 4/12	34094	Till	HCTZ 50 mg	#30	1 qd	5
2. 4/12	34095	Till	Slow-K 8 mEq	#C	1 t.i.d.	3
3. 5/23	37844	Wasser	Tylenol/Cod. No. 3	#60	1 t.i.d.	1
4. 5/28	38248	Till	Lotensin 10 mg	#30	1 daily	2

PHARMACIST'S NOTES AND OTHER PATIENT INFORMATION

Date	Comment
1. 4/21	100 Drixoral Sustained-Action Tablets (OTC)

DIRECTIONS (Questions 2a through 2l): Each of the numbered items or incomplete statements in this section is followed by answers or by completions of the statement. Select the ONE lettered answer or completion that is BEST in each case.

2a. Which of the following products would be equivalent to the HCTZ prescribed?

   I. Diuril

   II. Zaroxolyn

   III. Oretic

   (A) I only

   (B) III only

   (C) I and II only

   (D) II and III only

   (E) I, II, and III

2b. Which of the following best describes Slow-K?

   (A) Microencapsulation

   (B) Chewable tablet

   (C) Enteric coating

   (D) Spansule

   (E) Wax matrix

2c. Each Slow-K dosage unit contains 8 mEq of potassium as potassium chloride. How many mg of potassium chloride are in each Slow-K tablet? (Atom. wt. K = 39; Cl = 35)

(A) 740 mg

(B) 296 mg

(C) 312 mg

(D) 872 mg

(E) 592 mg

2d. Lotensin can best be described as a (an)

(A) angiotensin-II antagonist

(B) alpha$_1$-adrenergic blocker

(C) nonspecific beta-adrenergic blocker

(D) angiotensin-converting enzyme inhibitor

(E) direct-acting vasodilator

2e. Which of the following agents is most similar to HCTZ?

(A) Bumetanide

(B) Torsemide

(C) Acetazolamide

(D) Chlorthalidone

(E) Ethacrynic acid

2f. When requesting Drixoral from the pharmacist, the patient should be informed that Drixoral

(A) may interact with the Slow-K

(B) is contraindicated in patients with rheumatoid arthritis

(C) is contraindicated in patients allergic to codeine

(D) may not be sold without a prescription

(E) is contraindicated in hypertensive patients

2g. When Lotensin is added to this patient's regimen, there is an increased likelihood of

(A) hyperkalemia

(B) hypoglycemia

(C) hypokalemia

(D) hypernatremia

(E) hypocalcemia

2h. Lotensin is in the same pharmacological class as

   I. Univasc

   II. Monopril

   III. Cozaar

(A) I only

(B) III only

(C) I and II only

(D) II and III only

(E) I, II, and III

2i. Pruritis is a reported adverse effect related to the use of Lotensin. Pruritis can best be defined as

(A) hypermotility of the GI tract

(B) hearing difficulty

(C) itching

(D) taste impairment

(E) drooling

2j. The dose of codeine found in each dose of Tylenol/Codeine No. 3 is

(A) 3 mg

(B) 30 mg

(C) 120 mg

(D) 180 mg

(E) 0.3 mg

2k. The therapeutic category of brompheniramine maleate in the Drixoral product is

(A) H$_1$-receptor antagonist

(B) H$_2$-receptor agonist

(C) H$_1$-receptor agonist

(D) H$_2$-receptor antagonist

(E) alpha$_1$-adrenergic agonist

2l. An adverse effect expected with the use of Tylenol/Codeine No. 3 is

(A) diarrhea

(B) urinary urgency

(C) constipation

(D) respiratory stimulation

(E) CNS stimulation

■ ◦ PROFILE NO. 3

Community Pharmacy Medication Record

Patient Name: Carolyn Mann
Address: 45 N. High St.
Age: 27
Sex: F
Allergies: aspirin

Height: 5'3"
Weight: 120 lb

DIAGNOSIS

Primary	Secondary
1. grand mal seizures since age 8	1. constipation
2.	2.
3.	3.

MEDICATION RECORD

Date	Rx No.	Physician	Drug & Strength	Quantity	Sig	Refills
1. 2/2	34568	Mazur	Micronor			5
2. 3/1	34568	Mazur	Refill			
3. 3/21	35908	Wilson	Dilantin Kap. 0.1	#C	3 daily	2
4. 4/2	38998	Mazur	Theragran-M	#C	1 daily	2

PHARMACIST'S NOTES AND OTHER PATIENT INFORMATION

Date	Comment
1. 4/2	Semicid 1 pk (OTC)
2. 4/9	Colace 100 mg #100 (OTC)

DIRECTIONS (Questions 3a through 3m): Each of the numbered items or incomplete statements in this section is followed by answers or by completions of the statement. Select the ONE lettered answer or completion that is BEST in each case.

3a. Micronor can best be described as a (an)

(A) triphasic oral contraceptive
(B) progestin-only oral contraceptive
(C) biphasic oral contraceptive
(D) ovulation inducer
(E) vaginal deodorant product

3b. Semicid is employed as a vaginal

(A) douche solution
(B) lubricant
(C) cream
(D) silicone implant
(E) suppository

3c. A synonym for grand mal seizures is

(A) tonic–clonic seizures
(B) absence seizures
(C) focal seizures
(D) status epilepticus
(E) Jacksonian seizures

3d. The Dilantin product prescribed may be administered

I. in three divided daily doses
II. as a single daily dose
III. on a p.r.n. basis

(A) I only
(B) III only
(C) I and II only
(D) II and III only
(E) I, II, and III

3e. In the course of receiving Dilantin the patient develops gingival hyperplasia. This is a disorder of the

(A) gums
(B) cardiac wall
(C) nasal mucosa
(D) renal tubules
(E) vaginal lining

3f. The generic name of the Dilantin product prescribed is

(A) phenytoin sodium
(B) ethotoin
(C) phensuximide
(D) phenytoin
(E) mephenytoin

3g. A plasma phenytoin determination reveals a plasma concentration of 5 µg/mL. This indicates that

(A) hepatic impairment may exist
(B) the patient may be taking more doses than prescribed
(C) the concentration is within the therapeutic range
(D) the patient may have renal impairment
(E) the patient may not be taking all prescribed doses

3h. The prescriber should be called because of

(A) cross-sensitivity between aspirin and Dilantin
(B) carcinogenicity with Dilantin
(C) reduction in Dilantin effectiveness
(D) reduction in Micronor effectiveness
(E) improper Dilantin dose prescribed

3i. Which of the following is true of parenterally administered Dilantin?

I. Dilantin parenteral solutions must be kept refrigerated until just prior to administration.
II. Precipitation is likely to occur when Dilantin is combined with promethazine HCl in an IV admixture.
III. IM administration should generally be avoided.

(A) I only
(B) III only
(C) I and II only
(D) II and III only
(E) I, II, and III

3j. Patients receiving Dilantin may develop a morbilliform rash. Morbilliform refers to

(A) multicolored
(B) pus-containing
(C) unilateral
(D) symmetrical
(E) measles-like

3k. The active ingredient of Semicid is

(A) ethinyl estradiol
(B) oxyquinoline sulfate
(C) nonoxynol-9
(D) sodium lauryl sulfate
(E) boric acid

3l. The active ingredient in Colace is a (an)

(A) anionic surfactant
(B) stimulant
(C) cationic surfactant
(D) osmotic laxative
(E) bulk former

3m. Which of the following is true of Theragran-M?

(A) It is only available as a liquid.

(B) It is a sustained-release capsule product.

(C) Its use should be avoided in patients on Dilantin.

(D) Its use should be avoided in patients on Micronor.

(E) It is available without a prescription.

■ PROFILE NO. 4

Community Pharmacy Medication Record

Patient Name: Harry Walsh
Address: 17 Dyer Dr.
Age: 66   Height: 5′11″
Sex: M   Weight: 185 lb
Allergies:

DIAGNOSIS

Primary	Secondary
1. Parkinson's disease	1.
2.	2.
3.	3.

MEDICATION RECORD

Date	Rx No.	Physician	Drug & Strength	Quantity	Sig	Refills
1. 2/3	56445	Tillman	Sinemet 10/100	#C	1 t.i.d.	2
2. 3/1	56445	Tillman	Refill			
3. 3/19	59008	Tillman	Sinemet 25/250	#C	t.i.d.	2
4. 3/19	59009	Tillman	Cogentin 0.5 mg	#90	1 b.i.d.	2
5. 4/15	59008	Tillman	Refill			
6. 4/15	61122	Tillman	Symmetrel 100 mg	#60	1 b.i.d.	3

DIRECTIONS (Questions 4a through 4l): Each of the numbered items or incomplete statements in this section is followed by answers or by completions of the statement. Select the ONE lettered answer or completion that is BEST in each case.

4a. The function of carbidopa in the Sinemet formulation is to

(A) act as a precursor for levodopa

(B) act as a xanthine oxidase inhibitor

(C) act as a microsomal enzyme inhibitor

(D) inhibit decarboxylation of peripheral levodopa

(E) increase the absorption of levodopa from the GI tract

4b. Patients receiving levodopa should avoid using vitamin supplements that contain

(A) folic acid

(B) pyridoxine

(C) ascorbic acid

(D) riboflavin

(E) thiamine

4c. A patient using Sinemet complains of an appreciable darkening of the urine beginning about 3 days after starting Sinemet therapy. The pharmacist should tell the patient to

(A) disregard the discoloration because it is not harmful

(B) check the expiration date on the Sinemet container to make sure it has not expired

(C) immediately stop taking the Sinemet and call the prescriber

(D) avoid the use of acidic foods while on Sinemet

(E) avoid the use of alkaline foods while on Sinemet

4d. Cogentin has been prescribed because of its action as a (an)

(A) centrally acting skeletal muscle relaxant

(B) sedative

(C) peripheral vasodilator

(D) memory enhancer

(E) anticholinergic

4e. Which of the following is NOT employed in the treatment of Parkinson's disease?

(A) Biperiden (Akineton)

(B) Selegiline (Eldepryl)

(C) Pergolide (Permax)

(D) Tranylcypromine (Parnate)

(E) Bromocriptine (Parlodel)

4f. Symmetrel is also employed in the treatment of

(A) viral infections

(B) psychoses

(C) gout

(D) hypertension

(E) bronchial asthma

4g. Diplopia is an adverse effect related to the use of levodopa. This can best be described as

(A) urinary retention

(B) impaired muscular coordination

(C) hearing loss

(D) a cardiac tachyarrhythmia

(E) double vision

4h. When a patient on levodopa is to be switched to Sinemet, which of the following is (are) true?

I. Plasma levodopa levels must be measured each day for the first 5 days of Sinemet therapy.

II. Permit at least 8 hours to elapse between the last dose of levodopa and the first dose of Sinemet.

III. Reduce the dose of levodopa by 75%.

(A) I only

(B) III only

(C) I and II only

(D) II and III only

(E) I, II, and III

4i. Levodopa can best be described as a (an)

(A) cholinergic agonist

(B) dopamine antagonist

(C) skeletal muscle relaxant

(D) neurotransmitter

(E) dopamine precursor

4j. Which of the following products may be used to provide individually titrated doses of carbidopa?

(A) Intropin
(B) Dopar
(C) Larobec
(D) Lodosyn
(E) Permax

4k. The prolonged use of which of the following drugs is associated with the development of Parkinson-like symptoms?

(A) Ciprofloxacin
(B) Chlorpromazine
(C) Encainide
(D) Enalapril maleate
(E) Bupropion

4l. A patient with Parkinson's disease is likely to exhibit which of the following symptoms?

I. Muscle rigidity
II. Visual impairment
III. Thrombocytopenia

(A) I only
(B) III only
(C) I and II only
(D) II and III only
(E) I, II, and III

■ PROFILE NO. 5

Community Pharmacy Medication Record

Patient Name: Mildred North
Address: 721 Yager St.
Age: 64
Sex: F
Allergies: pollen, penicillin

Height: 5'5"
Weight: 155 lb

DIAGNOSIS

Primary	Secondary
1. open-angle glaucoma, primary	1. wheezing
2. emphysema	2.
3.	3.

MEDICATION RECORD

Date	Rx No.	Physician	Drug & Strength	Quantity	Sig	Refills
1. 7/29	59083	Weber	Pilocarpine 1%	15 mL	gtt 1 os t.i.d.	2
2. 8/20	59083	Weber	Refill			
3. 9/11	65002	Weber	Betoptic 0.5%	10 mL	gtt 1 os b.i.d.	2
4. 10/21	65002	Weber	Refill			

PHARMACIST'S NOTES AND OTHER PATIENT INFORMATION

Date	Comment
1. 9/14	Ecotrin Maximum Strength (OTC)
2. 10/7	Visine (OTC)

DIRECTIONS (Questions 5a through 5l): Each of the numbered items or incomplete statements in this section is followed by answers or by completions of the statement. Select the ONE lettered answer or completion that is BEST in each case.

5a. The primary action of pilocarpine in the treatment of glaucoma is as a (an)

(A) mydriatic
(B) cycloplegic
(C) miotic
(D) vasoconstrictor
(E) carbonic anhydrase inhibitor

5b. Pilocarpine is most similar in pharmacologic action to

(A) timolol
(B) carbachol
(C) physostigmine
(D) propafenone
(E) isoflurophate

5c. Several weeks after using pilocarpine, the patient's intraocular pressure is measured as 14 mm Hg. This indicates that

(A) the dose of pilocarpine should be increased
(B) the patient has narrow-angle glaucoma
(C) an error in measurement must have occurred
(D) the intraocular pressure is under control
(E) the dose of pilocarpine should be decreased

5d. Ocusert Pilo-20 is a system designed to release pilocarpine into the eye at a rate of

(A) 20 µg/day
(B) 20 µg/hr
(C) 20 mg/hr
(D) 20 mg/day
(E) 20 mg/week

5e. An Ocusert Pilo-20 system must be replaced

(A) every day
(B) every 20 days
(C) every month
(D) when burning of the eye is experienced
(E) every 7 days

5f. Betoptic is employed for the same purpose as

I. Ocupress
II. Timoptic
III. OptiPranolol

(A) I only
(B) III only
(C) I and II only
(D) II and III only
(E) I, II, and III

5g. Betoptic is believed to act in reducing intraocular pressure by

(A) increasing the outflow of aqueous humor
(B) causing cycloplegia
(C) causing miosis
(D) interfering with carbonic anhydrase action
(E) decreasing aqueous humor production

5h. Betoptic labeling indicates that the solution contains EDTA. This is used in this formulation as a (an)

(A) viscosity builder
(B) surfactant
(C) buffer
(D) antiseptic
(E) chelating agent

5i. The Visine purchased OTC by this patient contains

(A) physostigmine
(B) tropicamide
(C) oxymetazoline
(D) tetrahydrozoline
(E) ephedrine

5j. The prescriber should be contacted by the pharmacist to discuss the possibility of

   (A) blood dyscrasias
   (B) interaction between pilocarpine and Betoptic
   (C) urinary retention
   (D) respiratory distress
   (E) interaction between pilocarpine and Ecotrin

5k. The Ecotrin Maximum Strength formulation is most similar to which of the following?

   (A) Easprin
   (B) Bufferin
   (C) Disalcid
   (D) Dolobid
   (E) Alka-Seltzer

5l. Patients with glaucoma should avoid drugs that are

   (A) anticholinergics
   (B) broad-spectrum antimicrobial agents
   (C) metabolized in the liver
   (D) renally eliminated
   (E) peripheral vasodilators

■ PROFILE NO. 6

Community Pharmacy Medication Record

Patient Name: Lori Masters
Address: 34 Orchard St.
Age: 21
Sex: F
Allergies: penicillin

Height: 5'2"
Weight: 119 lb

DIAGNOSIS

Primary	Secondary
1. acne vulgaris—severe	1.
2.	2.
3.	3.

MEDICATION RECORD

Date	Rx No.	Physician	Drug & Strength	Quantity	Sig	Refills
1. 6/7	45023	Thomas	Benzac 5 Gel	45 g	ut dict	3
2. 6/22	48399	Wilson	Retin-A liquid	28 mL	Apply p.r.n.	2
3. 7/13	45023	Thomas	Refill			
4. 8/24	45023	Thomas	Refill			
5. 9/17	57888	Wilson	Cleocin T Gel	30 g	Apply topically	3
6. 10/5	59778	Thomas	Accutane 20 mg	#60	1 b.i.d.	5

PHARMACIST'S NOTES AND OTHER PATIENT INFORMATION

Date	Comment
1. 7/1	Brasivol Medium
2. 7/30	Pernox Scrub 60 mL

DIRECTIONS (Questions 6a through 6l): Each of the numbered items or incomplete statements in this section is followed by answers or by completions of the statement. Select the ONE lettered answer or completion that is BEST in each case.

6a. The active ingredient in Benzac is

(A) benzoyl peroxide
(B) benzyl alcohol
(C) isotretinoin
(D) tretinoin
(E) benzalkonium chloride

6b. Patients using Retin-A should avoid

I. having product come in contact with the eyes
II. excessive sunlight
III. use of antimicrobial agents

(A) I only
(B) III only
(C) I and II only
(D) II and III only
(E) I, II, and III

6c. Retin-A liquid contains butylated hydroxy-toluene. The function of this ingredient is as a (an)

(A) viscosity builder
(B) solvent
(C) coloring agent
(D) chelating agent
(E) antioxidant

6d. Which of the following adverse effects is associated with the use of Cleocin?

(A) Hepatic impairment
(B) Renal impairment
(C) Ataxia
(D) Diarrhea
(E) Aplastic anemia

6e. The Cleocin-T product contains 10 mg of clindamycin per milliliter and is available in a 30-mL package size. This means that the solution has a strength of clindamycin of

(A) 10%
(B) 3%
(C) 0.1%
(D) 1%
(E) 0.3%

6f. Accutane is most closely related to

(A) pantothenic acid
(B) ascorbic acid
(C) vitamin D
(D) lactic acid
(E) vitamin A

6g. Which of the following is (are) common adverse effects associated with the use of Accutane?

I. Hearing loss
II. Chelitis
III. Conjunctivitis

(A) I only
(B) III only
(C) I and II only

(D) II and III only
(E) I, II, and III

6h. On dispensing Accutane, the pharmacist must provide the patient with a (an)

(A) wooden applicator
(B) neutralizing solution
(C) "REFRIGERATE" auxiliary label
(D) accurate liquid measuring device
(E) patient package insert

6i. Prior to dispensing Accutane, the pharmacist should contact the prescriber to ascertain whether the patient is

(A) allergic to tetracycline
(B) allergic to penicillin
(C) a diabetic
(D) pregnant
(E) allergic to Novocain

6j. Brasivol contains aluminum oxide. This ingredient is employed in this product as a (an)

(A) lubricant
(B) antimicrobial agent
(C) vehicle
(D) abrasive
(E) desiccating agent

6k. Pernox scrub contains salicylic acid. This ingredient is employed in this product as a (an)

(A) antiseptic
(B) buffer
(C) antioxidant
(D) keratolytic
(E) astringent

6l. Patients with acne often secrete large amounts of

(A) cholesterol
(B) phosphodiesterase
(C) xanthine oxidase
(D) bilirubin
(E) sebum

PROFILE NO. 7

Community Pharmacy Medication Record

Patient Name: Harold Downy
Address: 199 Main St.
Age: 38   Height: 6'1"
Sex: M   Weight: 210 lb
Allergies:

DIAGNOSIS

Primary	Secondary
1. asthma	1.
2.	2.
3.	3.

MEDICATION RECORD

Date	Rx No.	Physician	Drug & Strength	Quantity	Sig	Refills
1. 6/19	40098	Tisch	Medihaler Iso	15 mL		5
2. 6/19	40099	Tisch	Theolair 250 mg	#90	1 t.i.d.	3
3. 7/7	40098	Tisch	Refill			
4. 7/7	40099	Tisch	Refill			
5. 8/1	46443	Tisch	Intal Soln 2 mL amps	# 30	ut dict	2
6. 8/1	46444	Tisch	Vanceril Aerosol Inhale	#1	ut dict	1

PHARMACIST'S NOTES AND OTHER PATIENT INFORMATION

Date	Comment
1.	Patient smokes 2 packs of cigarettes daily.
2. 8/3	Nytol Tablets (OTC)
3. 9/1	Nicoderm Patches #14—1 box OTC

DIRECTIONS (Questions 7a through 7m): Each of the numbered items or incomplete statements in this section is followed by answers or by completions of the statement. Select the ONE lettered answer or completion that is BEST in each case.

7a. The active ingredient in Medihaler-Iso is isoproterenol. This agent can best be described as a (an)

(A) nonselective alpha-adrenergic agonist

(B) selective beta$_2$-receptor agonist

(C) nonselective beta-adrenergic agonist ✓

(D) alpha-adrenergic antagonist

(E) beta-adrenergic antagonist

7b. In an acute asthmatic attack, the patient uses one inhalation of Medihaler-Iso and, after 5 minutes, still has not been relieved. The patient should be advised to

(A) go to the local emergency room immediately

(B) administer a second inhalation if relief is not evident

(C) administer a double dose (2 inhalations) within 30 minutes after the first if relief is not evident

(D) breathe into a paper bag for 6 minutes to increase the respiratory concentration of carbon dioxide

(E) inhale steam in order to increase the penetration of the isoproterenol into the respiratory tract

7c. The active ingredient in Theolair is theophylline. This agent may be described as a

(A) methylxanthine

(B) prodrug

(C) xanthine oxidase inhibitor

(D) sympathomimetic

(E) carbonic anhydrase inhibitor

7d. Which of the following is NOT a pharmacologic action of theophylline?

(A) Increased diuresis

(B) Bronchodilation

(C) Increased gastric acid secretion

(D) Increased heart rate

(E) CNS depression

7e. Which of the following theophylline derivatives is most appropriate to use in a rectal dosage form?

(A) Theophylline anhydrous

(B) Dyphylline

(C) Oxtriphylline

(D) Theophylline sodium glycinate

(E) Aminophylline

7f. The Intal solution prescribed for this patient is administered

(A) intravenously

(B) by inhalation

(C) subcutaneously

(D) intramuscularly

(E) rectally

7g. The active ingredient found in Intal is

(A) dopamine

(B) oxtriphylline

(C) cromolyn

(D) dexamethasone sodium phosphate

(E) flunisolide

7h. The active ingredient in Vanceril can best be described as a (an)

(A) corticosteroid

(B) mucolytic

(C) respiratory surfactant

(D) bronchodilator

(E) anticholinergic

7i. Vanceril should be administered

I. using a nebulizer

II. as needed to control acute asthmatic attacks

III. right after a bronchodilator has been inhaled

(A) I only

(B) III only

(C) I and II only

(D) II and III only

(E) I, II, and III

7j. The patient's heavy use of cigarettes may

(A) decrease the metabolism of theophylline

(B) increase the metabolism of isoproterenol

(C) increase the metabolism of the Intal

(D) decrease the metabolism of isoproterenol

(E) increase the metabolism of theophylline

7k. Which of the following is true of Nicoderm Patches?

    I. They are applied for a 24-hour period.

    II. They contain the same active ingredient as ProStep.

    III. The area to which they are to be applied should be moistened before use.

(A) I only

(B) III only

(C) I and II only

(D) II and III only

(E) I, II, and III

7l. An advantage of albuterol over isoproterenol is

(A) availability in a parenteral as well as an inhalation dosage form

(B) more rapid onset of action when inhaled

(C) fewer cardiac effects

(D) no need for refrigeration prior to use

(E) asthmatic control with single daily dosing

7m. Vanceril is most similar to

(A) Atrovent

(B) Beclovent

(C) Sustaire

(D) Maxair

(E) Tornalate

PROFILE NO. 8

Community Pharmacy Medication Record

Patient Name: Carlos Burgos
Address: 34 Redbird Lane
Age: 61   Height: 5'6"
Sex: M   Weight: 190 lb
Allergies:

DIAGNOSIS

Primary	Secondary
1. angina pectoris	1.
2. chronic alcoholism	2.
3.	3.

MEDICATION RECORD

Date	Rx No.	Physician	Drug & Strength	Quantity	Sig	Refills
1. 1/14	40952	Krajec	Nitrostat 0.4 mg	#C	p.r.n.	3
2. 1/30	42772	Krajec	Nitro-Dur 0.1	#30	apply daily	
3. 2/26	42772	Krajec	Refill			
4. 3/16	42772	Krajec	Refill			
5. 4/7	42772	Krajec	Refill			
6. 4/28	50632	Krajec	Nitrolingual Spray	#1	p.r.n.	2
7. 4/28	50633	Krajec	Tranxene 7.5 mg	#30	1 t.i.d.	2
8. 4/28	50634	Krajec	Persantine 25 mg	#90	1 t.i.d.	3

PHARMACIST'S NOTES AND OTHER PATIENT INFORMATION

Date	Comment
1. 3/2	Dristan Tabs (OTC)

DIRECTIONS (Questions 8a through 8k): Each of the numbered items or incomplete statements in this section is followed by answers or by completions of the statement. Select the ONE lettered answer or completion that is BEST in each case.

8a. An advantage of Nitrostat over other sublingual nitroglycerin products is that it is

(A) available in color-coded tablets
(B) longer acting
(C) more rapidly absorbed
(D) effective when used orally as well as sublingually
(E) less subject to potency loss

8b. Nitrostat should be dispensed

(A) in a tight, light-resistant plastic vial
(B) in quantities not greater than 25 tablets
(C) in its original container
(D) with a 6-month expiration date
(E) with a "REFRIGERATE" auxiliary label

8c. The patient should be advised to apply the Nitro-Dur to

    I. the distal parts of the extremities

    II. the same application site each time it is applied

    III. a hairless site

    (A) I only

    (B) III only

    (C) I and II only

    (D) II and III only

    (E) I, II, and III

8d. When discontinuing therapy with Nitro-Dur

    (A) headaches frequently occur

    (B) the dosage should be reduced gradually over a 3-day period

    (C) the number of hours per day that it is applied should be reduced gradually over 7 days

    (D) severe nausea and vomiting may occur

    (E) the dosage and frequency of application should be reduced gradually over a 4- to 6-week period

8e. An antianginal product administered by inhalation is

    (A) pentaerythritol tetranitrate

    (B) Nitrolingual Spray

    (C) erythritol tetranitrate

    (D) isosorbide dinitrate

    (E) amyl nitrite

8f. In addition to being employed in the treatment of angina, dipyridamole (Persantine) is also used as a (an)

    (A) antiplatelet agent

    (B) antiarrhythmic agent

    (C) analgesic

    (D) antihypertensive agent

    (E) nonsteroidal anti-inflammatory agent

8g. The reason why nitroglycerin products are generally NOT administered orally is because nitroglycerin

    (A) will decompose rapidly in stomach acid

    (B) undergoes rapid first-pass deactivation

    (C) is decomposed rapidly by pepsin

    (D) it is very irritating to GI membranes

    (E) is poorly absorbed from the GI tract

8h. Patients using nitroglycerin should be advised to AVOID the use of

    (A) dairy products

    (B) aspirin

    (C) tyramine-containing foods

    (D) foods with a high oxalate content

    (E) alcohol

8i. Solutions of nitroglycerin intended for IV administration should be

    (A) refrigerated until 30 min prior to administration

    (B) given using the administration set provided by the manufacturer

    (C) warmed for 15 min prior to infusion to dissolve crystalline material

    (D) given only by rapid IV injection

    (E) kept covered with an opaque shield to protect it from decomposition

8j. When nitroglycerin topical ointment is administered,

    I. it should be rubbed into the skin until no further ointment is evident on the skin surface

    II. the area to which it is applied is covered with plastic wrap

    III. the dose is measured in inches

    (A) I only

    (B) III only

    (C) I and II only

    (D) II and III only

    (E) I, II, and III

8k. The most rapid onset of action is likely to occur with the use of

(A) Nitro-Dur

(B) Nitrogard

(C) Minitran

(D) Nitrolingual Spray

(E) Nitrodisc

■ PROFILE NO. 9

Community Pharmacy Medication Record

Patient Name: Maria Balou
Address: 845 Walton Ave.
Age: 32
Sex: F
Allergies: tetracyclines

Height: 5'4"
Weight: 145 lb

DIAGNOSIS

Primary	Secondary
1. Type I diabetes mellitus	1.
2.	2.
3.	3.

MEDICATION RECORD

Date	Rx No.	Physician	Drug & Strength	Quantity	Sig	Refills
1. 9/11	29087	Madison	Humulin R 100 U	10 mL	24 U q AM	5
2. 9/11	29088	Madison	Humulin N 100 U	10 mL	30 U mixed with Humulin R q AM	5
3. 9/11	29089	Madison	B-D Lo-Dose Syringes	#100		5
4. 9/11	29090	Madison	AccuChek bG	#1	as directed	

PHARMACIST'S NOTES AND OTHER PATIENT INFORMATION

Date	Comment
1. 9/1	Optilets-M-500 Filmtabs #100
2. 9/11	Clinitest Tabs #100
3. 9/20	Contac 12-Hour Caplets (OTC)

DIRECTIONS (Questions 9a through 9m): Each of the numbered items or incomplete statements in this section is followed by answers or by completions of the statement. Select the ONE lettered answer or completion that is BEST in each case.

9a. The term "type I diabetes mellitus" is also referred to as

(A) diabetes insipidus

(B) brittle diabetes

(C) adult-onset diabetes

(D) insulin-resistant diabetes

(E) insulin-dependent diabetes

9b. Which of the following is (are) true of Humulin R?

    I. It is prepared by recombinant DNA technology.

    II. It is a clear solution.

    III. It is long acting.

(A) I only

(B) III only

(C) I and II only

(D) II and III only

(E) I, II, and III

9c. In order to measure 24 U of Humulin R, the patient must withdraw what quantity of insulin from the vial?

(A) 0.024 mL

(B) 2.4 mL

(C) It depends on the volume of the syringe.

(D) 0.24 mL

(E) Precise measurement of 24 U cannot be made with an insulin syringe.

9d. In examining the patient, the physician notes that the patient complains of polydipsia. This refers to

(A) blurred vision

(B) excessive appetite

(C) excessive weight gain

(D) excessive urination

(E) excessive thirst

9e. Which of the following would be considered a normal fasting blood glucose level for this patient?

(A) 100 mg/dL

(B) 100 µg/L

(C) 100 µg/dL

(D) 1 µg/mL

(E) 100 mg/L

9f. The only insulin that is suitable for administration by IV infusion is

(A) Lente

(B) globin

(C) PZI

(D) regular

(E) NPH

9g. In mixing the insulins prescribed, the patient should be advised

(A) to draw up the Humulin N first

(B) to draw up the Humulin R first

(C) that the mixture may be stored in the syringe for up to 1 month if kept refrigerated

(D) that the mixture may be stored in the syringe for up to 1 month if kept frozen

(E) that mixing these insulins is not advisable and the prescriber should be notified

9h. The patient's use of Optilets-M-500 Filmtabs may

(A) decrease the patient's insulin requirement

(B) cause a hyperglycemic episode

(C) cause a hypoglycemic episode

(D) increase the patient's insulin requirement

(E) interfere with Clinitest testing

9i. The Clinitest test operates by the same mechanism as

(A) Diastix

(B) Clinistix

(C) Chemstrip bG

(D) Benedict's test

(E) Chemstrip K

9j. The patient's use of Contac 12-hour Caplets may

(A) precipitate ketoacidosis

(B) decrease the patient's insulin requirement

(C) increase the chance of lipodystrophy

(D) increase the chance of lipoatrophy

(E) increase the patient's insulin requirement

9k. B-D Lo-Dose syringes have a capacity of

(A) 2 mL

(B) 5 mL

(C) 1.0 mL

(D) 0.25 mL

(E) 0.5 mL

9l. Which of the following antidiabetic agents is a second-generation sulfonylurea?

(A) Tolazamide

(B) Chlorpropamide

(C) Acetohexamide

(D) Glipizide

(E) Tolbutamide

9m. A serious complication in the use of metformin HCl (Glucophage) in the treatment of diabetes mellitus is

(A) hyperbilirubinemia

(B) lactic acidosis

(C) pancreatitis

(D) encephalopathy

(E) aplastic anemia

■ PROFILE NO. 10

Community Pharmacy Medication Record

Patient Name: Rowena Adams
Address: 99 East Ave.
Age: 51
Sex: F
Allergies:

Height: 5'7"
Weight: 155 lb

DIAGNOSIS

Primary	Secondary
1. venous thrombosis	1.
2. hypothyroidism	2.
3.	3.

MEDICATION RECORD

Date	Rx No.	Physician	Drug & Strength	Quantity	Sig	Refills
1. 5/3	89322	Graves	Warfarin 5 mg	#10	1 daily	
2. 5/12	90109	Graves	Warfarin 7.5 mg	#30	1 daily	
3. 5/21	91202	Graves	Warfarin 7.5 mg	#30	1 daily	
4. 6/18	91202	Graves	Refill			2
5. 7/15	91202	Graves	Refill			
6. 8/1	94388	Wilson	Synthroid 100 µg	#60	1 daily	5
7. 8/29	99733	Waxman	Empirin/Cod. No. 3	#30	1 b.i.d.	

DIRECTIONS (Questions 10a through 10l): Each of the numbered items or incomplete statements in this section is followed by answers or by completions of the statement. Select the ONE lettered answer or completion that is BEST in each case.

10a. Warfarin is most closely related chemically to

(A) heparin
(B) alteplase
(C) dicumarol
(D) ticlopidine
(E) streptokinase

10b. Administration of which of the following drugs is likely to increase warfarin activity in this patient?

(A) Phenobarbital
(B) Cimetidine
(C) Rifampin
(D) Phenytoin
(E) Glutethimide

10c. An appropriate antidote for the treatment of warfarin overdose is

(A) phytonadione
(B) EDTA
(C) protamine
(D) potassium permanganate
(E) zinc sulfate

10d. This patient asks the pharmacist for a recommendation for an OTC analgesic for her tennis elbow. Which of the following agents would be appropriate to recommend?

I. Datril
II. Advil
III. Ecotrin

(A) I only
(B) III only
(C) I and II only
(D) II and III only
(E) I, II, and III

10e. If the pharmacist wished to dispense a generic form of Synthroid, which of the following would be used?

(A) Liotrix
(B) Liothyronine
(C) Levothyroxine
(D) Thyroglobulin
(E) Propylthiouracil

10f. A dose of 100 μg of Synthroid is approximately equivalent to

(A) 100 mg of Thyrar
(B) 25 μg of Proloid
(C) 10 μg of Cytomel
(D) 25 μg of Levothroid
(E) 65 mg of Thyroid USP

10g. Which of the following may be used to treat hyperthyroidism?

I. Propylthiouracil
II. Methimazole
III. Sodium iodide ^{131}I

(A) I only
(B) III only
(C) I and II only
(D) II and III only
(E) I, II, and III

10h. The use of Synthroid by this patient is likely to

(A) increase the dosage requirement for warfarin
(B) prevent the oral absorption of warfarin
(C) increase the likelihood of renal damage
(D) decrease the dosage requirement for warfarin
(E) increase the likelihood of hepatic damage

10i. In a radiation emergency, which of the following would be appropriate to administer?

(A) Propylthiouracil
(B) Liothyronine
(C) Liotrix
(D) Thyroglobulin
(E) Potassium iodide

10j. Thyroid hormone synthesis is controlled by

(A) human chorionic gonadotropin

(B) oxytocin from the posterior pituitary

(C) FSH from the anterior pituitary

(D) TSH from the anterior pituitary

(E) LH from the anterior pituitary

10k. The use of Empirin/Codeine No. 3 by this patient is likely to

(A) increase the action of the Synthroid

(B) decrease the action of Synthroid

(C) decrease the action of warfarin

(D) increase the action of warfarin

(E) cause agranulocytosis

10l. Which of the following laboratory determinations may be used to monitor the patient's progress on warfarin?

(A) BUN

(B) Bilirubin

(C) Amylase

(D) INR

(E) Creatine kinase

■ PROFILE NO. 11

Hospital Pharmacy Medication Record

Patient Name: Wilma Best
Room Number: 742
Age: 24
Sex: F
Allergies: aspirin, codeine

Height: 5'1"
Weight: 135 lb

DIAGNOSIS

Primary	Secondary
1. chronic UTI	1. migraines
2.	2. PMS
3.	3.

LAB TESTS

Date	Test & Results
1. 7/14	Urinalysis pyuria, C&S = 1×10^6 *E coli*
2.	
3.	

MEDICATION RECORD

Date	Drug & Strength	Sig	DC'd
1. 7/15	Keflin 2 g IV	2 g q.i.d. × 7 days	
2. 7/15	Pyridium 100 mg	1 t.i.d.	
3. 7/23	TMP–SMX	1 q12h	

PHARMACIST'S NOTES AND OTHER PATIENT INFORMATION

Date	Comment
1. 7/25	Patient discharged with following Rxs: Septra DS #20 1 q12h When completed, use Mandelamine 0.5 g q.i.d. for 2 weeks

DIRECTIONS (Questions 11a through 11n): Each of the numbered items or incomplete statements in this section is followed by answers or by completions of the statement. Select the ONE lettered answer or completion that is BEST in each case.

11a. The term "pyuria" indicates the presence of what substance in the urine?

(A) Pyruvate
(B) Pyridoxine
(C) Pus
(D) Red blood cells
(E) Pyrogens

11b. *Escherichia coli* may be described as

(A) pneumococci
(B) gram-negative bacilli
(C) gram-positive bacilli
(D) a systemic fungal organism
(E) a virus

11c. Drugs of choice for a UTI due to *E coli* include

I. trimethoprim–sulfamethoxazole
II. ciprofloxacin
III. ofloxacin

(A) I only
(B) III only
(C) I and II only
(D) II and III only
(E) I, II, and III

11d. The physician's order for TMP–SMX may be filled using

I. Septra
II. Bactrim
III. Trimox

(A) I only
(B) III only
(C) I and II only
(D) II and III only
(E) I, II, and III

11e. A physician wishes to prescribe a fluoro-quinolone-class drug. The pharmacist should suggest any of the following EXCEPT

(A) Cipro
(B) Cinobac
(C) Floxin
(D) Negram
(E) Noroxin

11f. Patients consuming drugs such as Septra should be advised to

I. drink a large amount of fluids
II. maintain a very acidic urine
III. avoid the use of folic acid–containing products

(A) I only
(B) III only
(C) I and II only
(D) II and III only
(E) I, II, and III

11g. A patient wishes to test her urine to determine the presence of bacteriuria. Which of the following products would be suitable for this purpose?

(A) Ictotest
(B) Azostix
(C) Microstix-3
(D) Predict
(E) Chemstrip K

11h. The Pyridium ordered for this patient can most accurately be classified as a (an)

(A) urinary antiseptic
(B) antimicrobial agent
(C) buffer
(D) antispasmodic
(E) analgesic

11i. This patient should be advised that Pyridium may cause

(A) temporary weight gain
(B) migraines
(C) discoloration of the urine
(D) dizziness
(E) temporary infertility

11j. Pyridium should not be administered for longer than

(A) 2 days
(B) 5 days
(C) 10 days
(D) 14 days
(E) 30 days

11k. Symptoms of premenstrual syndrome (PMS) may include all of the following EXCEPT

(A) backache
(B) cramping
(C) edema
(D) irritability
(E) weight loss

11l. Which of the following ingredients is (are) included in over the counter (OTC) PMS products?

I. Caffeine
II. Pamabrom
III. HCTZ

(A) I only
(B) III only
(C) I and II only
(D) II and III only
(E) I, II, and III

11m. Which of the following drugs may the physician prescribe if the UTI is not clearing?

I. Ciprofloxacin
II. Imipenem/cilastatin
III. Penicillin VK

(A) I only
(B) III only
(C) I and II only
(D) II and III only
(E) I, II, and III

11n. On 7/16, the patient was catheterized. Which of the following are appropriate urinary catheters?

I. Foley
II. Broviac
III. Hickman

(A) I only
(B) III only
(C) I and II only
(D) II and III only
(E) I, II, and III

PROFILE NO. 12

Hospital Pharmacy Medication Record

Patient Name: Marvin Lessard
Room Number: 241-2
Age: 64   Height: 5'11"
Sex: F   Weight: 188 lb
Allergies: none reported

DIAGNOSIS

Primary	Secondary
1. chronic myelocytic leukemia	1. oral candida
2.	2.
3.	3.

LAB TESTS

Date	Test & Results
1. 6/4	WBC $(\times 10^3)$ = 180; K = 4.5; Na = 138
2. 6/6	WBC $(\times 10^3)$ = 115; K = 3.18; Na = 136
3. 6/8	WBC $(\times 10^3)$ = 75; K = 3.1; Na = 134
4. 6/10	WBC $(\times 10^3)$ = 6.5; K = 2.6; Na = 128
5. 6/12	WBC $(\times 10^3)$ = 0.9; K = 3.0; Na = 132

MEDICATION RECORD

Date	Drug & Strength	Sig	DC'd
1. 6/4	Colace 100 mg	1 or 2 daily	
2. 6/4	Dalmane 15 mg	1 hs	
3. 6/4	Daunorubicin	45 mg/m²/day on days 1 to 3	
4. 6/4	Cytarabine	100 mg/m²/day on days 1 to 7	
5. 6/4	Allopurinol	300 mg b.i.d. × 10 days	
6. 6/7	Mycostatin Liq.	q3h × 10 days	
7. 6/7	Mitrolan tabs	chew 1 q4h p.r.n.	

DIRECTIONS (Questions 12a through 12n): Each of the numbered items or incomplete statements in this section is followed by answers or by completions of the statement. Select the ONE lettered answer or completion that is BEST in each case.

12a. The patient's body surface area in square meters can best be determined with the use of a

(A) caliper
(B) tape measure
(C) picogram
(D) nomogram
(E) micrometer

12b. Daunorubicin is available in vials containing 20 mg of the drug. Assuming that the patient's body surface area was determined to be 1.85 m², how many vials of daunorubicin need to be supplied for each day's administration?

(A) 5
(B) 1
(C) 10
(D) 2
(E) 3

12c. Cytarabine can best be described as a (an)

(A) antibiotic
(B) mitotic inhibitor
(C) antimetabolite
(D) alkylating agent
(E) antiestrogen

12d. From the laboratory data provided, it appears that the patient is experiencing

(A) hypokalemia
(B) infection
(C) hyperkalemia
(D) myelosuppression
(E) hypernatremia

12e. In which age range is acute lymphocytic leukemia most prevalent?

(A) <15 yrs
(B) 20–30 yrs
(C) 30–50 yrs
(D) 50–70 yrs
(E) >70 yrs

12f. Chemotherapeutic drugs classified as antimetabolites include

I. cyclophosphamide } alkylating agents
II. carmustine
III. methotrexate

(A) I only
(B) III only
(C) I and II only

(D) II and III only
(E) I, II, and III

12g. Allopurinol is pharmacologically classified as a (an)

(A) beta-adrenergic agonist
(B) MAO inhibitor
(C) xanthine oxidase inhibitor
(D) antimetabolite
(E) alkylating agent

12h. Patients using allopurinol should be advised to

(A) drink adequate fluids
(B) avoid dairy products
(C) expect urine discoloration
(D) avoid bruising
(E) take at least 1 g of vitamin C daily

12i. In order to monitor the use of allopurinol, determinations should be made of

(A) serum potassium
(B) serum folate
(C) urinary glucose
(D) serum uric acid
(E) urinary 5-HT

12j. An appropriate instruction for the use of Mycostatin liquid would be to

(A) take with a large glass of water
(B) swish and swallow
(C) take on an empty stomach
(D) mix it with fruit juice before administration
(E) allow product to stand until it thickens

12k. If extravasation occurred with the administration of daunorubicin, which of the following would be recommended?

(A) Inject subcutaneous epinephrine into the area.
(B) Insert a catheter into the injection site.

(C) Apply a corticosteroid cream to the injection site.

(D) Inject sodium bicarbonate solution into the injection site.

(E) Apply cold compresses to the injection site.

12l. A serious adverse effect associated with daunorubicin administration is

   I. cardiotoxicity

  II. nephrotoxicity

 III. ocular degeneration

(A) I only

(B) III only

(C) I and II only

(D) II and III only

(E) I, II, and III

12m. Although he sleeps well at night, Mr. Lessard appears to be unstable during the day and has fallen several times. The pharmacist should suggest that the Dalmane order be switched to

   I. temazepam

  II. triazolam

 III. clorazepate - $t_{1/2}$ 30 -100hs

(A) I only

(B) III only

(C) I and II only

(D) II and III only

(E) I, II, and III

12n. Mr. Lessard has been purchasing products from his local health food store. Which of the following ingredients have been advertised as sleep aids?

   I. Ginseng

  II. Melatonin

 III. L-tryptophan

(A) I only

(B) III only

(C) I and II only

(D) II and III only

(E) I, II, and III

PROFILE NO. 13

Hospital Pharmacy Medication Record

Patient Name: Claudia Masterson
Room Number: 708-A
Age: 20   Height: 5'4"
Sex: F   Weight: 125 lb
Allergies: tetracyclines

DIAGNOSIS

Primary	Secondary
1. PUD since age 18	1. recurrent diarrhea since 6/5
2. iron deficiency anemia	2.
3.	3.

LAB TESTS

Date	Test & Results
1. 6/4	Hgb = 7.5 g%, Hct = 32.4% MCHC = 26%, MCV = 76 μm^3, serum iron 440 μg%, TIBC = 450 μg% 4+ stool guaiac
2.	
3.	

MEDICATION RECORD

Date	Drug & Strength	Sig	DC'd
1. 6/4	Mylanta Liq.	30 mL 1 hr & 3 hr pc	
2. 6/4	Tagamet 300 mg	1 q.i.d.	
3. 6/4	Xanax 0.5 mg	1 t.i.d.	
4. 6/5	Kaopectate	15 mL p each loose BM	
5. 6/5	Feosol 200 mg	1 t.i.d.	

PHARMACIST'S NOTES AND OTHER PATIENT INFORMATION

Date	Comment
1.	Patient has been on Xanax since age 19.

DIRECTIONS (Questions 13a through 13n): Each of the numbered items or incomplete statements in this section is followed by answers or by completions of the statement. Select the ONE lettered answer or completion that is BEST in each case.

13a. After 6 months of iron therapy, the patient's hemoglobin level should ideally be

(A) 2–4 g/dL
(B) 5–7 g/dL
(C) 8–10 g/dL
(D) 11–13 g/dL
(E) 15–18 g/dL

13b. Which one of the following drugs is most useful for increasing erythropoiesis?

(A) Epogen
(B) Folex
(C) INH
(D) Intron-A
(E) Lozol

13c. A possible cause of this patient's diarrhea is the use of

(A) Mylanta
(B) Tagamet
(C) Feosol
(D) Xanax
(E) Kaopectate

13d. The patient's aunt has suggested the use of alendronate, which has helped improve her general well being. Which of the following statement(s) concerning this drug is (are) true?

  I. It is intended for the treatment of osteoporosis, especially after menopause.
  II. The drug must be taken with a full glass of plain water.
  III. The drug is best taken at bedtime.

(A) I only
(B) III only
(C) I and II only
(D) II and III only
(E) I, II, and III

13e. A drug interaction is likely to occur with the concomitant use of

  I. Tagamet and Mylanta
  II. Feosol and Mylanta
  III. Tagamet and Xanax

(A) I only
(B) III only
(C) I and II only
(D) II and III only
(E) I, II, and III

13f. Iron absorption may be increased by administering which of the following agents to this patient?

(A) Docusate sodium
(B) Ascorbic acid
(C) Benzalkonium chloride
(D) Pyridoxine hydrochloride
(E) Desferal mesylate

13g. Feosol contains

(A) ferrous gluconate
(B) ferrous fumarate
(C) ferrous sulfate
(D) ferric chloride
(E) ferric ammonium citrate

13h. Ferrous sulfate is available in all of the following dosage forms EXCEPT

(A) elixir
(B) oral drops
(C) oral liquid
(D) parenteral injection
(E) tablets

13i. Examination of this patient's red blood cells is likely to reveal cells that are

  I. microcytic
  II. hypochromic
  III. megaloblastic

(A) I only
(B) III only
(C) I and II only
(D) II and III only
(E) I, II, and III

13j. A drug that may be more appropriate than Tagamet for use in this patient is

(A) Zantac
(B) Imodium
(C) Cephulac
(D) Dialose
(E) Doxinate

13k. Causes of megaloblastic anemia include a deficiency of

    I. cyanocobalamin
    II. folic acid
    III. iron

(A) I only
(B) III only
(C) I and II only
(D) II and III only
(E) I, II, and III

13l. Dietary sources rich in vitamin B_{12} include

    I. apples
    II. broccoli
    III. liver

(A) I only
(B) III only
(C) I and II only
(D) II and III only
(E) I, II, and III

13m. Which of the following statements concerning pernicious anemia is (are) true?

    I. The condition is caused by a deficiency in folic acid.
    II. Higher incidence occurs in women than in men.
    III. Occurrence appears to be both genetically and geographically based.

(A) I only
(B) III only
(C) I and II only
(D) II and III only
(E) I, II, and III

13n. When discharged from the hospital, Ms. Masterson has been advised to start a smoking cessation program. Which of the following OTC products are marketed as transdermal patches?

    I. Nicorette
    II. Nicotrol
    III. Nicoderm

(A) I only
(B) III only
(C) I and II only
(D) II and III only
(E) I, II, and III

■ PROFILE NO. 14

Community Pharmacy Medication Record

Patient Name: Joe Gaines
Address: 43 Pine St.
Age: 38
Sex: M
Allergies: chocolate

Height:
Weight: 180 lb

DIAGNOSIS

Primary
1. mild hypertension
2. noninsulin-dependent diabetes
3.

Secondary
1. fits of depression
2.
3.

MEDICATION RECORD

Date	Rx No.	Physician	Drug & Strength	Quantity	Sig	Refills
1. 6/4	132887	Long	HCTZ q25 mg	#60	1 qd	5
2.	132888	Long	Inderal 40 mg	#120	1 b.i.d.	5
3.	132889	Long	Diabinese 250 mg	#60	1 bid	5
4.	132890	Long	Slow-K 8 mEq	#60	1 qd	5

PHARMACIST'S NOTES AND OTHER PATIENT INFORMATION

Date	Comment
1.	Joe enjoys his beer; be sure to warn about possible drug/alcohol interactions.
2. 6/12	Sold Joe some diet tablets (containing PPA). Check his progress next time in store.

DIRECTIONS (Questions 14a through 14o): Each of the numbered items or incomplete statements in this section is followed by answers or by completions of the statement. Select the ONE lettered answer or completion that is BEST in each case.

Questions 14a through 14f: On June 15, Joe Gaines brings into the pharmacy a new prescription for penicillin VK 500 mg #40 with a Sig: 1 tablet q.i.d. until gone. He has been instructed by his physician to soak his swollen and infected thumb in alternate solutions of pHisoHex and epsom salts every 2 hours.

14a. The prescriber probably prescribed penicillin because an infection was suspected to have been caused by

(A) *Chlamydia*
(B) *Staphylococcus epidermidis*
(C) *Pseudomonas*
(D) *Streptococcus*
(E) a fungus

14b. The previous prescription could be filled by using any of the following EXCEPT

(A) Betapen
(B) Pentids
(C) Pen Vee
(D) Veetids
(E) V-Cillin

14c. pHisoHex is considered effective in treating infections caused by

I. fungi
II. gram-negative microorganisms
III. gram-positive microorganisms

(A) I only
(B) III only
(C) I and II only
(D) II and III only
(E) I, II, and III

14d. The active ingredient in Hibiclens is

(A) benzalkonium chloride
(B) chlorhexidine gluconate
(C) glutaraldehyde
(D) hexachlorophene
(E) iodine

14e. Which one of the following pairings of active ingredient to product is INCORRECT?

(A) Chlorhexidine–Hibistat
(B) Chlorhexidine–Peridex
(C) Iodine–Betadine
(D) Iodine–Cidex
(E) Benzalkonium chloride–Ionax

14f. Chemically, epsom salts is

(A) aluminum sulfate
(B) aluminum acetate
(C) calcium sulfate
(D) magnesium sulfate
(E) a mixture of calcium and magnesium sulfates

14g. The solubility of epsom salts in water is 1 g in 0.8 mL of water. How many grams of the salts should be added to 4 fluid ounces of water to make a saturated solution?

(A) 17 g
(B) 38 g
(C) 67 g
(D) 120 g
(E) 150 g

14h. Mr. Gaines requests a bottle of Percogesic. Which one of the following statements concerning Percogesic is true?

(A) The active ingredient is acetaminophen only.
(B) The active ingredients are acetaminophen and aspirin.
(C) One of the active ingredients is phenyltoloxamine.
(D) A prescription is required for dispensing.
(E) One of the active ingredients is an antacid.

14i. Mr. Gaines and his wife are planning a trip to an area of Central America that has poor sanitary facilities. Which one of the following products may both prevent and treat travelers' diarrhea?

(A) Kaopectate
(B) Metronidazole
(C) Mylanta
(D) Rolaids
(E) Pepto-Bismol

14j. Prescription drugs that are effective for travelers' diarrhea include

I. fluoroquinolone
II. trimethoprim and sulfamethoxazole
III. penicillin

(A) I only
(B) III only

(C) I and II only

(D) II and III only

(E) I, II, and III

14k. Mr. Gaines has returned from his trip with an infection of giardiasis. Which of the following drugs may successfully treat this condition?

I. Cefadroxil

II. Metronidazole

III. Quinacrine

(A) I only

(B) III only

(C) I and II only

(D) II and III only

(E) I, II, and III

14l. A week after deer hunting, Mr. Gaines exhibits symptoms of Lyme disease. Which of the following statements is (are) true of this condition?

I. Early signs are a skin rash and malaise.

II. Late stages often result in chronic arthritis.

III. The disease is caused by a protozoon.

(A) I only

(B) III only

(C) I and II only

(D) II and III only

(E) I, II, and III

14m. Successful treatment of Lyme disease includes

I. doxycycline 100 mg b.i.d.

II. ceftriaxone 2 g IV daily

III. metronidazole 500 mg daily

(A) I only

(B) III only

(C) I and II only

(D) II and III only

(E) I, II, and III

14n. Mr. Gaines has read that aspirin will decrease the chance of heart attacks. How many 325 mg tablets should be suggested to him as a realistic dose?

(A) 1 or less tablets daily

(B) 1 or 2 tablets daily

(C) 1 tablet twice a day

(D) 1 tablet three times a day

(E) 1 tablet four times a day

14o. The active ingredient in Kaopectate liquid that acts as an absorbent is

(A) attapulgite

(B) bentonite

(C) kaolin

(D) charcoal

(E) simethicone

■ PROFILE NO. 15

Hospital Pharmacy Medication Record

Patient Name: James Gurley
Room Number: 420-2
Age: 26   Height: 6′2″
Sex: M   Weight: 142 lb
Allergies: pollen, dust

DIAGNOSIS

Primary	Secondary
1. duodenal ulcer	1. epilepsy (stabilized)
2.	2.
3.	3.

MEDICATION RECORD

Date	Drug & Strength	Sig	DC'd
1. 2/4	Dilantin 100 mg	3 daily	
2.	Isuprel Mistometer 15 mL	1 to 2 puffs p.r.n.	
3.	Mylanta	15 mL q2h	
4. 2/6	Tagamet 400 mg	1 q.i.d.	

PHARMACIST'S NOTES AND OTHER PATIENT INFORMATION

Date	Comment
1.	Patient's mild asthma controlled by occasional use of Tedral tablets and Mistometer. Dr. okays use of home supply of each.

DIRECTIONS (Questions 15a through 15p): Each of the numbered items or incomplete statements in this section is followed by answers or by completions of the statement. Select the ONE lettered answer or completion that is BEST in each case.

15a. The nursing staff reports that Mr. Gurley is experiencing dizziness and has fallen down several times. It is advisable to

   (A) continue the drug regimen as the side effects are transient

   (B) increase the dose of Dilantin

   (C) decrease the dose of Tagamet

   (D) decrease the dose of Dilantin

   (E) take Tagamet with food to increase its absorption and decrease stomach irritation

15b. The medical term for Mr. Gurley's poor muscle coordination is

   (A) ataxia

   (B) atresia

   (C) aphasia

   (D) dementia

   (E) dysarthria

15c. Which of the following drugs have therapeutic activity similar to that of Tagamet?

   I. Diflunisal

   II. Famotidine

   III. Nizatidine

   (A) I only

   (B) III only

(C) I and II only

(D) II and III only

(E) I, II, and III

15d. Zollinger–Ellison syndrome is the result of adenomas in the

(A) gallbladder

(B) liver

(C) stomach

(D) pancreas

(E) small intestine

15e. Mr. Gurley's physician calls the pharmacy for information concerning benzodiazepines that will not be affected by cimetidine. Which one of the following agents is most appropriate?

(A) Chlordiazepoxide

(B) Diazepam

(C) Flurazepam

(D) Alprazolam

(E) Oxazepam

15f. If a physician decides to maintain Mr. Gurley on lithium therapy as an outpatient, which of the following guidelines should be followed?

I. An oral dosing range of 900 to 1500 mg daily

II. Plasma lithium levels between 2 and 4 mEq/L

III. Blood sampling 2 h after dosing

(A) I only

(B) III only

(C) I and II only

(D) II and III only

(E) I, II, and III

15g. After 1 week of lithium therapy with a dosage regimen of 600 mg b.i.d., the patient is experiencing mild hand tremors and polyuria. The pharmacist should consult with the prescriber concerning the possibility of

(A) giving the drug on a 300 mg q.i.d. schedule

(B) increasing the dosage to 1500 mg daily

(C) decreasing the dosage to 600 mg daily

(D) giving the drug once a day in the morning

(E) discontinuing the drug

15h. Lithium is probably being prescribed

(A) to treat acute manic episodes

(B) as an anti-Parkinson drug

(C) as a hypnotic agent

(D) to treat status epilepticus

(E) to treat schizophrenia

15i. Five days after discharge from the hospital, Mr. Gurley brings an antibiotic prescription into the pharmacy. He asks for an explanation of "nosocomial infection." The pharmacist can best explain nosocomial as being

(A) communicable

(B) hospital related

(C) drug related

(D) unknown origin

(E) noncommunicable

15j. Mr. Gurley has a new prescription for Prozac 20 mg, which has the generic name of

(A) amoxapine

(B) desipramine

(C) fluoxetine

(D) trazodone

(E) phenelzine

15k. The antidepressant activity of Prozac is thought to be due to

(A) binding to beta-adrenergic receptors

(B) prevention of reuptake of serotonin

(C) blockage of reuptake of norepinephrine

(D) blockage of reuptake of dopamine

(E) being a dopamine antagonist

15l. Which of the following is (are) potential side effects of Prozac?

    I. Anorexia

    II. Insomnia

    III. Increase in heart rate

    (A) I only

    (B) III only

    (C) I and II only

    (D) II and III only

    (E) I, II, and III

15m. Prozac is available in which of the following dosage forms?

    I. Capsules

    II. Oral liquid

    III. Parenteral liquid

    (A) I only

    (B) III only

    (C) I and II only

    (D) II and III only

    (E) I, II, and III

15n. Which of the following is (are) true of the antipsychotic drug olanzapine?

    I. It is available under the tradename of Zyprexa

    II. The patient should be warned of possible orthostatic hypotension

    III. The drug should be taken only with meals

    (A) I only

    (B) III only

    (C) I and II only

    (D) II and III only

    (E) I, II, and III

15o. Mr. Gurley is very apprehensive about using an antidepressant drug. The pharmacist may inform him that

    I. the incidence of individuals becoming addicted or dependent on this class of drugs is very low

    II. the drug may not show beneficial effects for several weeks

    III. as soon as beneficial effects are observed, he will then be able to stop taking the drug

    (A) I only

    (B) III only

    (C) I and II only

    (D) II and III only

    (E) I, II, and III

15p. Which of the following descriptions of Zoloft is (are) true when comparing it to Prozac?

    I. The patient can be dosed either in the morning or at night.

    II. The drug has a shorter elimination half-life.

    III. Lower mg doses are needed.

    (A) I only

    (B) III only

    (C) I and II only

    (D) II and III only

    (E) I, II, and III

■ PROFILE NO. 16

Community Pharmacy Medication Record

Patient Name: Agnes Johnson
Address: 27 Green St.
Age: 38   Height: 5'8"
Sex: F   Weight: 150 lb
Allergies: sulfa drugs, tartrazine, bee stings

DIAGNOSIS

Primary   Secondary
1. mild hypertension   1.
2. UTI   2.
3.   3.

MEDICATION RECORD

Date	Rx No.	Physician	Drug & Strength	Quantity	Sig	Refills
1. 6/12	87773	Flynn	Ortho-Novum 1/35	3 pack	1 daily ut dict	2×
2. 6/12	87774	Flynn	HCTZ 25 mg	#100	1 daily	1×
3. 7/1	89940	Collins	Ampicillin 500 mg	#40	1 q6h	1×

PHARMACIST'S NOTES AND OTHER PATIENT INFORMATION

Date   Comment
1. 8/5   Ms. Johnson returns to the pharmacy and complains that her urinary tract infection has returned. She asks if she should take the remaining 20 capsules from her 7/1 prescription or call her doctor. She admits that the pills seemed to help.

DIRECTIONS (Questions 16a through 16o): Each of the numbered items or incomplete statements in this section is followed by answers or by completions of the statement. Select the ONE lettered answer or completion that is BEST in each case.

16a. The pharmacist should advise Ms. Johnson to

(A) finish the remaining capsules

(B) call the doctor for an increase in the ampicillin dose

(C) ask the doctor for another, more effective drug

(D) get a partial refill of ampicillin and use a total of 40 capsules

(E) use up the remaining 20 capsules but drink cranberry juice at the same time

16b. Bacteriuria is considered present when the bacteria count in the urine reaches _____ cfu/mL.

(A) 100

(B) 1000

(C) 10,000

(D) 100,000

(E) >100,000

16c. Dr. Collins calls the pharmacy on Sept. 2 stating that Ms. Johnson has been noncompliant in completing regimens of therapy for her UTIs. Which of the following single-dose regimens is (are) appropriate?

  I. Amoxil 500 mg 6 capsules
  II. TMP–SMX 2 tablets
  III. Furadantin 50 mg 1 capsule

(A) I only
(B) III only
(C) I and II only
(D) II and III only
(E) I, II, and III

16d. Acidification of the urine may be accomplished by the oral ingestion of

  I. ascorbic acid 6 g/day
  II. ammonium chloride 2–3 g/day
  III. calcium carbonate, 10 tab/day

(A) I only
(B) III only
(C) I and II only
(D) II and III only
(E) I, II, and III

16e. Ms. Johnson is concerned about the obesity of her 15-year-old daughter, Jenny, and requests a bottle of Dexatrim. Which of the following is (are) present in this OTC product?

  I. Benzocaine
  II. Caffeine
  III. Phenylpropanolamine

(A) I only
(B) III only
(C) I and II only
(D) II and III only
(E) I, II, and III

16f. Obesity has been attributed to which of the following factors?

  I. Anxiety but not depression
  II. Derangement in the satiety center
  III. Genetic

(A) I only
(B) III only
(C) I and II only
(D) II and III only
(E) I, II, and III

16g. Which of the following drugs may be prescribed for the treatment of a patient with bulimia?

  I. Desipramine
  II. Fluoxetine
  III. Methylphenidate

(A) I only
(B) III only
(C) I and II only
(D) II and III only
(E) I, II, and III

16h. Bulimia is characterized by all of the following behavior patterns EXCEPT

(A) consumption of large amounts of food at one sitting
(B) patient believes that he or she is too fat even when individual is underweight
(C) patient-induced vomiting
(D) compulsion for vigorous exercise to prevent overweight
(E) frequent use of laxatives

16i. Besides its use as an anorexigenic agent, phenylpropanolamine is included in pharmaceutical products as a (an)

(A) antihistamine
(B) antihypertensive agent
(C) local anesthetic
(D) nasal decongestant
(E) sleep aid

16j. Side effects of phenylpropanolamine may include any of the following EXCEPT

(A) constipation
(B) dry mouth
(C) hypertension
(D) mydriasis
(E) sedation

Questions 16k through 16o are based on the following prescription presented to the pharmacist by Ms. Johnson.

Rx	
Menthol	
Camphor	aa qs 1%
LCD	2%
Lubriderm	qs 120 mL

16k. The physical form of the final compounded prescription is most likely to be a (an)

(A) ointment
(B) lotion
(C) topical solution
(D) gel
(E) paste

16l. The amount of menthol required for this prescription is

(A) 0.3 g
(B) 0.5 g
(C) 0.6 g
(D) 1.0 g
(E) 1.2 g

16m. When preparing this ointment, the pharmacist may choose to

I. make a eutectic of the menthol and camphor
II. add isopropyl alcohol to dissolve the menthol and camphor
III. add polysorbate 80 (Tween 80) to solubilize the LCD

(A) I only
(B) III only
(C) I and II only
(D) II and III only
(E) I, II, and III

16n. The previous prescription is most likely written for the treatment of

(A) dermatitis due to poison ivy
(B) insect bites
(C) acne
(D) localized abscesses
(E) psoriasis

16o. Patients using coal tar products should be cautioned that such products

I. may cause photosensitization
II. may have carcinogenic potential if placed on the rectal, genital, or groin area
III. should not be used as a shampoo

(A) I only
(B) III only
(C) I and II only
(D) II and III only
(E) I, II, and III

■ PROFILE NO. 17

Hospital Pharmacy Medication Record

Patient Name: Edward Coster
Room Number: 612-2
Age: 62   Height: 5'11"
Sex: M   Weight: 122 lb
Allergies: NK

DIAGNOSIS

Primary	Secondary
1. CA colon	1. hypertension
2.	2. lung rales
3.	3.

LAB TESTS

Date	Test & Results
1. 10/6	WBC 8000
2.	Hemoglobin 15 g/dL Hematocrit 40%
3.	Glucose 100 mg/dL
4. 10/6	BUN 10 mg/dL
5.	Serum creatinine 1 mg/dL
6.	Albumin 4 g/dL
7. 10/7	Electrolytes: Na = 138 mEq; K = 4 mEq; Cl = 120 mEq/L

MEDICATION RECORD

Date	Drug & Strength	Sig	DC'd
1. 10/5	Digoxin 0.25 mg	1 qd p.o.	
2.	Propranolol 40 mg	1 b.i.d. p.o.	
3.	Colace 100 mg	p.r.n.	
4.	Dalmane 30 mg	1 hs p.r.n.	
5. 10/6	GoLytely	Bt 24 h pre-surgery	
6. 10/7	usual preop per Dr. Lachman		
7. 10/8	Start TPN 1 L postop 1st day then 3 L daily; after 1st day start 500 mL Liposyn III 20% q.o.d		

PHARMACIST'S NOTES AND OTHER PATIENT INFORMATION

Date	Comment	
1. 10/8	Start following TPN as directed	
	Amino acid sol. 8.5%	500 mL
	D40W	500
	Calcium chloride	8.6 mEq
	Potassium Cl	40
	NaCl	40
	MVI	1 vial
	Insulin	10 units
	Rate—50 mL 1st hr then 100 mL per hour	

DIRECTIONS (Questions 17a through 17o): Each of the numbered items or incomplete statements in this section is followed by answers or by completions of the statement. Select the ONE lettered answer or completion that is BEST in each case.

17a. Based on the reported lab tests, Mr. Coster is likely to have

(A) a systemic infection
(B) an anemic condition
(C) diabetes
(D) renal impairment
(E) none of the above

17b. Usually, antibiotic prophylaxis for surgical patients is started

(A) 4 h presurgery
(B) 1–2 h presurgery
(C) during surgery
(D) 1 hr postsurgery
(E) 4 h postsurgery

17c. The most appropriate presurgical antibiotic prophylaxis for a patient undergoing intestinal surgery will be oral

(A) gentamicin + tetracycline
(B) erythromycin + neomycin
(C) cephalosporin + neomycin
(D) penicillin + gentamicin
(E) amoxicillin + clavulanate potassium

17d. The order for GoLytely (PEG/Electrolyte solution) is intended to

(A) supply additional electrolytes to the blood
(B) supply electrolytes to the GI tract
(C) cleanse the GI tract
(D) provide bulk in the GI tract
(E) provide water as a refreshing beverage

17e. When selecting a commercial amino acid solution for the TPN order, the pharmacist would consider which of the following?

I. Aminosyn (Abbott)
II. FreAmine (Kendall McGaw)
III. NephrAmine (Kendall McGaw)

(A) I only
(B) III only
(C) I and II only
(D) II and III only
(E) I, II, and III

17f. Suitable route(s) of administration for Mr. Coster's TPN solution include(s)

I. central infusion
II. peripheral infusion
III. enteral infusion

(A) I only
(B) III only
(C) I and II only
(D) II and III only
(E) I, II, and III

17g. Before compounding the ordered TPN formula, the prescriber should be consulted concerning the

I. high level of chlorides
II. level of dextrose
III. amount of multivitamins desired

(A) I only
(B) III only
(C) I and II only
(D) II and III only
(E) I, II, and III

17h. The amount of nitrogen provided by each liter of the TPN formula will be approximately _____ g.

(A) 6.8
(B) 14
(C) 36
(D) 42.5
(E) 85

17i. The number of nonprotein calories present in each bottle will be approximately _____ kcal.

(A) 680
(B) 800
(C) 1200
(D) 1540
(E) 1800

17j. The target ratio of nonprotein calories to grams of nitrogen for TPN formulas in a non-stressed patient is approximately

(A) 1:1
(B) 50:1
(C) 150:1
(D) 250:1
(E) 500:1

17k. The administration of Liposyn III is intended to prevent

(A) agranulocytosis
(B) decubitus ulcers
(C) EFAD
(D) BEE
(E) phlebitis

17l. The number of calories provided by each bottle of Liposyn III will be

(A) 100
(B) 500
(C) 1000
(D) 1200
(E) 1500

17m. After 4 days, the patient's surgical scar has not healed and a bedsore has developed on the buttocks. Which one of the following ingredients has been shown to speed wound healing processes?

(A) Ascorbic acid
(B) Folic acid
(C) Iron
(D) Selenium
(E) Zinc

17n. On the fifth day, the patient exhibits symptoms of Legionnaires' disease. Which of the following statements is (are) true concerning this disease?

I. Causative agent is a fungus.
II. Transmission is by airborne inhalation.
III. Smokers are more susceptible than the general population.

(A) I only
(B) III only
(C) I and II only
(D) II and III only
(E) I, II, and III

17o. The drug of choice in the treatment of Legionnaires' disease is

(A) cefaclor
(B) erythromycin
(C) gentamicin
(D) penicillin VK
(E) acyclovir

■ PROFILE NO. 18

Hospital Pharmacy Medication Record

Patient Name: Frances Costello
Room Number: 621
Age: 42   Height: 5'4"
Sex: F   Weight: 132 lb
Allergies: aspirin, penicillin?

DIAGNOSIS

Primary	Secondary
1. Hodgkin's disease	1. Graves' disease
2.	2. essential hypertension (under control with diet)
3.	3. allergies

LAB TESTS

Date	Test & Results
1. 6/12	SMA-12

MEDICATION RECORD

Date	Drug & Strength	Sig	DC'd
1. 6/12	propylthiouracil 50 mg	2 b.i.d. — GD	
2.	mechlorethamine	6 mg/m² on day 1 — HD	
3.	procarbazine	100 mg/m² — HD	
4.	prednisone	40 mg daily	
5.	vincristine	2 mg on day 1	
6.	Dalmane 30 mg	1 hs p.r.n.	
7.	Colace 100 mg	1 qd — S.S	
8.	APAP	2 tabs p.r.n. fever	

PHARMACIST'S NOTES AND OTHER PATIENT INFORMATION

Date	Comment
1. 6/12	Start MOPP therapy on 6/14 if blood work results are normal.

DIRECTIONS (Questions 18a through 18o): Each of the numbered items or incomplete statements in this section is followed by answers or by completions of the statement. Select the ONE lettered answer or completion that is BEST in each case.

18a. Which one of the following drugs is NOT a part of the chemotherapeutic regimen known as MOPP?

(A) Mechlorethamine
(B) Prednisone
(C) Procarbazine
(D) Propylthiouracil
(E) Vincristine

18b. Which of the following drugs is (are) given orally during MOPP treatment?

    I. Mechlorethamine

    II. Procarbazine

    III. Prednisone

    (A) I only

    (B) III only

    (C) I and II only

    (D) II and III only

    (E) I, II, and III

18c. Which one of the following forms of cancer is least responsive to chemotherapy?

    (A) Hepatocellular

    (B) Hodgkin's

    (C) Ovarian

    (D) Prostate

    (E) Testicular

18d. Vincristine is available under the tradename of

    (A) Adriamycin

    (B) Oncovin

    (C) Platinol

    (D) Blenoxane

    (E) Novantrone

18e. The intern reports that Mrs. Costello is experiencing extravasation of the mechlorethamine (Mustargen). Which one of the following courses of treatment should be initiated?

    (A) Apply warm compresses immediately

    (B) Infiltrate sodium thiosulfate $^1/_6$th N into area and apply cold compresses.

    (C) Infiltrate sodium thiosulfate $^1/_6$th N into area and apply warm compresses.

    (D) Infuse heparin sodium 20,000 units into area.

    (E) Withdraw infusion needle and apply compresses of sodium thiosulfate 10% W/V.

18f. How many grams of sodium thiosulfate USP ($Na_2S_2O_3 \cdot 5\ H_2O$; mol. wt. form = 248) are needed to prepare 100 mL of 1/6 normal solution?

    (A) 2.1 g

    (B) 4.1 g

    (C) 7.5 g

    (D) 14.9 g

    (E) 24.8 g

18g. The pharmacy has only the anhydrous form of the chemical mentioned in Question 18f. How many grams are needed to prepare the solution? ($Na_2S_2O_3 \cdot 5\ H_2O$ = 248; H_2O = 18)

    (A) 1.3 g

    (B) 2.6 g

    (C) 3.8 g

    (D) 5.6 g

    (E) 0 (because anhydrous form cannot be used)

18h. Adverse effects of chemotherapeutic agents, such as bone marrow depression, pass through three stages—onset, maximum depression, and recovery to normal. Which one of the following terms is used to indicate the time for maximum depression?

    (A) Climb

    (B) Lag time

    (C) Retention time

    (D) Nadir

    (E) Suppression time

18i. Which one of the following drugs can be included in chemotherapy with little expectation of bone marrow depression?

    (A) Cyclophosphamide

    (B) Ifosfamide

    (C) Cisplatin

    (D) Doxorubicin

    (E) Vincristine

18j. Which of the following criteria is (are) used when selecting antineoplastic drugs for combination therapy?

    I. Different mechanisms of cytotoxic activity

    II. Different spectra of toxicity

    III. Prefer drugs with low therapeutic indices

(A) I only
(B) III only
(C) I and II only
(D) II and III only
(E) I, II, and III

18k. The physician orders weekly injections of cyanocobalamin (vitamin B_{12}). Which of the following routes of administration are appropriate?

    I. Subcutaneous

    II. Intramuscular

    III. Intravenous

(A) I only
(B) III only
(C) I and II only
(D) II and III only
(E) I, II, and III

18l. Postmenopausal females may prevent the development of osteoporosis by daily intake of

    I. calcium

    II. estrogens

    III. psyllium

(A) I only
(B) III only
(C) I and II only
(D) II and III only
(E) I, II, and III

18m. Mrs. Costello's allergies have returned. Which of the following antihistamines may the pharmacist dispense without a prescription?

    I. Brompheniramine

    II. Chlorpheniramine

    III. Clemastine

(A) I only
(B) III only
(C) I and II only
(D) II and III only
(E) I, II, and III

18n. Which of the following antihistamines is (are) not likely to cause drowsiness?

    I. Astemizole

    II. Terfenadine

    III. Clemastine

(A) I only
(B) III only
(C) I and II only
(D) II and III only
(E) I, II, and III

18o. Which of the following statements concerning Estraderm transdermal patches is (are) true?

    I. Patch must be replaced once every week.

    II. Lower dosing is possible because drug administration avoids first-pass effect.

    III. Drug is as effective as Premarin in prophylaxis of osteoporosis and postmenopausal syndrome.

(A) I only
(B) III only
(C) I and II only
(D) II and III only
(E) I, II, and III

■ PROFILE NO. 19

Hospital Pharmacy Medication Record

Patient Name: Janice Lattimer
Room Number: 604-2
Age: 48   Height: 5'10"
Sex: F   Weight: 140 lb
Allergies: None known

DIAGNOSIS

Primary	Secondary
1. CA ovaries	1. essential hypertension
2.	2.
3.	3.

MEDICATION RECORD

Date	Drug & Strength	Sig	DC'd
1. 5/2	HCTZ 50 mg	1 qd	
2.	Colace 100 mg	1 every am	
3.	Lasix 40 mg	1 daily p.o.	
4.	Dalmane 15 mg	1 hs p.r.n.	
5. 5/6	Start following therapy in morning and discharge patient:		
	(1) Valium 10 mg p.o. 4 hr. pre-op;		
	(2) Doxorubicin 50 mg IV;		
	(3) Cisplatin 50 mg IV;		
	(4) Cyclophosphamide 700 mg IV		

PHARMACIST'S NOTES AND OTHER PATIENT INFORMATION

Date	Comment
1. 5/7	Scheduled follow-up therapy every 4 weeks for total of five more sessions with usual blood work.

DIRECTIONS (Questions 19a through 19p): Each of the numbered items or incomplete statements in this section is followed by answers or by completions of the statement. Select the ONE lettered answer or completion that is BEST in each case.

19a. Doxorubicin is available as

(A) Adriamycin

(B) CeeNu

(C) Cytosar-U

(D) Vepesid

(E) Cytoxan

19b. Ms. Lattimer should be warned of the possibility of alopecia when using which of the following drugs?

   I. Cisplatin

  II. Cyclophosphamide

 III. Doxorubicin

(A) I only

(B) III only

(C) I and II only

(D) II and III only

(E) I, II, and III

19c. Significant side effects of doxorubicin include

   I. cardiomyopathy

  II. leukopenia

 III. hepatotoxicity

(A) I only
(B) III only
(C) I and II only
(D) II and III only
(E) I, II, and III

19d. The dose of cyclophosphamide being administered to Ms. Lattimer is

(A) 5 mg/kg
(B) 11 mg/kg
(C) 24 mg/kg
(D) 700 mg/lb
(E) 700 mg/kg

19e. The pharmacist may wish to suggest the addition of metoclopramide to Ms. Lattimer's therapy. This drug is used as a (an)

(A) antiemetic
(B) antihistamine
(C) local anesthetic
(D) antidepressant
(E) antivesicant

19f. After two courses of therapy, Ms. Lattimer's serum creatinine level is 3 mg/dL. The physician should be consulted to

(A) increase Lasix dose
(B) decrease cisplatin dose
(C) decrease cyclophosphamide dose
(D) decrease doxorubicin dose
(E) decrease Lasix dose

19g. A major toxic effect commonly observed in patients receiving cyclophosphamide (Cytoxan) therapy is

(A) anemia
(B) leukopenia
(C) hidrosis
(D) hepatotoxicity
(E) mental confusion

19h. Leucovorin (folinic acid) may be required after the administration of high doses of

(A) cisplatin
(B) doxorubicin
(C) cyclophosphamide
(D) methotrexate
(E) vincristine

19i. For which of the following drugs is the intrathecal route of administration acceptable?

I. Thiotepa
II. Methotrexate
III. Vincristine

(A) I only
(B) III only
(C) I and II only
(D) II and III only
(E) I, II, and III

19j. A potential side effect(s) of long-term treatment with methotrexate is (are)

I. hepatotoxicity
II. rheumatoid arthritis
III. nephrotoxicity

(A) I only
(B) III only
(C) I and II only
(D) II and III only
(E) I, II, and III

19k. Methotrexate is available in which of the following dosage forms?

I. Oral solution
II. Oral tablets
III. Lyophilized powder for injection

(A) I only
(B) III only
(C) I and II only
(D) II and III only
(E) I, II, and III

19l. Antiemetics available in both oral and injectable dosage forms include

    I. dronabinol (Marinol)
    II. granisetron (Kytril)
    III. ondansetron (Zofran)

(A) I only
(B) III only
(C) I and II only
(D) II and III only
(E) I, II, and III

19m. Which of the following chemotherapeutic agents is (are) appropriate for the indicated disease?

    I. Etoposide (Vepesid) for testicular tumors
    II. Mercaptopurine (Purinethol) for leukemia
    III. Paclitaxel (Taxol) for breast cancer

(A) I only
(B) III only
(C) I and II only
(D) II and III only
(E) I, II, and III

19n. Ms. Lattimer brings a new prescription into your pharmacy for Vasotec. The generic name for this drug product is

(A) enalapril
(B) lisinopril
(C) labetalol
(D) captopril
(E) verapamil

19o. The mode of action of Vasotec for hypertension is as a (an)

(A) alpha-adrenergic blocking agent
(B) alpha-beta-adrenergic blocking agent
(C) angiotensin-converting enzyme inhibitor
(D) calcium channel blocking agent
(E) centrally acting alpha agonist

19p. When dispensing the Vasotec prescription, the pharmacist should counsel the client that the drug may cause

    I. dry coughing
    II. precipitous fall in blood pressure during initial dosing
    III. reflex tachycardia

(A) I only
(B) III only
(C) I and II only
(D) II and III only
(E) I, II, and III

PROFILE NO. 20

Community Pharmacy Medication Record

Patient Name: James Tralor
Address: RD 4
Age: 55
Sex: M
Allergies: NK

Height:
Weight:

DIAGNOSIS

Primary
1. mild hypertension
2. suspected high cholesterol
3.

Secondary
1. arthritis left hand
2. peptic ulcer (under control)
3.

MEDICATION RECORD

	Date	Rx No.	Physician	Drug & Strength	Quantity	Sig	Refills
1.	2/2	43568	Lange	Digoxin 0.025	#30	1 q AM	6 mos
2.		43569	Lange	Furosemide 20 mg	#60	1 q AM	6 mos
3.		43570	Lange	Slow-K 8 mEq 1 qd	100	with food	1×
4.	3/1	44490	Lange	HCTZ 25 mg	#30	1 qod	6 mos
5.		43568	Lange	Digoxin 0.025	#30	1 qd	
6.		45004	Lange	Colestipol	500 g	tsp daily ut dict	Refill
7.	4/5	44242	Levy	Zyloprim 100 mg	#100	b.i.d.	2×
8.	5/6	45037	Lange	Verapamil 80 mg	#100	1 qd	1×
9.		45038	Lange	Mevacor	#30	qd	1×

PHARMACIST'S NOTES AND OTHER PATIENT INFORMATION

	Date	Comment
1.	4/1	Client complained about difficulty in taking the colestipol. Suggest he talk to MD about another product. Also that he should have his swollen hand checked—acute gout?
2.	4/6	Patient purchased slow-release niacin 250 mg.

DIRECTIONS (Questions 20a through 20n): Each of the numbered items or incomplete statements in this section is followed by answers or by completions of the statement. Select the ONE lettered answer or completion that is BEST in each case.

20a. The pharmacist should consult Dr. Lange concerning

 I. Mr. Tralor's compliance with HCTZ

 II. the desired strength of Mevacor

 III. a potential interaction between digoxin and verapamil

 (A) I only
 (B) III only
 (C) I and II only
 (D) II and III only
 (E) I, II, and III

20b. Verapamil is best classified as a (an)

   (A) adrenergic blocking agent
   (B) calcium entry blocker
   (C) ganglionic blocking agent
   (D) saluretic
   (E) vasopressor

20c. Which one of the following controlled-release forms of verapamil is claimed to align with the patient's circadian rhythm?

   (A) Calan SR
   (B) Covera-HS
   (C) Isoprin SR
   (D) Verelan
   (E) Isoptin injection

20d. Oral doses of verapamil undergo significant first-pass effect. This fact can be deduced from which of the following true statements?

   I. The dose required for parenteral administration is much lower than oral dosing.
   II. The apparent volume of distribution is high (420 L).
   III. The drug is approximately 90% protein bound in the blood.

   (A) I only
   (B) III only
   (C) I and II only
   (D) II and III only
   (E) I, II, and III

20e. The pharmacist will counsel Mr. Tralor to consume the Mevacor

   (A) before breakfast
   (B) with breakfast
   (C) after breakfast
   (D) with any meal
   (E) in the evening

20f. When selecting a generic brand of furosemide tablets, the pharmacist reviews the following relationships between brands A, B, C, and D:

   Disintegration times $A > B > C > D$
   Dissolution times $C < B < A < D$

Which brand should the pharmacist select as probably having the greatest bioavailability?

   (A) A
   (B) B
   (C) C
   (D) D
   (E) Either A or B

20g. Niacin (nicotinic acid) is probably being consumed

   (A) to reduce stress
   (B) to prevent or treat peripheral neuritis
   (C) to prevent or treat beriberi
   (D) to improve the absorption of digoxin
   (E) to reduce cholesterol levels

20h. Patients receiving niacin may experience

   I. constipation
   II. GI disorders
   III. flushing

   (A) I only
   (B) III only
   (C) I and II only
   (D) II and III only
   (E) I, II, and III

20i. A desirable and realistic level of total cholesterol in the blood for an adult is

   (A) <100 mg/dL
   (B) <200 mg/dL
   (C) <250 mg/dL
   (D) <300 mg/dL
   (E) <500 mg/dL

20j. A significant increased risk of heart disease occurs when which of the following is (are) elevated?

   I. HDLP
   II. LDLP
   III. VLDLP

(A) I only
(B) III only
(C) I and II only
(D) II and III only
(E) I, II, and III

20k. Which one of the following antihyperlipidemic agents is considered the most potent?

(A) Cholestyramine
(B) Colestipol
(C) Gemfibrozil
(D) Lovastatin
(E) Simvastatin

20l. Cholestyramine has the tendency to bind

   I. components of bile
   II. weakly acidic drugs
   III. weakly basic drugs

(A) I only
(B) III only
(C) I and II only
(D) II and III only
(E) I, II, and III

20m. Which of the following statements concerning alcohol are true?

   I. Marked mental impairment occurs when blood levels are >100 mg/dL.
   II. Alcohol is oxidized to acetaldehyde in the liver.
   III. The metabolism of alcohol follows first-order kinetics exclusively.

(A) I only
(B) III only
(C) I and II only
(D) II and III only
(E) I, II, and III

20n. Deficiencies in which of the following vitamins are especially dangerous in the alcoholic patient?

   I. Folic acid
   II. Thiamine
   III. Ascorbic acid

(A) I only
(B) III only
(C) I and II only
(D) II and III only
(E) I, II, and III

■ PROFILE NO. 21

Community Pharmacy Medication Record

Patient Name: Irma Jackson
Address: 12 Comfort Lane
Age: 77   Height:
Sex: F   ✓   ✓   Weight: 112 lb
Allergies: sensitive to aspirin, sulfas; limit chocolates

DIAGNOSIS

Primary	Secondary
1. parkinsonism	1. mild anemia
2. glaucoma	2. stroke (1 yr ago)
3. CHF	3.

MEDICATION RECORD

Date	Rx No.	Physician	Drug & Strength	Quantity	Sig	Refills
1. 8/4	82542	Puleo	Fe Sulfate 250 mg	60	1 q AM	2×
2.	82543	Puleo	Synthroid 50 μg	60	1 q AM	2×
3.	82544	Puleo	Digoxin 0.25 mg	100	1 qd	1×
4. 9/28	82543	Puleo	Ref. Synthroid 50 μg	60	1 q AM	1×
5.	89680	Puleo	Fe Sulfate 250 mg	100	2 q AM	2×
6. 10/4	89890	Collins	Amantadine 8 oz	2 tsp	b.i.d.	1×

PHARMACIST'S NOTES AND OTHER PATIENT INFORMATION

Date	Comment
1.	Do not use poison prevention closures.
2.	Irma is sometimes confused; explain all medicines to her. Whenever possible, suggest she take medications first thing in the AM with breakfast.
3.	OTCs-Mylanta 15 mL q AM and PM
	Tums—1 every night
	Vitamin C-500 mg q AM

DIRECTIONS (Questions 21a through 21n): Each of the numbered items or incomplete statements in this section is followed by answers or by completions of the statement. Select the ONE lettered answer or completion that is BEST in each case.

21a. Synthroid was prescribed to control

(A) hypothyroidism
(B) hyperthyroidism
(C) Graves' disease
(D) hyperparathyroidism
(E) hypoparathyroidism

21b. If Mrs. Jackson misses a dose of Synthroid, she should be instructed to

(A) double the following morning's dose

(B) take 1 $1/2$ tablets the following morning

(C) increase her intake of iodized salt

(D) call her physician for advice

(E) continue with normal dosing the following morning

21c. When questioned about her recent weight loss, Mrs. Jackson admitted that her breakfast and lunch consisted of two pieces of toast and herbal tea sweetened with Equal. The active ingredient in Equal is

(A) acesulfam

(B) aspartame

(C) fructose

(D) saccharin

(E) sucrose

21d. Factors contributing to Mrs. Jackson's poor blood iron levels may be

I. dietary intake

II. antacid consumption

III. daily consumption of vitamin C

(A) I only

(B) III only

(C) I and II only

(D) II and III only

(E) I, II, and III

21e. Amantadine may have been prescribed

I. as a protectant against influenza B

II. as a protectant against influenza A

III. to treat the parkinsonism

(A) I only

(B) III only

(C) I and II only

(D) II and III only

(E) I, II, and III

21f. Mrs. Jackson's daughter is worried that her mother is showing symptoms of Alzheimer's disease. Which one of the following is the earliest symptom of this disease?

(A) Incontinence

(B) Inability to learn new skills

(C) Loss of recent memory

(D) Loss of remote memory

(E) Wandering

21g. Drugs currently in use for Alzheimer's include

I. selegiline

II. ergoloid mesylates

III. tacrine

(A) I only

(B) III only

(C) I and II only

(D) II and III only

(E) I, II, and III

21h. Which of the following is true of tacrine?

I. Nephrotoxicity is a major side effect.

II. Oral dosing is four times a day.

III. It should be given on an empty stomach.

(A) I only

(B) III only

(C) I and II only

(D) II and III only

(E) I, II, and III

21i. When dispensing the original prescriptions on 8/4, the pharmacist should have counseled the patient to take the digoxin

(A) first thing in the morning before food

(B) with breakfast

(C) after breakfast

(D) with lunch

(E) in the evening with the Mylanta

21j. For this patient, the evening dose of Tums is probably intended to

(A) decrease gastric secretions
(B) decrease gastroesophageal reflux
(C) prevent osteoporosis
(D) provide magnesium ions
(E) improve the absorption of digoxin

21k. Pharmacokinetic changes in the elderly often include increases in

I. proportional amount of body fat
II. plasma albumin levels
III. renal clearance

(A) I only
(B) III only
(C) I and II only
(D) II and III only
(E) I, II, and III

21l. Based on the following data, determine the milliliters of digoxin elixir needed to replace a daily 0.25-mg dose of digoxin tablets.

	Strength	"F value"
Digoxin tablet	0.25 mg	0.6
Digoxin elixir	0.05 mg/mL	0.75

(A) 3 mL
(B) 3.8 mL
(C) 4 mL
(D) 5 mL
(E) 6.4 mL

21m. An early sign of digoxin toxicity in Mrs. Jackson is likely to be

(A) hazy vision
(B) hearing impairment
(C) tinnitus
(D) yellowish skin
(E) increase in appetite

21n. The pharmacist may need to suggest an adjustment in the dosing of digoxin if the patient is placed on which of the following drugs?

I. Amiodarone
II. Quinidine
III. Verapamil

(A) I only
(B) III only
(C) I and II only
(D) II and III only
(E) I, II, and III

PROFILE NO. 22

Hospital Pharmacy Medication Record

Patient Name: Kathy Riley
Room Number: ER
Age: 28
Sex: F
Allergies: penicillin, sulfas

Height: 5′6″
Weight: 145 lb

DIAGNOSIS

Primary	Secondary
1. gravid	1. colitis
2. severe cramps	2. COPD (since childhood)
3.	3.

LAB TESTS

Date	Test & Results
1. 7/12	SMA-12
2.	blood profile
3.	blood typing

MEDICATION RECORD

Date	Drug & Strength	Sig	Refills
1. 7/13	D5W 1 L daily	KVO	
2.	Terbutaline 25 µg/min then .5 mg sc q4hr		
3.	Restoril	1 hs p.r.n.	
4.	Colace 100 mg	1 qd	
5.	APAP	2 tabs p.r.n. fever	
6. 7/15	KCl 40 mEq in D5NS 1 L t.i.d.		
7.	Barium sulfate admin per usual/Dr. Cooper orders		
8. 7/16	Atropine 4 mg/chlorpromazine 12.5 mg preop		

PHARMACIST'S NOTES AND OTHER PATIENT INFORMATION

Date	Comment
1. 7/13	Patient being transfered to room 434b. Continue tocolytic therapy.

DIRECTIONS (Questions 22a through 22n): Each of the numbered items or incomplete statements in this section is followed by answers or by completions of the statement. Select the ONE lettered answer or completion that is BEST in each case.

22a. Terbutaline is being used as a tocolytic agent. The term tocolytic refers to a drug that

(A) increases GI tract tone
(B) reduces GI tract motility
(C) reduces uterine contractility
(D) prevents emesis
(E) dilates bronchioles

22b. A tradename product of terbutaline is

(A) Alupent
(B) Brethine
(C) Pamelor
(D) Proventil
(E) Terazol

22c. The pharmacist places 2 mL of terbutaline injection (1 mg/mL) into 250 mL of D_5W. How many drops per minute will be needed to deliver the terbutaline if the administration set delivers 15 drops to the mL?

(A) 6
(B) 11
(C) 23
(D) 46
(E) 120

22d. As compounded, for how many minutes will the solution in Question 22c last on the patient?

(A) 40 min
(B) 80 min
(C) 100 min
(D) 160 min
(E) 480 min

22e. Provided that the concentration of drug solution is adjusted, which of the following devices may be used to infuse the terbutaline?

I. Elastomeric bottle
II. Syringe pump
III. PCA device

(A) I only
(B) III only
(C) I and II only
(D) II and III only
(E) I, II, and III

22f. Barium sulfate is best described as a (an)

(A) antacid
(B) antidiarrheal
(C) diagnostic agent
(D) cleansing laxative
(E) protectant against colitis

22g. Which of the following concerning barium sulfate is (are) true?

I. Practically insoluble in water
II. Administered by the oral route
III. Administered by the rectal route

(A) I only
(B) III only
(C) I and II only
(D) II and III only
(E) I, II, and III

22h. The purpose of the preop atropine is to

(A) relieve the patient's anxiety
(B) reduce secretions
(C) cause vasoconstriction of small blood vessels
(D) constrict the bronchioles
(E) lessen presurgical nervousness

22i. The pharmacist should question the atropine/chlorpromazine order because of

I. an acid–base reaction between the two ingredients
II. the combination is irrational
III. the high dose of atropine requested

(A) I only
(B) III only
(C) I and II only
(D) II and III only
(E) I, II, and III

Questions 22j through 22n: Mrs. Riley is discharged from the hospital on 7/21 with prescriptions for a Foley catheter, ostomy pouches, transderm dressings, Slo-Bid 100 mg t.i.d., Valium 2 mg 1 t.i.d. p.r.n., Metamucil plain 1 tbsp AM, and a multivitamin for pregnancy.

22j. For which of the following items is a prescription actually needed?

  I. Foley catheter
  II. Ostomy pouches
  III. Translucent drain dressings

  (A) I only
  (B) III only
  (C) I and II only
  (D) II and III only
  (E) I, II, and III

22k. Ingredients in Metamucil include

  I. docusate
  II. polycarbophil
  III. psyllium

  (A) I only
  (B) III only
  (C) I and II only
  (D) II and III only
  (E) I, II, and III

22l. Mrs. Riley should be counseled to consume the Metamucil by

  (A) mixing the granules with 8 oz of water, stirring, and drinking immediately
  (B) mixing the granules with 1 pt of water, stirring, and drinking immediately
  (C) mixing the granules with 8 oz water, stirring, letting mixture sit for 20 min before drinking

  (D) swallowing the granules, then drinking 8 oz of water
  (E) allowing the granules to effervesce in 8 oz of water before consuming

22m. Products with therapeutic activity similar to that of Slo-Bid include

  I. Klor-Con
  II. Slow-K
  III. Theo-Dur

  (A) I only
  (B) III only
  (C) I and II only
  (D) II and III only
  (E) I, II, and III

22n. If Mrs. Riley's physician decides to initiate antihypertensive therapy, which one of the following antihypertensive agents is probably the best choice for use during pregnancy?

  (A) Captopril
  (B) Enalapril
  (C) Hydrochlorothiazide
  (D) Methyldopa
  (E) Nifedipine

■ PROFILE NO. 23

Community Pharmacy Medication Record

Patient Name: Jane Parker
Address: 3518 Central Blvd.
Age: 28   Height: 5'6"
Sex: F   Weight: 135 lb
Allergies:

DIAGNOSIS

Primary	Secondary
1. vaginal infection	1. anemia
2. endometriosis	2. PMS (painful)
3.	3. anxiety

MEDICATION RECORD

Date	Rx No.	Physician	Drug & Strength	Quantity	Sig	Refills
1. 4/4	34765	Coughlin	Monistat-7 Insert	#30	1 qn	1x
2.	34766	"	Valium 5 mg 1 bid		p.r.n.	1x
3.	34767	"	Ovcon-50 ut dict	2683x		
4. 4/27	34765	"	Monistat-7 same as before		0	
4.	34766	"	Valium 5 mg #30 same		0	

PHARMACIST'S NOTES AND OTHER PATIENT INFORMATION

Date	Comment
1. 4/27	Jane complains that the birth control pills made her nauseous, so she stopped taking them after 1 week.
2. 6/14	Change records to Jane's new married name—Mrs. Frederick Nolan.

DIRECTIONS (Questions 23a through 23o): Each of the numbered items or incomplete statements in this section is followed by answers or by completions of the statement. Select the ONE lettered answer or completion that is BEST in each case.

23a. The Monistat prescription is probably being used to treat

(A) aspergillosis
(B) candidiasis
(C) gonorrhea
(D) genital herpes
(E) syphilis

23b. The most common causative microorganism of nongonococcal urethritis is

(A) *Candida cryptococcus*
(B) *Chlamydia trachomatis*
(C) *Klebsiella aerogenes*
(D) *Proteus mirabilis*
(E) *Treponema pallidum*

23c. The drug usually considered the first choice to treat all stages of syphilis is

(A) doxycycline
(B) erythromycin

(C) fluconazole

(D) penicillin

(E) ciprofloxacin

23d. The drug(s) usually considered as first choice(s) in the treatment of chlamydia infections include

I. doxycycline

II. azithromycin

III. fluconazole

(A) I only

(B) III only

(C) I and II only

(D) II and III only

(E) I, II, and III

23e. Ms. Parker asks what form of contraception is as effective as oral contraceptive tablets. The pharmacist should mention

(A) condoms

(B) diaphragms

(C) IUDs

(D) rhythm method

(E) spermicidal jellies

23f. Which of the following are acceptable lubricants for use with a condom or diaphragm?

I. K-Y jelly

II. Spermicidal cream

III. White Vaseline

(A) I only

(B) III only

(C) I and II only

(D) II and III only

(E) I, II, and III

23g. Which one of the following is inserted under the skin and offers up to 5 years of contraceptive protection?

(A) Depo-Provera

(B) Nonoxynol-9

(C) Norplant

(D) ParaGard

(E) Progestasert

23h. Ms. Parker's endometriosis is best treated by the use of

(A) Danocrine

(B) Deltasone

(C) Naprosyn

(D) Sansert

(E) Zantac

Questions 23i through 23o: Jane's husband confides in you that he is concerned by his wife's recent behavior. Fearing that she is going to become infected by bacteria, she wears a mask around the house, washes her hands every hour, and checks to make sure all windows are closed.

23i. Jane's behavior is characteristic of persons suffering from

(A) generalized anxiety disorder (GAD)

(B) obsessive–compulsive disorder (OCD)

(C) panic disorder

(D) posttraumatic stress disorder

(E) social phobia

23j. A drug used in the treatment of OCD is

(A) Anafranil

(B) Ativan

(C) Compazine

(D) Haldol

(E) Orudis

23k. Benzodiazepines are often used to treat generalized anxiety disorders. Which one of the following is NOT a benzodiazepine?

(A) Alprazolam (Xanax)

(B) Chlordiazepoxide (Librium)

(C) Methylphenidate (Ritalin)

(D) Clorazepate (Tranxene)

(E) Lorazepam (Ativan)

23l. The mechanism of action of the benzodi-azepines is believed to be

(A) alpha$_1$ blockage
(B) beta-adrenergic blockage
(C) blockage of dopamine receptor sites
(D) blockage of the reuptake of dopamine
(E) potentiation of the inhibitory neuro-transmitter GABA

23m. True statements concerning clozapine (Clozaril) include

I. The drug is a dopamine-receptor antagonist.
II. There is a lower incidence of extrapyramidal effects than with chlorpromazine.
III. The drug should be discontinued if white blood cell levels fall below 2000/mm^3.

(A) I only
(B) III only
(C) I and II only
(D) II and III only
(E) I, II, and III

23n. Side effects occurring with clozapine include all of the following EXCEPT

(A) drowsiness
(B) hypersalivation
(C) weight gain
(D) tardive dyskinesia
(E) anticholinergic effects

23o. Which one of the following drugs is similar in action to clozapine?

(A) Clonazepam (Klonopin)
(B) Venlafaxine (Effexor)
(C) Nortripyline (Aventyl)
(D) Risperidone (Risperdal)
(E) Paroxetine (Paxil)

PROFILE NO. 24

Community Pharmacy Medication Record

Patient Name: Jason White
Address: 869 Elm St.
Age: 3   Height: 36″
Sex: M   Weight: 40 lb
Allergies: chocolate?, salicylates

DIAGNOSIS

Primary	Secondary
1. recurrent earaches	1. frequent colds
2. strep. throat	2. allergies?
3. colitis	3.

MEDICATION RECORD

Date	Rx No.	Physician	Drug & Strength	Quantity	Sig	Refills	
1. 9/2	83043	McLaughlin	Azulfidine Susp	0.5 tsp b.i.d.	Disp 6 oz	3x	
2. 10/6	84665	McLaughlin	Pen Vee K Susp 250	200 mL	1 tsp q.i.d.		1x
3. 11/5	86956	Steen	Cromolyn sodium eye drops		2 gtts os t.i.d.		

PHARMACIST'S NOTES AND OTHER PATIENT INFORMATION

Date	Comment
1.	
2.	
3.	

DIRECTIONS (Questions 24a through 24o): Each of the numbered items or incomplete statements in this section is followed by answers or by completions of the statement. Select the ONE lettered answer or completion that is BEST in each case.

24a. Causative organisms of otitis media include

   I. *Helicobacter pylori*
  II. *Haemophilus influenzae*
 III. *Streptococcus pneumoniae*

(A) I only
(B) III only
(C) I and II only
(D) II and III only.
(E) I, II, and III

24b. Drugs of choice for otitis media include

    I. ampicillin

    II. amoxicillin

    III. cefaclor

    (A) I only

    (B) III only

    (C) I and II only

    (D) II and III only

    (E) I, II, and III

24c. When asked to suggest a drug to reduce Jason's fever and headache, the pharmacist could select products containing

    I. aspirin

    II. ibuprofen

    III. acetaminophen

    (A) I only

    (B) III only

    (C) I and II only

    (D) II and III only

    (E) I, II, and III

24d. Chemically, ibuprofen is a derivative of

    (A) fibric acid

    (B) phenylacetic acid

    (C) propionic acid

    (D) salicylic acid

    (E) xanthines

24e. When used to reduce fever, ibuprofen should not be used

    (A) for more than 3 days

    (B) for more than 10 days

    (C) for less than 3 days

    (D) for less than 10 days

    (E) if the fever is greater than 104° F

Questions 24f through 24h: The eyedrop prescription filled on 11/5 reads as follows:

Rx

Cromolyn sodium 2.5%   30 mL

Dispense a sterile isotonic solution
Sig: gtt ii OS TID

24f. The pharmacist dilutes the commercially available 4% cromolyn solution with purified water. How many milligrams of sodium chloride are needed to render the solution isotonic, assuming that the 4% solution was isotonic?

    (A) 100 mg

    (B) 170 mg

    (C) 330 mg

    (D) 540 mg

    (E) 900 mg

24g. If the pharmacist decides to prepare the original prescription using cromolyn capsules and purified water, the final solution must be passed through a _____-micron filter into a sterile dropper bottle.

    (A) .22

    (B) .45

    (C) 1.0

    (D) 5.0

    (E) 10

24h. The directions on the prescription label should include "OS," meaning

    (A) single eye

    (B) each eye

    (C) left eye

    (D) both eyes

    (E) affected eye

24i. Cromolyn solutions are used in the eyes to

I. treat *Pseudomonas* infections

II. relieve glaucoma

III. treat conjunctivitis

(A) I only

(B) III only

(C) I and II only

(D) II and III only

(E) I, II, and III

24j. Which one of the following tricyclic antidepressants has been used successfully in treating bedwetting by children?

(A) Amitriptyline (Elavil)

(B) Doxepin (Sinequan)

(C) Imipramine (Tofranil)

(D) Nortriptyline (Pamelor)

(E) Trimipramine (Surmontil)

24k. Ms. White requests a mild sleep aid for herself. The pharmacist is likely to suggest products containing which one of the following ingredients?

(A) Flurazepam

(B) Diphenhydramine

(C) Dimenhydrinate

(D) Estazolam

(E) Triazolam

24l. When Ms. White asks how to administer the ophthalmic solution to Jason, the pharmacist may suggest

I. quickly place the 2 drops directly onto the cornea

II. place 1 drop into the lower inside lid of the eye then follow with the second drop after a few minutes

III. after instillation, gently squeeze inner corner of eye nearest the nose for a minute

(A) I only

(B) III only

(C) I and II only

(D) II and III only

(E) I, II, and III

24m. Which one of the following devices would allow the most convenient and accurate determination of Jason's body temperature in the clinic?

(A) Oral thermometer

(B) Basal thermometer

(C) Tympanic thermometer

(D) TENS device

(E) Rectal thermometer

24n. Buildup of cerumen in the ear may be removed with the aid of which of the following OTC products?

I. Debrox

II. S.T. 37

III. Anbesol

(A) I only

(B) III only

(C) I and II only

(D) II and III only

(E) I, II, and III

24o. The allergist believes that Jason may be sensitive to tartrazine. Tartrazine is present in some pharmaceuticals as a (an)

(A) antioxidant

(B) antimicrobial preservative

(C) antiseptic

(D) buffer

(E) coloring agent

PROFILE NO. 25

Nursing Home Pharmacy Medication Record

Patient Name: Richard Meyers
Room Number: 312
Age: 68   Height: 6′
Sex: M   Weight: 160 lb
Allergies:

DIAGNOSIS

Primary
1. gout
2. Parkinson's
3. borderline hypertension
4. ankylosing spondylitis

Secondary
1. recovering alcoholic
2. smoker
3. asthma

MEDICATION RECORD

Date	Physician	Drug & Strength	Sig	DC'd
1. 2/6	Leader	Allopurinol 300 mg	i daily	6 mos
2.	Leader	Slo-Phyllin 250 mg	b.i.d.	2 mos
3.	Leader	Brethaire	1 puff p.r.n.	2 mos
4.	Leader	Sinemet 10/100	1 t.i.d.	3 mos
5. 2/8	Leader/per phone	Give Maalox	15 mL p.r.n.	
6. 2/20	Leader	Start IV amino-phylline 0.6 mg/kg/h for 2 days		

PHARMACIST'S NOTES AND OTHER PATIENT INFORMATION

Date	Comment
1. 2/9	Evaluated Mr. Meyers—asthma appears under control. Refuses to stop smoking.
2. 2/19	Patient appears to have difficulty breathing and is taking excessive amt's of Brethaire.

DIRECTIONS (Questions 25a through 25o): Each of the numbered items or incomplete statements in this section is followed by answers or by completions of the statement. Select the ONE lettered answer or completion that is BEST in each case.

25a. The immediate prime goal for the treatment of acute gout will be to

   I. relieve the pain of the attack

  II. administer high doses of an uricosuric agent

 III. reduce uric acid levels

(A) I only

(B) III only

(C) I and II only

(D) II and III only

(E) I, II, and III

25b. Drugs of choice for treating acute attacks of gout include

    I. allopurinol
    II. colchicine
    III. NSAIDs

(A) I only
(B) III only
(C) I and II only
(D) II and III only
(E) I, II, and III

25c. Drugs of choice for controlling hyperuricemia include

    I. allopurinol
    II. colchicine
    III. prednisone

(A) I only
(B) III only
(C) I and II only
(D) II and III only
(E) I, II, and III

25d. Nursing should be advised that the allopurinol

    I. should be consumed with a large amount of fluid
    II. may initially precipitate an attack of gout
    III. must be taken on an empty stomach to assure absorption

(A) I only
(B) III only
(C) I and II only
(D) II and III only
(E) I, II, and III

25e. The new order for Maalox may result in

(A) increased absorption of Sinemet
(B) decreased absorption of Sinemet
(C) decreased absorption of Zyloprim
(D) increase risk of constipation
(E) calcium binding of the Sinemet

25f. Maalox contains which of the following antacids?

(A) Aluminum hydroxide only
(B) Magnesium hydroxide only
(C) Aluminum and magnesium hydroxides
(D) Calcium carbonate
(E) Sodium bicarbonate

25g. Mr. Meyers is despondent because he is almost bald and asks about the drug that grows hair. The pharmacist should inform him that the drug is effective mainly in patients

    I. with small balding areas
    II. younger than age 40
    III. whose hair has thinned within the past 10 years

(A) I only
(B) III only
(C) I and II only
(D) II and III only
(E) I, II, and III

25h. Minoxidil is available in which of the following dosage forms?

    I. Topical solution
    II. Tablets
    III. Topical ointment

(A) I only
(B) III only
(C) I and II only
(D) II and III only
(E) I, II, and III

25i. Based on the order on 2/20, the pharmacist prepares an admixture of aminophylline 500 mg in 1 L D5W. What flow rate (gtt/min) should be set if the administration set delivers 15 drops to the mL?

(A) 2 gtt/min
(B) 10 gtt/min
(C) 15 gtt/min
(D) 22 gtt/min
(E) 46 gtt/min

25j. When prescribing the dose for Question 25i, the prescriber took into consideration which of the following?

    I. Smoking decreases the half-life of theophylline.

    II. Aminophylline is more potent, mg to mg, than theophylline.

    III. The targeted theophylline serum level is 1 to 2 μg/mL.

    (A) I only

    (B) III only

    (C) I and II only

    (D) II and III only

    (E) I, II, and III

25k. All of the following drugs will significantly increase the half-life of theophylline EXCEPT

    (A) erythromycin

    (B) cimetidine

    (C) ciprofloxacin

    (D) isoniazid

    (E) ranitidine

25l. Theophylline's pharmacokinetics follow a two-compartment model when administered by IV bolus. Which of the following statements is (are) true?

    I. The drug has faster initial distribution than elimination.

    II. When graphed, there will be two slopes.

    III. The half-lives of drugs following two-compartment modeling are longer than those following one-compartment modeling.

    (A) I only

    (B) III only

    (C) I and II only

    (D) II and III only

    (E) I, II, and III

25m. Early symptoms of theophylline toxicity include nausea, anorexia, and

    (A) bradycardia

    (B) bleeding gums

    (C) hypotension

    (D) hypertension

    (E) tachycardia

25n. Drugs that significantly increase the clearance of theophylline in the body include

    (A) interferon

    (B) allopurinol

    (C) phenytoin

    (D) propranolol

    (E) cimetidine

25o. Drugs that have the tendency to impart an orange color to urine, sweat, and tears include

    (A) carbamazepine

    (B) isoniazid

    (C) verapamil

    (D) phenolphthalein

    (E) rifampin

◾ PROFILE NO. 26

Community Pharmacy Medication Record

Patient Name: Henry Smythe
Address: 34 Webster Drive
Age: 45
Sex: M
Allergies:

Height: 5'10"
Weight: 180 lb

DIAGNOSIS

Primary	Secondary
1. manic-depressive illness	1.
2.	2.
3.	3.

MEDICATION RECORD

Date	Rx No.	Physician	Drug & Strength	Quantity	Sig	Refills
1. 8/9	78977	Kramer	Elavil 25 mg	#90	1 t.i.d.	3
2. 9/4	78977	Kramer	Refill			
3. 10/1	78977	Kramer	Refill			
4. 10/24	80434	Kramer	Lithobid 300 mg	#60	1 b.i.d.	4
5. 11/12	81773	Davis	HydroDIURIL 25 mg	#60	1 b.i.d.	
6. 11/24	82140	Davis	Azulfidine 500 mg	q.i.d.	#100	3

PHARMACIST'S NOTES AND OTHER PATIENT INFORMATION

Date	Comment
1. 11/12	low-sodium diet

DIRECTIONS (Questions 26a through 26p): Each of the numbered items or incomplete statements in this section is followed by answers or by completions of the statement. Select the ONE lettered answer or completion that is BEST in each case.

26a. Which of the following drugs is most similar in action to Elavil?

(A) Compazine
(B) Pamelor
(C) Nardil
(D) Loxitane
(E) Clozaril

26b. Which of the following is NOT a common adverse effect of Elavil?

(A) Orthostatic hypotension
(B) Sedation
(C) Dry mouth
(D) Urinary retention
(E) Hirsutism

26c. Patients receiving Lithobid should be advised to

(A) avoid taking the drug at bedtime
(B) avoid taking the drug with milk
(C) drink 8 to 12 glasses of water per day while on the drug
(D) consume a low-sodium diet
(E) consume a low-potassium diet

26d. In using lithium products, toxicity commonly occurs when serum lithium levels exceed

(A) 1.5 mEq/L
(B) 1.5 mg/dL
(C) 1.5 mg/L
(D) 15 mg/L
(E) 300 μg/mL

26e. The addition of hydrochlorothiazide to the patient's regimen is likely to

(A) increase serum lithium levels
(B) decrease serum lithium levels
(C) decrease the absorption of lithium
(D) increase the absorption of lithium
(E) have no effect on lithium action

26f. In monitoring serum lithium levels, blood samples are usually drawn

(A) in the morning
(B) at bedtime
(C) just prior to taking a dose
(D) 1 to 3 h after taking a dose
(E) at the midpoint between two doses

26g. Lithobid 300 mg capsules contain how many milliequivalents (mEq) of lithium? [$Li_2CO_3 = 74$; $Li = 7$]

(A) 4 mEq
(B) 8 mEq
(C) 16 mEq
(D) 21 mEq
(E) 43 mEq

26h. HydroDIURIL can best be described as a (an)

(A) loop diuretic
(B) osmotic diuretic
(C) mercurial diuretic
(D) carbonic anhydrase inhibitor
(E) thiazide diuretic

26i. Which one of the following drugs has the greatest potential for causing new memory impairment (anterograde amnesia)?

(A) Flurazepam
(B) Temazepam
(C) Quazepam
(D) Estazolam
(E) Triazolam

26j. Mr. Smythe is having difficulty in falling asleep but doesn't wake up during the night. Which one of the following is probably the best choice of hypnotic?

(A) Estazolam (Prosom)
(B) Temazepam (Restoril)
(C) Molindone (Moban)
(D) Flurazepam (Dalmane)
(E) Zolpidem (Ambien)

26k. The most recent prescription for Mr. Smythe is used in the treatment of

(A) respiratory infection
(B) constipation
(C) systemic infection
(D) colitis
(E) impotence

26l. A therapeutic substitute for sulfasalazine is

(A) Bentyl
(B) Buspar
(C) Dipentum
(D) Imodium
(E) Lomotil

26m. Which of the following diuretics is a good therapeutic alternative to HydroDIURIL in order to reduce lithium accumulation?

   I. Amiloride

   II. Esidrex

   III. Oretic

   (A) I only

   (B) III only

   (C) I and II only

   (D) II and III only

   (E) I, II, and III

26n. Diphenhydramine should not be suggested if an elderly patient is suffering from

   I. incontinence

   II. diarrhea

   III. prostatitis

   (A) I only

   (B) III only

   (C) I and II only

   (D) II and III only

   (E) I, II, and III

26o. A lab test that aids in the diagnosis of cancer of the prostate is

   (A) ESR

   (B) GGT

   (C) ABG

   (D) blood differential

   (E) PSA

26p. Mitrolan is prescribed for which of the following effects?

   I. Antacid

   II. Antidiarrheal

   III. Treat constipation

   (A) I only

   (B) III only

   (C) I and II only

   (D) II and III only

   (E) I, II, and III

■ PROFILE NO. 27

Community Pharmacy Medication Record

Patient Name: Sylvia Cajole
Address: 233 Adler Court
Age: 64   Height: 5'3"
Sex: F   Weight: 155 lb
Allergies:

DIAGNOSIS

Primary	Secondary
1. rheumatoid arthritis	1.
2.	2.
3.	3.

MEDICATION RECORD

Date	Rx No.	Physician	Drug & Strength	Quantity	Sig	Refills
1. 2/27	34987	Garth	Oxaprozin 600 mg	#60	2 b.i.d.	5
2. 2/27	34988	Garth	Mylanta Liq.	12 oz	as needed	5
3. 3/15	35875	Garth	Piroxicam 20 mg	#40	1 q.i.d.	5

PHARMACIST'S NOTES AND OTHER PATIENT INFORMATION

Date	Comment
1. 3/6	Advil Tablets (OTC)
2. 3/17	Anacin Tablets

DIRECTIONS (Questions 27a through 27j): Each of the numbered items or incomplete statements in this section is followed by answers or by completions of the statement. Select the ONE lettered answer or completion that is BEST in each case.

27a. In dispensing the prescription for oxaprozin, the pharmacist could have dispensed which of the following products?

(A) Daypro
(B) Orudis
(C) Ansaid
(D) Toradol
(E) Lodine

27b. Oxaprozin is believed to act by

(A) antagonizing dopamine receptors
(B) stimulating dopamine receptors
(C) inhibiting xanthine oxidase
(D) increasing the production of prostaglandins
(E) decreasing the production of prostaglandins

27c. Which of the following statements is true?

I. The active ingredient of Advil is ibuprofen.
II. Advil should be administered three to four times daily.

III. Antacids should not be used within 2 hours of taking Advil.

(A) I only
(B) III only
(C) I and II only
(D) II and III only
(E) I, II, and III

27d. Mylanta Liquid contains

(A) calcium carbonate
(B) propylene glycol
(C) polyethylene glycol
(D) simethicone
(E) cation exchange resin

27e. When dispensing piroxicam, the pharmacist could dispense

(A) Nalfon
(B) Orudis
(C) Feldene
(D) Torodol
(E) Anaprox

27f. When the piroxicam prescription was filled the pharmacist should have advised the physician that

(A) it is not available in a 20-mg strength
(B) it is only used on a prn basis for acute pain
(C) it should not be used for more than 10 days
(D) it is not to be used in patients with rheumatoid arthritis
(E) it should not be administered four times daily

27g. Patients with rheumatoid arthritis who do not respond to NSAIDS may be given

(A) fluorouracil
(B) famotidine

(C) methysergide maleate
(D) auranofin
(E) allopurinol

27h. Misoprostol (Cytotec) can best be described as a (an)

I. synthetic prostaglandin analog
II. inhibitor of gastric acid secretion
III. H_2-receptor antagonist

(A) I only
(B) III only
(C) I and II only
(D) II and III only
(E) I, II, and III

27i. Misoprostol (Cytotec) is contraindicated for use in

(A) pregnant women
(B) patients using aspirin
(C) patients with osteoarthritis
(D) the elderly
(E) patients with hypertension

27j. Which of the following is an ingredient in Anacin?

I. Acetaminophen
II. Aspirin
III. Caffeine

(A) I only
(B) III only
(C) I and II only
(D) II and III only
(E) I, II, and III

PROFILE NO. 28

Community Pharmacy Medication Record

Patient Name: Michael Teller
Address: 902 West 1st St.
Age: 71
Sex: M
Allergies:

Height: 5'7"
Weight: 182 lb

DIAGNOSIS

Primary	Secondary
1. hypertension	1.
2. congestive heart disease	2.
3.	3.

MEDICATION RECORD

Date	Rx No.	Physician	Drug & Strength	Quantity	Sig	Refills
1. 6/23	90988	Wilson	Digoxin 0.25	#30	1 daily	3
2. 6/23	90989	Wilson	Lasix 40 mg	#60	1 b.i.d.	3
3. 6/23	90990	Wilson	Klorvess 20 mEq	#60	1 daily	3
4. 8/10	90988	Wilson	Refill			
5. 8/10	90989	Wilson	Refill			
6. 8/10	93889	Thomas	Amiloride 5 mg tab	#30	1 daily in AM	3

PHARMACIST'S NOTES AND OTHER PATIENT INFORMATION

Date	Comment
1. 7/15	Baking soda to settle stomach

DIRECTIONS (Questions 28a through 28j): Each of the numbered items or incomplete statements in this section is followed by answers or by completions of the statement. Select the ONE lettered answer or completion that is BEST in each case.

28a. Digoxin can be described as an agent that produces a

    I. vagomimetic effect
    II. positive inotropic effect
    III. positive chronotropic effect

(A) I only
(B) III only
(C) I and II only
(D) II and III only
(E) I, II, and III

28b. Patients with congestive heart disease who begin using digoxin are likely to experience

(A) tardive dyskinesia
(B) edema
(C) decreased force of cardiac contraction
(D) slowed heart rate
(E) orthostatic hypotension

28c. Which of the following drugs is most closely related to digoxin?

(A) Hydralazine
(B) Mexiletine
(C) Flecainide
(D) Cyclandelate
(E) Amrinone

28d. Which of the following would be suitable to use in a patient who needs a cardiac glycoside but has severe renal impairment?

(A) Amiodarone
(B) Disopyramide
(C) Digoxin
(D) Digitoxin
(E) Isradipine

28e. If this patient's medication were changed from digoxin tablets to Lanoxicaps, what would be an appropriate equivalent dose?

(A) 2.5 mg
(B) 25 µg
(C) 200 µg
(D) 0.25 mg
(E) 0.125 mg

28f. Which of the following are effects associated with digoxin toxicity?

I. Diarrhea
II. Ventricular tachycardia
III. Agranulocytosis

(A) I only
(B) III only
(C) I and II only
(D) II and III only
(E) I, II, and III

28g. In dispensing Midamor, the pharmacist should recommend to the prescriber that

(A) the dose of digoxin be increased by 50%
(B) the Klorvess be discontinued
(C) the dose of Klorvess be raised by 50%
(D) the dose of digoxin be decreased by 50%
(E) the dose of Klorvess be reduced by 50%

28h. Klorvess is available as a (an)

I. effervescent granules
II. effervescent tablet
III. solution

(A) I only
(B) III only
(C) I and II only
(D) II and III only
(E) I, II, and III

28i. Bumex is most similar to

(A) Demadex
(B) HydroDIURIL
(C) Midamor
(D) Dyrenium
(E) Diamox

28j. The profile for Mr. Teller reveals the possibility of

I. substance abuse
II. potential complexation
III. a dosage error

(A) I only
(B) III only
(C) I and II only
(D) II and III only
(E) I, II, and III

■ PROFILE NO. 29

Community Pharmacy Medication Record

Patient Name: David Marchese
Address: 1904 Murray St.
Age: 10   Height: 4'4"
Sex: M   Weight: 78 lb
Allergies: ragweed pollen

DIAGNOSIS

Primary	Secondary
1. bronchial asthma	1.
2. head lice	2.
3.	3.

MEDICATION RECORD

Date	Rx No.	Physician	Drug & Strength	Quantity	Sig	Refills
1. 7/9	38383	Charmin	Benadryl 25 mg caps	#30	b.i.d.	1
2. 7/9	38384	Charmin	RID Shampoo	2 oz	Apply ut dict	1
3. 7/15	39439	Charmin	Diprosone Cream 0.05%	15 g	Apply as needed	

PHARMACIST'S NOTES AND OTHER PATIENT INFORMATION

Date	Comment
1. 7/9	Hydrocortisone cream 0.5% (OTC)

DIRECTIONS (Questions 29a through 29j): Each of the numbered items or incomplete statements in this section is followed by answers or by completions of the statement. Select the ONE lettered answer or completion that is BEST in each case.

29a. Benadryl may have been prescribed for this patient as a (an)

   I. antipruritic
  II. sedative
 III. antihistamine

  (A) I only
  (B) III only
  (C) I and II only
  (D) II and III only
  (E) I, II, and III

29b. An active ingredient of RID Shampoo is/are

  (A) lindane
  (B) pyrethrins
  (C) piperonyl butoxide
  (D) undecylenic acid
  (E) crotamiton

29c. In counseling the parent of the patient receiving RID Shampoo, the pharmacist should stress the importance of avoiding

   I. the use of vitamin A–containing foods
  II. the use of metallic combs
 III. contact with the eyes

  (A) I only
  (B) III only

(C) I and II only

(D) II and III only

(E) I, II, and III

29d. Another name for head lice is

(A) *Sarcoptes scabiei*

(B) *Pediculus pubis*

(C) tinea capitis

(D) *Pediculus capitis*

(E) tinea versicolor

29e. RID Shampoo is usually administered

(A) once daily for 3 days

(B) once daily for 5 days

(C) twice daily for 3 days

(D) twice daily for 2 days

(E) once in 7 days

29f. Diprosone Cream contains

(A) hydrocortisone

(B) fluocinonide

(C) dexamethasone

(D) triamcinolone acetonide

(E) betamethasone dipropionate

29g. Diprosone Cream should not be used in patients with

I. bacterial infection

II. herpes simplex infection

III. *Candida* infection

(A) I only

(B) III only

(C) I and II only

(D) II and III only

(E) I, II, and III

29h. Which of the following products for the treatment of head lice may be purchased over the counter (OTC)?

I. A-200 Pyrinate

II. Nix

III. Eurax

(A) I only

(B) III only

(C) I and II only

(D) II and III only

(E) I, II, and III

29i. Patients with ragweed allergy should avoid lice remedies that contain

(A) pyrethrins

(B) organic solvents

(C) lindane

(D) parabens

(E) pyrogens

29j. Scabies is a condition caused by a

(A) fungus

(B) mite

(C) flea

(D) protozoan

(E) virus

PROFILE NO. 30

Community Pharmacy Medication Record

Patient Name: Laura Machless
Address: 89 Noah Road
Age: 25
Sex: F
Allergies:

Height: 5'3"
Weight: 105 lb

DIAGNOSIS

Primary	Secondary
1. heroin abuse	1. PCP
2. AIDS-HIV	2.
3.	3.

MEDICATION RECORD

Date	Rx No.	Physician	Drug & Strength	Quantity	Sig	Refills
1. 5/16	39998	Malhous	Retrovir Caps 100 mg	#100	2 q4h	2
2. 5/28	39999	Malhous	Pentam 300	10	Bring to office	

PHARMACIST'S NOTES AND OTHER PATIENT INFORMATION

Date	Comment
1. 6/1	Robitussin DM (OTC)

DIRECTIONS (Questions 30a through 30j): Each of the numbered items or incomplete statements in this section is followed by answers or by completions of the statement. Select the ONE lettered answer or completion that is BEST in each case.

30a. Which of the following agents would be appropriate to use in treating a patient with acute heroin overdose?

(A) Naprosyn
(B) Tolazamide
(C) Naloxone
(D) Physostigmine
(E) Cuprimine

30b. Another name for heroin is

(A) methylmorphine
(B) oxycodone
(C) ethylmorphine
(D) oxymorphone
(E) diacetylmorphine

30c. "PCP" in the profile refers to

(A) phencyclidine
(B) pronounced cardiac pronation
(C) pneumocystis carinii pneumonia
(D) postcoronary patient
(E) precancerous psoriasis

30d. Another name for Retrovir is

    I. ribavirin

   II. zidovudine

  III. AZT

  (A) I only

  (B) III only

  (C) I and II only

  (D) II and III only

  (E) I, II, and III

30e. Patients receiving Retrovir must be monitored carefully for the development of

  (A) pneumothorax

  (B) malignant hypertension

  (C) edema

  (D) hematologic suppression

  (E) pulmonary fibrosis

30f. Retrovir capsules must be administered

  (A) for not longer than 1 week

  (B) on an empty stomach

  (C) for not longer than 1 month

  (D) with milk or antacids

  (E) around the clock

30g. Patients on Retrovir should avoid the use of

  (A) penicillins

  (B) beta-adrenergic blockers

  (C) acetaminophen

  (D) iron products

  (E) vitamin A

30h. Pentamidine (Pentam) is available in which of the following dosage forms?

    I. Injection

   II. Aerosol

  III. Capsules

  (A) I only

  (B) III only

  (C) I and II only

  (D) II and III only

  (E) I, II, and III

30i. Patients using Pentam must be monitored for the development of

  (A) GI ulceration

  (B) *Pseudomonas* infection

  (C) kidney failure

  (D) liver failure

  (E) severe hypotension

30j. Which of the following are active ingredients in Robitussin DM?

    I. Codeine

   II. Dextromethorphan HBr

  III. Guaifenesin

  (A) I only

  (B) III only

  (C) I and II only

  (D) II and III only

  (E) I, II, and III

Answers and Explanations

1a. **(A)** The tinea fungus lives in dead, keratinous tissue. Athlete's foot is caused by tinea pedis. Candidal fungal infections generally involve warm, dark, and moist areas of the body such as the vagina, anus, and oral cavity. Candidiasis involving the oral cavity is called thrush. *(6:1606)*

1b. **(D)** Tinea cruris is a fungal organism that survives only on dead, keratinized tissue. *(6:1184)*

1c. **(E)** The active ingredient of Fulvicin P/G (griseofulvin) is ultramicrosized; that is, its particle size is dramatically reduced to improve its absorption. *(3:358b)*

1d. **(D)** Polyethylene glycol is employed in the Fulvicin P/G formulation in order to help form the microcrystalline form of griseofulvin. *(3:358b)*

1e. **(D)** Patients who are using griseofulvin products need to be advised to avoid ultraviolet light because this drug may be a photosensitizing agent. Griseofulvin must be used consistently throughout the prescribed period in order to permit adequate levels of griseofulvin to accumulate in areas of the skin that are affected by the fungus. *(3:358a)*

1f. **(A)** Griseofulvin is derived from the same organism as penicillin. Patients who have a history of hypersensitivity reactions to penicillin, therefore, should use caution in the use of griseofulvin. *(3:358)*

1g. **(B)** Grisactin Ultra also contains ultramicrosized griseofulvin as the active ingredient. Grifulvin V contains microsized griseofulvin, that is, griseofulvin particles that are larger in size than are the particles in ultramicrosized products. *(3:358b)*

1h. **(E)** Clotrimazole (Lotrimin) cream is indicated for the topical treatment of tinea infections. It is available as an OTC product. *(3:578a)*

1i. **(C)** The use of potent topical corticosteroids on the skin reduces the defense mechanisms that the body has against fungi, bacteria, and viruses. This can result in worsening of the infection. *(6:1471)*

1j. **(C)** Pyrethrins and permethrins are agents related to certain plant components. Patients sensitive to ragweed should avoid these agents. *(2a:658)*

1k. **(D)** Dry lesions often benefit from the use of an occlusive product such as an ointment. *(2a:546)*

2a. **(B)** Oretic is a brand of hydrochlorothiazide. Diuril is a brand of chlorothiazide. Zaroxolyn is metolazone, a thiazide-like diuretic. *(3:135a)*

2b. **(E)** Slow-K is a formulation that contains potassium chloride crystals dispersed in a wax matrix. The wax matrix serves to provide a slow release for the potassium chloride and thereby reduces the irritant effect of the salt. *(3:16b)*

2c. **(E)** The molecular weight of potassium chloride is 74. One milliequivalent of potassium chloride, therefore, contains 74 mg of potassium chloride. Eight milliequivalents of potassium chloride will contain 8 mEq × 74 mg/mEq = 592 mg of potassium chloride. *(1:91)*

2d. **(D)** Benazepril (Lotensin) is an angiotensin-converting enzyme (ACE) inhibitor that is indicated for the treatment of hypertension. *(5:208)*

2e. **(D)** Chlorthalidone (Hygroton) and HCTZ are thiazide diuretics. Bumetanide, torsemide, and ethacrynic acid are loop diuretics, whereas acetazolamide is a carbonic anhydrase inhibitor. *(3:135a–137d)*

2f. **(E)** Drixoral is a product that contains the antihistamine brompheniramine maleate and the decongestant pseudoephedrine. Because pseudoephedrine is a vasoconstrictor, its use in hypertensive patients is undesirable. *(2a:143)*

2g. **(A)** Lotensin decreases aldosterone production and, as a result, may increase serum potassium levels. The concomitant use of Lotensin with potassium-sparing diuretics and/or potassium supplements may therefore result in hyperkalemia. *(5:208)*

2h. **(C)** Moexepril HCl (Univasc) and fosinopril sodium (Monopril) are ACE inhibitors. Losartan potassium (Cozaar) is an angiotensin-II antagonist. *(5:208)*

2i. **(C)** Pruritis is itching. *(27:1277)*

2j. **(B)** Each Tylenol/Codeine No. 3 tablet contains 30 mg of codeine and 300 mg of acetaminophen. *(3:243r)*

2k. **(A)** Brompheniramine maleate is an H_1-receptor antagonist, which is in the alkylamine class of antihistaminic agents. *(2a:140)*

2l. **(C)** Codeine produces an antiperistaltic action on the GI tract and commonly causes constipation. *(6:532)*

PROFILE NO. 3

3a. **(B)** Micronor is a progestin-only oral contraceptive. Such products are somewhat less effective than combination products that contain both an estrogen and progestin. Progestin-only products are taken daily rather than cyclically. *(5:1606)*

3b. **(E)** Semicid is a contraceptive vaginal suppository that contains the spermicidal agent nonoxynol-9. *(3:535a)*

3c. **(A)** Grand mal seizures are currently more popularly referred to as tonic–clonic seizures. They are characterized by the initial presence of tonic muscle contractions, shortly followed by clonic contractions. *(5:1183)*

3d. **(C)** Dilantin Kapseals contain phenytoin sodium extended. This product is suitable for single daily dosing or divided daily dosing. Products that contain phenytoin sodium, prompt, are suitable only for divided daily dosing. *(5:1190)*

3e. **(A)** Gingival hyperplasia is characterized by an overgrowth of gum tissue within the oral cavity. This predisposes the patient to oral infection and loss of tooth integrity. Good oral hygiene is therefore absolutely essential for patients using phenytoin. *(5:1190)*

3f. **(A)** Dilantin Kapseals are manufactured by Parke-Davis and contain phenytoin sodium, extended, as their active ingredient. *(3:383b)*

3g. **(E)** The therapeutic plasma concentration of phenytoin is 10 to 20 μg/mL. A phenytoin plasma concentration of 5 μg/mL several weeks after initiating therapy is indicative of inadequate dosing or noncompliance. *(5:1189)*

3h. **(D)** Phenytoin use may decrease the pharmacologic effect of the Micronor by increasing the hepatic metabolism of the progestin in Micronor. Because progestin-only products such as Micronor tend to be somewhat less effective in preventing pregnancy, this may result in an unwanted pregnancy. *(8:333)*

3i. **(D)** The IM route for phenytoin sodium is generally avoided because the precipitation of phenytoin at the injection site may be painful and result in erratic absorption. Phenytoin is easily precipitated in the presence of an acidic substance in the IV admixture. The addition of phenytoin sodium to an IV infusion is therefore generally not recommended. *(3:283)*

3j. **(E)** A morbilliform rash is one that resembles that of measles. *(27:981)*

3k. **(C)** Nonoxynol-9 is a surfactant spermicide that is the active ingredient of Semicid. *(3:535a)*

3l. **(A)** Docusate sodium, the active ingredient of the stool softener Colace, is an anionic surfactant that promotes the penetration of water into the intestinal contents. This softens the contents and facilitates their evacuation. *(2a:232)*

3m. **(E)** Theragran-M is a therapeutic multivitamin product that also contains minerals. *(3:32)*

PROFILE NO. 4

4a. **(D)** Carbidopa serves as a dopadecarboxylase inhibitor that prevents the peripheral decarboxylation of levodopa and permits a greater proportion of the levodopa dose to enter the brain in its intact form. The use of carbidopa in combination with levodopa permits the use of lower levodopa doses than would be used without carbidopa. *(5:1251)*

4b. **(B)** Pyridoxine promotes the peripheral conversion of levodopa to dopamine, thereby decreasing the activity of the administered levodopa. *(3:290)*

4c. **(A)** Darkening of the urine with the use of levodopa or Sinemet is normal and is a product of levodopa metabolism. It may be disregarded by the patient. *(3:290a)*

4d. **(E)** Benztropine mesylate (Cogentin) is an anticholinergic agent used in the treatment of Parkinson's disease. Such agents reduce the incidence and severity of akinesia, rigidity, and tremor in patients with Parkinson's. Anticholinergic drugs are used as adjuncts to levodopa in the treatment of Parkinson's disease. *(5:1249–50)*

4e. **(D)** The other choices are anticholinergic agents or dopaminergic agents used in treating Parkinson's disease. Tranylcypromine (Parnate) is a monoamine oxidase (MAO) inhibitor used in treating depression. *(5:1253)*

4f. **(A)** Amantadine (Symmetrel), in addition to being employed in the treatment of Parkinson's disease, is also used in the prevention and treatment of respiratory tract infections caused by influenza A virus. *(3:406)*

4g. **(E)** Diplopia, or double vision, is sometimes experienced by patients receiving levodopa therapy. *(27:441)*

4h. **(D)** When a patient on levodopa is to be switched to Sinemet, at least 8 hours must be allowed to elapse from the last dose of levodopa to the first dose of Sinemet in order to decrease the likelihood of toxicity. Because the carbidopa in the Sinemet increases the proportion of intact levodopa that enters the brain, the dose of levodopa administered via Sinemet should be 75% to 80% less than that administered prior to the initiation of Sinemet therapy. *(3:290e)*

4i. **(E)** Levodopa is a precursor of dopamine, an agent that seems to be lacking in the brain of patients with Parkinson's disease. *(5:1250)*

4j. **(D)** Carbidopa is available by itself as Lodosyn. It should be employed in combination with levodopa to create a dosage combination for patients with Parkinson's disease. *(3:290c)*

4k. **(B)** Chlorpromazine is a phenothiazine antipsychotic agent that acts as a dopamine antagonist. With prolonged use, it can cause a variety of Parkinson-like effects. *(5:1244)*

4l. **(A)** Parkinson's disease generally causes muscle rigidity, tremor, and postural disturbances. *(5:1244)*

PROFILE NO.5

5a. **(C)** Pilocarpine acts to produce constriction of the pupil (miosis). This helps to increase the outflow of aqueous humor from the eye and lower intraocular pressure. *(5:1791)*

direct acting miotic

5b. **(B)** Carbachol, like pilocarpine, is a direct-acting miotic agent. Physostigmine and isoflurophate are also miotics; however, they work by inhibiting the enzyme acetylcholinesterase. *(5:1792)*

5c. **(D)** Intraocular pressure may vary considerably in the same individual, depending on the time of day the measurement is taken as well as many other factors. A measurement of 14 mm Hg is well within the normal range of 10 to 20 mm Hg. *(5:1783)*

5d. **(B)** The Ocusert Pilo-20 system is designed to release 20 µg of pilocarpine per hour for 1 week. This slow but steady drug administration permits better control of intraocular pressure and fewer adverse effects when compared to the use of pilocarpine eye drops. *(3:481)*

5e. **(E)** The Ocusert Pilo-20 system must be replaced every 7 days. When first inserted, the pilocarpine is released from the system at about three times the rate indicated on the package. After about 6 hours, the rate of drug release diminishes to the labeled rate and re-

mains within 20% of this rate for the rest of the 7 days. *(3:481)*

5f. **(E)** Betaxolol (Betoptic), timolol (Timoptic), carteolol (Ocupress), and metipranolol (OptiPranolol) are beta-adrenergic blocking agents used ophthalmically in the treatment of glaucoma. They appear to act by decreasing the output of aqueous humor within the eye. *(5:1790)*

5g. **(E)** Betaxolol (Betoptic) is a beta-adrenergic blocking agent that appears to be useful in the treatment of glaucoma because of its ability to reduce aqueous humor production within the eye. It is usually administered twice daily. *(5:1790)*

5h. **(E)** EDTA, or ethylenediamine tetraacetic acid, is a chelating agent that has the ability to remove trace quantities of metals that might promote the decomposition of the active drug. *(2a:455)*

5i. **(D)** Visine contains tetrahydrozoline as its active ingredient. This agent is an imidazoline decongestant that tends to exhibit alpha-adrenergic agonist activity. Its use in the eye causes vasoconstriction and relief of "red eyes" and ophthalmic congestion. *(2a:457)*

5j. **(D)** The use of a beta-adrenergic blocking agent such as betaxolol (Betoptic) by a patient with a history of respiratory illness and breathing difficulty may be hazardous because beta blockers may cause bronchoconstriction. Even the relatively small amount of drug that enters the systemic circulation via an ophthalmic administration has been reported to cause breathing difficulty in susceptible patients. *(5:1791)*

5k. **(A)** Both Ecotrin Maximum Strength and Easprin are enteric-coated aspirin formulations. They each have an enteric coat on the surface of the tablet that dissolves only when the tablet reaches the more neutral-to-alkaline region of the small intestine. *(3:248f)*

51. **(A)** Anticholinergic drugs may cause mydriasis (pupillary dilation). This is likely to result in increased intraocular pressure. *(5:1798)*

PROFILE NO. 6

6a. **(A)** The active ingredient in Benzac is benzoyl peroxide, an agent that appears to act by providing antibacterial activity, especially against *Propionibacterium acnes*, the predominant organism in acne lesions. *(2a:575)*

6b. **(C)** Patients using tretinoin (Retin-A) products should be advised to avoid the use of the product near the eyes, mouth, angles of the nose, and mucous membranes because tretinoin may irritate these tissues. Patients using this product should also be advised to avoid excessive exposure to sunlight and sunlamps because the drug may increase the patient's susceptibility to burning. Although tretinoin is a vitamin A derivative, its topical use makes it unnecessary for patients to limit their intake of vitamin A-containing foods. *(3:543)*

6c. **(E)** Butylated hydroxytoluene, or BHT, is an antioxidant that is commonly employed in food and topical products in order to reduce the likelihood of spoilage. *(1:1380)*

6d. **(D)** The use of clindamycin, the active ingredient of Cleocin, has been associated with the development of diarrhea in some patients. If the diarrhea is severe and/or persistent, the patient's physician should be contacted because such a response may indicate the development of pseudomembranous enterocolitis, a serious and potentially life-threatening condition. *(5:2130)*

6e. **(D)** A product that contains 10 mg of drug per milliliter will contain 1000 mg, or 1.0 g/100 mL. This is equivalent to a 1% (w/v) solution of the drug. *(1:82)*

6f. **(E)** Accutane contains isotretinoin as its active ingredient. This is an isomer of retinoic acid, a metabolite of retinol (vitamin A). *(3:543d)*

6g. **(D)** Many adverse effects are associated with the use of Accutane. Cheilitis, an inflammation around the margins of the lips, is very common. Conjunctivitis (inflammation of the conjunctival lining of the eye) is also a common adverse effect associated with the use of this drug. *(3:543d)*

6h. **(E)** Because of the many adverse effects associated with the use of Accutane, a patient package insert must be dispensed by the pharmacist to any patient receiving this drug. *(3:543d)*

6i. **(D)** The use of Accutane in patients who are or may become pregnant is contraindicated because the use of this drug in pregnant patients has been shown to cause fetal abnormalities. Accutane has been given a pregnancy category X rating by the FDA because of this hazard. *(3:543d)*

6j. **(D)** Aluminum oxide is a water-insoluble material that is employed in the Brasivol formulation as an abrasive. When rubbed onto the affected area, the abrasive property is meant to help remove the comedone plugs and allow better drainage of the comedone. *(2a:574)*

6k. **(D)** Salicylic acid is a keratolytic agent; that is, it helps to remove keratin from the skin surface. This faciliates the opening of plugged comedones and decreases the likelihood of new comedone formation. *(2a:574)*

6l. **(E)** Sebum is a lipid secretion of the sebaceous glands, which are associated with the hair follicle. Sebum acts as a protectant on the skin surface. When the esterified fatty acids of sebum are broken down to free fatty acids by microorganisms, the inflammatory lesion of acne may be formed. *(2a:569)*

PROFILE NO. 7

7a. **(C)** Isoproterenol is a nonspecific beta-adrenergic agonist. It is capable of stimulating beta$_2$-receptors found in the respiratory tract to produce bronchodilation. It is also capable of stimulating beta$_1$-adrenergic receptors found in the heart, thereby producing cardiac stimulation. *(6:212)*

7b. **(B)** If the initial inhalation of Medihaler-Iso has not been successful in relieving an acute asthmatic attack, a second inhalation should be attempted 2 to 5 min after the first. If relief still does not occur, the patient should be advised to seek medical assistance. *(3:176)*

7c. **(A)** Theophylline is a methylxanthine, as is theobromine and caffeine. Methylxanthines tend to stimulate the CNS and the heart as well as increase diuresis. *(5:571)*

7d. **(E)** Theophylline, as well as most other methylxanthines, tends to cause stimulation of the CNS. *(5:571)*

7e. **(E)** Aminophylline, the ethylenediamine derivative of theophylline, is generally preferred for use in rectal suppository dosage forms because it is more water soluble than is theophylline and will tend to be absorbed more readily through membranes. *(6:673)*

7f. **(B)** Intal solution contains cromolyn sodium, an agent that inhibits the degranulation of mast cells and thereby decreases the likelihood of an asthmatic attack. It is administered by inhalation. Intal is also available in a powder form that is administered by inhalation using a special device known as a Spinhaler. *(5:576)*

7g. **(C)** Cromolyn is the active ingredient in Intal. It is a drug that acts to decrease the degranulation of mast cells in the respiratory tract, thereby decreasing the likelihood of an asthmatic attack. *(5:576)*

7h. **(A)** The active ingredient in Vanceril is beclomethasone dipropionate, a corticosteroid. When administered by inhalation to asthmatic patients, Vanceril reduces the likelihood of future acute asthmatic attacks. Vanceril is not suitable for use during an acute attack. *(5:579)*

7i. **(B)** Patients who are to use Vanceril as well as a bronchodilator by inhalation such as Medihaler-Iso should be advised to use the bronchodilator several minutes before the corticosteroid is administered in order to facilitate penetration of the steroid into the bronchial tree. Vanceril is only to be used to prevent an acute asthmatic attack, not to abort an existing acute attack. Vanceril is administered only by inhalation. *(5:583)*

7j. **(E)** Cigarette and marijuana smoking tend to induce hepatic metabolism of theophylline, thereby decreasing its action in the body. Smokers may therefore require a 50% to 100% greater dose of theophylline than nonsmokers in order to control their disease. *(6:677)*

7k. **(C)** Nicotine (Nicoderm) patches are applied for a 24-hour period. A new site should be used for each application. *(3:736f)*

7l. **(C)** Albuterol is a beta-adrenergic agonist, which is more specific in its action for beta$_2$-receptors in the respiratory tract than for beta$_1$-adrenergic receptors in the heart. Isoproterenol is relatively nonspecific in its effect. Albuterol is therefore less likely to cause unwanted cardiac stimulation than is isoproterenol. *(5:568)*

7m. **(B)** Both Beclovent and Vanceril are inhalation products containing beclomethasone dipropionate. *(3:180b)*

PROFILE NO. 8

8a. **(E)** Nitrostat is a nitroglycerin sublingual tablet that has been stabilized with polyethylene glycol in order to decrease the likelihood that volatilization of the nitroglycerin will take place. As a result, Nitrostat has a considerably longer shelf-life than do nonstabilized nitroglycerin tablets. *(3:143g)*

8b. **(C)** Nitrostat, as well as other oral nitroglycerin products, should be dispensed by the pharmacist in its original container because such containers are designed to minimize the loss of nitroglycerin during storage. *(3:143e)*

8c. **(B)** Transdermal nitroglycerin patches should be applied onto a hairless site. Site rotation is important with each administration in order to decrease the likelihood of skin irritation. Transdermal patches should not be applied to distal portions of the extremities because these areas do not permit as reliable absorption of the nitroglycerin as do other areas of the body. *(3:144)*

8d. **(E)** When discontinuing therapy with nitroglycerin transdermal systems, gradual reduction of both the dosage and frequency of application over a 4- to 6-week period is advisable in order to minimize the likelihood of sudden withdrawal reactions. *(3:143c)*

8e. **(E)** Amyl nitrite is the only antianginal product administered by inhalation. It is available as a liquid packaged in small glass capsules covered by protectant cotton or gauze material. When required, the capsule is crushed and the vapors released are inhaled by the patient. A rapid response is generally evident. Dosage control is, however, a major drawback in the use of this drug. *(3:143g)*

8f. **(A)** Dipyridamole (Persantine), in addition to being used in the treatment of angina, is also employed as an antiplatelet agent. It appears to act in this regard by inhibiting cyclic nucleotide phosphodiesterase activity. *(6:1353)*

8g. **(B)** Nitroglycerin administered orally undergoes extensive first-pass hepatic deactivation, thereby limiting the usefulness of this route of administration. *(6:764)*

8h. **(E)** The use of alcohol in combination with nitroglycerin may produce a hypotensive response because of the vasodilating action of both of these drugs. The hypotensive response may be manifested as dizziness, fainting, and/or weakness. *(6:765)*

8i. **(B)** Nitroglycerin may be adsorbed onto the polyvinyl chloride (PVC) tubing used in most IV administration sets. This may result in loss of drug and inadequate dosing. Manufacturers of nitroglycerin for IV use supply non-PVC infusion tubing, which minimizes the adsorption of nitroglycerin. Such special tubing is generally recommended for use with nitroglycerin products. *(3:143f)*

8j. **(D)** The dose of nitroglycerin topical ointment is measured in inches. It is applied to the skin with minimal rubbing, and the area to which it has been applied is covered with plastic wrap to facilitate drug absorption and to prevent staining of clothing. *(3:144a)*

8k. **(D)** Nitrolingual Spray and sublingual forms of nitroglycerin provide the most rapid onset of action, ranging from 1 to 3 minutes. Transdermal patches have a 30- to 60-min onset time. *(3:143g)*

PROFILE NO. 9

9a. **(E)** Patients with type I diabetes mellitus are generally insulin dependent. Their disease generally begins early in life and is characterized by little or no insulin production by the pancreas. *(5:1489)*

9b. **(C)** Humulin R insulin is human regular insulin that is prepared by recombinant DNA technology. As is the case with all regular insulin products, Humulin is a clear solution. *(3:129f)*

9c. **(D)** The Humulin R insulin contains 100 units of activity per milliliter. Twenty-four units of insulin activity will therefore be contained in 0.24 mL of the product. *(3:129f)*

9d. **(E)** Polydypsia refers to excessive thirst. This is frequently seen in type I diabetics because of the excessive urination (polyuria) that is associated with the body's attempt to eliminate excessive glucose in the blood. *(5:1491)*

9e. **(A)** A fasting blood sugar of 100 mg/dL is well within the normal range of 70 to 110 mg/dL. *(5:1491)*

9f. **(D)** Regular insulin is the only form of insulin available as a clear solution. The other forms are suspensions, which would be unsuitable for IV administration. *(3:130a)*

9g. **(B)** When mixing two types of insulin, the clear regular insulin is always drawn into the syringe first in order to reduce the likelihood of contamination of the regular insulin with suspended particles of the second insulin. Insulin mixtures may be stored in a prefilled syringe for up to 1 week with refrigeration. *(3:130a)*

9h. **(E)** Ascorbic acid found in multivitamin mixtures such as Optilets-M may interfere with Clinitest testing because the presence of a reducing substance, such as ascorbic acid, may be detected by the nonspecific test for reducing substances employed in the Clinitest. *(5:1505)*

9i. **(D)** Clinitest employs the copper reduction mechanism for the detection of reducing substances. This is the same mechanism employed by the Benedict's test. The other tests listed all use the glucose oxidase mechanism for detecting glucose. Because they are more specific for detecting glucose, they are less susceptible to interference by other reducing substances that may be in the urine. *(5:1504)*

9j. **(E)** Contac 12-Hour Caplets contain phenylpropanolamine, a sympathomimetic decongestant that is capable of inducing the conversion of glycogen to glucose in the body. This may increase glucose levels in the blood and increase the patient's insulin requirement. *(5:1491)*

9k. **(E)** Lo-Dose syringes have a capacity of 0.5 mL. They are useful in situations where a low dose (<50 units) of insulin must be administered. *(1:1856)*

9l. **(D)** Glipizide (Glucotrol) is a second-generation sulfonylurea. Such agents are administered in lower doses than are first-generation agents and tend to produce somewhat fewer adverse effects than do first-generation agents. *(3:130f)*

9m. **(B)** Lactic acidosis is a rare but serious complication in the use of metformin HCl. It may be fatal in 50% of patients who develop it. *(3:130p)*

PROFILE NO. 10

10a. **(C)** Both warfarin and dicumarol are oral anticoagulants that interfere with vitamin K–dependent clotting factors. They are both derivatives of 4-hydroxycoumarin. *(6:1347)*

10b. **(B)** The administration of cimetidine to a patient stabilized on warfarin is likely to result in increased warfarin activity because of the ability of cimetidine to inhibit the metabolism of warfarin. The other choices listed are agents that promote the hepatic metabolism of warfarin and would therefore decrease warfarin activity. *(6:906)*

10c. **(A)** Phytonadione (vitamin K_1) is a specific antidote for warfarin toxicity. Treatment of hemorrhage caused by oral anticoagulant therapy generally consists of the administration of 10 to 20 mg of phytonadione. *(5:416)*

10d. **(A)** Datril contains acetaminophen, an analgesic/antipyretic that does not appear to displace warfarin from plasma protein–binding sites. Ecotrin contains aspirin and Advil contains ibuprofen. Both of these agents are capable of displacing warfarin from protein-binding sites and increasing warfarin activity. *(2a:65)*

10e. **(C)** Synthroid contains levothyroxine, or T_4, as its active ingredient. *(3:132i)*

10f. **(E)** 100 μg of Synthroid is approximately equivalent to 65 mg of Thyroid USP and Thyrar, 65 mg of Proloid, and 25 μg of Cytomel. *(3:132)*

10g. **(E)** Propylthiouracil and methimazole each inhibit the synthesis of thyroid hormones. Sodium iodide ^{131}I is a radioactive isotope that is concentrated in thyroid tissue and emits radiation that destroys thyroid tissue. Any of these agents may be used to treat hyperthyroidism. *(5:1529)*

10h. **(D)** Synthroid and other thyroid hormone products appear to increase the catabolism of vitamin K–dependent clotting factors. This potentiates the action of warfarin and decreases the warfarin dosage requirement. *(6:1393)*

10i. **(E)** In a radiation emergency, the administration of potassium iodide would saturate the thyroid with nonradioactive iodide, thereby making it less likely that radioactive iodides created in the emergency would accumulate in thyroid tissue. *(6:1188)*

10j. **(D)** Thyroid hormone production in the body is controlled by the level of thyroid-stimulating hormone (TSH) produced by the anterior pituitary. *(5:1522)*

10k. **(D)** Empirin/Codeine No. 3 contains aspirin. The aspirin may displace warfarin from protein-binding sites and may increase warfarin activity in the body. *(6:629)*

10l. **(D)** The international normalized ratio (INR) is a measure that takes into consideration the prothrombin time (PT) and the International Sensitivity Index (ISI), which is a measure of the sensitivity of the thromboplastin reagent used to determine the PT. *(5:413)*

PROFILE NO. 11

11a. **(C)** The term "pyuria" refers to pus in the urine. Such a condition is often associated with a urinary tract infection (UTI). *(27:1302)*

11b. **(B)** *E coli* organisms are gram-negative bacilli commonly associated with the GI tract. They are commonly a causative organism in urinary tract infections as well as institutionally borne infections. *(6:1036)*

11c. **(E)** All of the listed drugs are considered for treatment of urinary tract infections. Several of the cephalosporins are also used. There are increasing incidences of drug resistant strains that may necessitate switching to another antimicrobial agent. *(6:1036,1064)*

11d. **(C)** Both Septra and Bactrim are combination products of trimethoprim–sulfamethoxazole that have synergic action against many microorganisms. The advantage of using such a combination as opposed to single-drug therapy is the ability of this combination to block two consecutive steps used by bacteria to produce tetrahydrofolic acid. Blocking two steps greatly diminishes the likelihood that bacterial resistance will develop. Trimox is one of the brand names for amoxicillin. *(19:63–64)*

11e. **(D)** Negram is nalidixic acid, which is a quinolone but not a fluoroquinolone. Its use in the treatment of UTIs has decreased because of the rapid development of bacterial resistance to the drug. The other choices are fluoroquinolones, which are all effective orally and exhibit relatively few side effects. Their respective brand versus tradenames are Cipro (ciprofloxacin), Cinobac (cinoxacin), Floxin (ofloxacin), and Noroxin (norfloxacin). *(6:1065,1070)*

11f. **(A)** Patients using either Septra or other sulfa drugs should be advised to maintain adequate fluid intake in order to facilitate the urinary antimicrobial action of the product as well as to prevent precipitation of poorly soluble drugs in the urinary tract. Urinary acidification may accelerate the precipitation of sulfa drugs. There is no need for patients to avoid the use of folic acid–containing foods. *(1:1276; 10)*

11g. **(C)** Microstix-3 (formerly Microstix Nitrite Strips) are designed to test for nitrite in the urine. Elevated nitrite levels are indicative of the presence of bacteria in the urine (ie, bacteriuria). *(3:745)*

11h. **(E)** Phenazopyridine (Pyridium) is an azo dye employed as a urinary analgesic. It has no antiseptic activity. Phenazopyridine is often used to reduce pain in patients with urinary tract infections prior to the successful control of bacteria by antimicrobial agents. *(6:1070)*

11i. **(C)** Phenazopyridine (Pyridium) is excreted unchanged into the urine. In doing so, it may cause a red-orange discoloration of the urine. *(6:1070; 19:63–69)*

11j. **(A)** When used with antimicrobial agents for the treatment of urinary tract infections, Pyridium should not be used for more than 2 days. This permits Pyridium's analgesic action to be employed during the early period of therapy when the infection is not yet under control. After 2 days, the infection should be under control and the continued use of Pyridium should not be required. In addition, the use of Pyridium beyond 2 days would mask pain that might be an indication of the failure of the antimicrobial therapy. *(1:1270)*

11k. **(E)** Probably the most common psychological symptom of premenstrual syndrome is tension characterized by irritability and depression which occur in 70% to 90% of all women. Weight gains of several pounds may be observed due to water retention. Several OTC products contain diuretics to combat this "bloating." However, the hydrochlorothiazides currently still require prescriptions. *(2a:104)*

11l. **(C)** Caffeine in doses of 100 to 200 mg every 3 to 4 h is a safe and effective diuretic but may cause sleeplessness. Pamabrom, a derivative of theophylline, is also effective in doses of 50 mg up to four times a day. Pamabrom is the active ingredient in Midol PMS and Pamprin. *(2a:105)*

11m. **(C)** Ciprofloxacin (Cipro) is effective for treating urinary tract infections and for prostatitis. Usual dose ranges are 250 to 500 mg every 12 h. The drug should not be used in pregnant women because it can cause permanent lesions in the weight-bearing joints. A second choice would be imipenem–cilastatin which allows a broad-spectrum coverage. *(5:742; 19:63–8)*

11n. **(A)** The Foley or balloon catheter is an indwelling urinary catheter. After insertion, it is inflated to prevent slippage out of the urinary tract. The other choices, the Broviac and the Hickman, are venous catheters intended for nutritional intravenous therapy. *(1:1866; 22:167)*

PROFILE NO. 12

12a. **(D)** A nomogram is a chart that permits the determination of a patient's body surface area (BSA) in square meters from the patient's known height and weight data. Nomograms are frequently employed in calculating doses for potent agents such as the antineoplastic drugs. *(11:1339)*

12b. **(A)** The patient is to receive 45 mg of daunorubicin per square meter of body surface area per day. Because the patient's BSA has been found to be 1.85 m^2, then 1.85 m^2 × 45 mg/m^2 = 83.25 mg of drug per administration. Because each vial contains 20 mg of drug, five vials will be required to supply the amount of drug needed. *(10; 23:68)*

12c. **(C)** Cytarabine (Arac) is a pyrimidine analog that is employed as an antimetabolite either alone or in combination with other antineoplastic drugs. Other pyrimidine antagonists include fluorouracil (5-FU) and the antiviral compound idoxuridine. *(6:1251)*

12d. **(D)** Myelosuppression, or suppression of the bone marrow, usually results in a sharp decrease in white blood cells as is seen on the patient's profile. This may be life-threatening because of the patient's increased susceptibility to infection. (11:1501)

12e. (A) Acute lymphocytic leukemia is a common malignancy in children and is rarely observed in persons older than age 15. Long-term survival rates of greater than 70% are now obtained with chemotherapy. (11:1501)

12f. (B) One of methotrexate's main uses is in psoriasis therapy. It is available in both oral and parenteral dosage forms. Carmustine (BCNN) inhibits synthesis of DNA and RNA and is classified as an alkylating agent, as is cyclophosphamide. (6:1242–43,1249; 11:1500)

12g. (C) Allopurinol is a xanthine oxidase inhibitor. Inhibition of xanthine oxidase enzyme results in a reduction in the formation of uric acid, a common metabolite formed in patients being treated with antineoplastic drugs. Allopurinol is, therefore, commonly employed in the prevention or management of hyperuricemia. (6:649)

12h. (A) When allopurinol therapy is initiated, large quantities of uric acid are mobilized in the body and enter the urinary tract. Without adequate hydration, urates are likely to precipitate in the tract, causing pain and inflammation. (6:650)

12i. (D) Because allopurinol is employed in managing uric acid levels in the body, the monitoring of serum urate levels will provide a means of determining the success of therapy. (6:650)

12j. (B) When nystatin (Mycostatin) oral suspension is employed in the treatment of oral candidiasis infection, it is important that sufficient contact time be allowed between the drug and the mucosal surface of the oral cavity. This can be accomplished by having the patient swish the suspension in the mouth for several minutes prior to swallowing it. (11:1432)

12k. (E) Extravasation is the leakage of injection fluid into tissue surrounding the injection site. When this occurs with the use of potent drugs such as daunorubicin, irritation and inflammation commonly occur. Once extravasation has occurred, the application of cold compresses to the injection site will relieve pain and minimize further dissemination of the drug into neighboring tissue. (19:91–12)

12l. (A) A serious adverse effect associated with the use of daunorubicin is cardiotoxicity. This is commonly manifested as congestive heart failure (CHF) and requires early diagnosis and aggressive treatment with sodium restriction, diuretics, and digoxin. (10; 11:1500)

12m. (C) The active metabolite of Dalmane has a long half-life, and thereby accumulates over time. It also suppresses REM sleep even at low doses. The net result is impaired daytime functioning, especially in the elderly. Temazepam (Restoril) and triazolam (Halcion) both have shorter half-lives and are less likely to cause side effects mentioned in the question. Clorazepate (Tranxene) should not be suggested because its half-life is 30 to 100 h. (11:1146)

12n. (D) Melatonin is an endogenous hormone that may effect human sleep patterns. Tryptophan has been advocated as a sleep aid, but its effectiveness has not been clearly established. (2a:184)

PROFILE NO. 13

13a. (D) A normal hemoglobin level is considered to be 12 g/dL for females and 13 g/dL for males. When values drop below 10 g/dL, symptoms of iron deficiency anemia become evident. Six months of iron therapy is generally sufficient to raise hemoglobin levels to within a normal range. A better estimate of iron therapy effectiveness would be an increase in hemoglobin of 2 g/dL in the first 3- to 4-week period. (11:197,208)

13b. (A) Epogen is Amgen's brand of erythropoietin, which is effective for the prevention of anemia and in reducing the need for blood transfusions. It is administered either intravenously or subcutaneously in doses of 50 to 150 units/kg to normalize body hemocrit counts. Folex is methotrexate, the drug of choice for several types of tumors. INH is the acronym for isoniazid, a tuberculostatic antibacterial. Intron-A (interferon alfa-2a is a biotech drug used in the therapy of hairy cell leukemia and AIDS-related Kaposi's sarcoma. Lozol (indapamide) is an antihypertensive agent. *(1:939; 6:1312)*

13c. **(A)** Mylanta Liquid contains magnesium hydroxide, aluminum hydroxide, and simethicone. The use of magnesium hydroxide–containing products is commonly associated with the development of diarrhea because the magnesium ion creates an osmotic effect in the GI tract. Mylanta gelcaps and chewable tablets contain magnesium hydroxide and calcium carbonate. *(2a:208; 2b:131,138)*

13d. **(C)** Alendronate (Fosamax) is intended to stop bone loss or rebuild new bone, especially in women after menopause. The drug is irritating especially to the esophagus, which is why it is taken with 8 oz of water before food is consumed. The patient should remain standing or sitting for at least 30 min after taking the dose. It is not taken at bedtime because of possible irritation. *(10)*

13e. **(E)** The concomitant use of Tagamet and Mylanta may result in a decrease of Tagamet absorption. At least 1 hour should elapse between the administration of these two drug products. The use of antacids such as Mylanta with iron products is likely to result in a decrease in absorption of the iron because iron tends to precipitate in an alkaline medium. The concomitant use of cimetidine (Tagamet) and alprozolam (Xanax) will likely increase the activity of the Xanax because Tagamet has been shown to inhibit the metabolism of many of the benzodiazepines, including Xanax. *(2a:211; 7:991)*

13f. **(B)** Iron absorption may be somewhat increased by the coadministration of approximately 200 mg of ascorbic acid per 30 mg of elemental iron administered. This appears to be the result of ascorbic acid's ability to maintain iron in the ferrous state, a form that is more absorbable than the ferric state. *(2a:382)*

13g. **(C)** Feosol tablets contain exsiccated (dried) ferrous sulfate. The exsiccated form of ferrous sulfate contains approximately 30% elemental iron, considerably higher than that contained in hydrous ferrous sulfate or ferrous gluconate. *(5:1859,1865)*

13h. **(D)** Because of potential local irritation, the only form of injectable iron is iron dextran injection available as InFeD and Dexferrum. Dosage forms of ferrous sulfate include tablets (Feosol), oral drops (Mol-Iron and Fer-In-Sol), oral liquid (Mol-Iron), and an elixir (Feosol). *(3:69;7:495; 11:207)*

13i. **(C)** Patients who have iron deficiency anemia tend to have red blood cells that are microcytic, smaller than normal—and hypochromic, lacking in normal color. Megaloblastic cells are larger than normal cells. These are frequently seen in patients who have pernicious anemia. *(11:199)*

13j. **(A)** Ranitidine (Zantac) is also an H_2-receptor antagonist that diminishes acid secretion in the stomach. An advantage of ranitidine over cimetidine is its relative lack of effect on hepatic metabolism of other drugs. Because this patient is using alprazolam (Xanax), a drug metabolized by hepatic enzymes, the use of ranitidine is more logical. *(2a:213)*

13k. **(C)** A deficiency or impaired utilization of vitamin B_{12} and especially of folic acid may result in megaloblastic anemia. Other causes of the anemia include use of cytotoxins, such as the antineoplastics, or the immunosuppressive agents. *(11:209)*

13l. **(B)** Foods from animal sources such as eggs, dairy products, and especially liver contain vitamin B_{12}. Another source is shellfish. Vegetables and fruit do not contain the vitamin. Strict vegetarians may eventually experience vitamin B_{12} deficiency. *(7:501; 19:88–8)*

13m. (D) Pernicious anemia is a progressive disease caused by a lack of the intrinsic factor resulting in malabsorption of vitamin B_{12}. The condition affects more adult women, especially African American women, than men. Individuals living in temperate regions (North America or northern Europe) are more susceptible than are people living in the tropics. There also appears to be an increased rate in certain families, suggesting a genetic factor. *(11:212)*

13n. (D) Nicotrol transdermal patches are designed for 6 weeks of therapy. Nicoderm CQ patches are marketed in three strengths (21, 14, and 7 mg) with the intention of the patient decreasing the strength used over a 10-week course. Nicorette is a gum containing either 2- or 4-mg nicotine polacrilex. *(2a:719; 2b:411)*

PROFILE NO. 14

14a. (D) Most *Streptococcus* infections are sensitive to penicillin whereas *Staphylococcus* infections are not, with the exception of non-penicillinase-producing *Staphylococcus aureus*. *Pseudomonas*, fungus, and *Chlamydia* are not sensitive to either penicillin G or V. The main advantage of penicillin V when compared to penicillin G is its greater absorption from the GI tract. When given in comparable doses, penicillin V will reach plasma concentration levels two to five times those of penicillin G. *(6:1081)*

14b. (B) Pentids is Squibb's brand name for products containing penicillin G potassium. *(10)*

14c. (B) Routine use of pHisoHex has reduced the incidence and severity of pyogenic skin infections, especially those caused by gram-positive microorganisms, such as staphylococci. However, there is the possibility of superinfection of gram-negative microorganisms and *Candida*. *(1:1266; 10)*

14d. (B) Chlorhexidine gluconate is the active ingredient in Hibiclens and Hibistat. It possesses bacteriocidal activity against both gram-positive and gram-negative bacteria and the 4% solution is popular as a surgical scrub. It is a faster acting agent than is hexachlorophene. *(1:1265)*

14e. (D) The active ingredient in Cidex is glutaraldehyde, used mainly as a disinfectant. Chlorhexidine is present in Hibiclens, which is used as a skin cleanser. Peridex also contains chlorhexidine. It is an oral rinse for the prevention of oral infections in immunocompromised patients. *(1:1266; 10)*

14f. (D) Magnesium sulfate has been used internally as a saline laxative. Topically, hot-concentrated solutions are used as soaks or poultices in treating deep-seated infections. *(1:898)*

14g. (E) If 0.8 mL of water will dissolve 1 g of magnesium sulfate, one must simply determine how many grams 120 mL of water will dissolve.

$$\frac{1\,g}{0.8\,mL} = \frac{x\,g}{120\,mL}$$

$$x = 150\,g$$

(23:98)

14h. (C) Percogesic contains 325 mg acetaminophen and 30 mg phenyltoloxamine citrate per tablet. Phenyltoloxamine is classified as an antihistamine. *(2b:30)*

14i. (E) Pepto-Bismol contains bismuth subsalicylate, which appears to exert an antisecretory effect on intestinal mucosa and also binds both cytotoxins and enterotoxins. Doses of 60 mL or 2 tablets four times a day have been used prophylactically. If diarrhea occurs, doses of 30 mL every one-half hour for eight doses is used. *(2a:255; 11:528)*

14j. (C) The fluoroquinolones are very effective agents and are used when the causative microorganism has not been identified. TMP–SMZ and doxycycline are still used, although there are increased incidences of microbial resistance. *(11:528)*

14k. **(D)** Giardiasis is a protozoal infection caused by *Giardia lamblia*. It mainly affects the intestinal tract, causing diarrhea, other GI disorders, and profound malaise. The drug of choice is metronidazole, which is better tolerated than the alternative quinacrine. *(1:251; 19:71–8)*

14l. **(C)** The disease is caused by the spirochete *Borrelia burgdorferi*, carried by a tick. Serious cases can result in crippling arthritis. *(19:72–1)*

14m. **(C)** Doxycycline or tetracycline are first-line antibiotics in the treatment of Lyme disease. However, more serious cases are treated with intravenous ceftriaxone. *(19:17–3)*

14n. **(A)** Aspirin is an antiplatelet drug that blocks the production of thromboxane A2. Several studies have shown that daily doses of 320 mg or less are effective in reducing the incidence of transient ischemic attacks and myocardial infarctions, especially in men. Doses above 320 mg are not advocated because side effects such as bleeding may occur. *(6:1355,57)*

14o. **(A)** Many products have converted from kaolin to attapulgite because of its greater absorbent properties. *(2b:158)*

PROFILE NO. 15

15a. **(D)** The rate of metabolism for Dilantin has decreased, probably because of Tagamet's ability to inhibit the hepatic oxidative enzyme system. The symptoms reported by the medical staff are consistent with high blood levels of phenytoin. The daily doses of phenytoin should be reduced. Another solution would be the replacement of Tagamet with another H_2-receptor antagonist. *(5:991)*

15b. **(A)** Ataxia is the inability to coordinate muscles controlling voluntary movement. Atresia is the absence of a hole; aphasia indicates an impaired ability to communicate; dysarthria is a difficulty of speech; and dementia indicates mental deterioration. *(27:104, 147,149,410,474)*

15c. **(D)** Famotidine is Merck's Pepcid. Although the onset of action is similar to that of cimetidine, nizatidine, and ranitidine, it is more potent and has a longer duration of activity. It is effective in the treatment of duodenal ulcers, acute gastric ulcers, and Zollinger–Ellison syndrome. Both 20 and 40 mg tablets are available as well as a suspension and an injection. Nizatidine (Axid) is available as 150 and 300 mg capsules. Diflunisal is marketed as an anti-inflammatory agent under the tradename of Dolobid. *(1:1211; 19:23–6)*

15d. **(D)** Zollinger–Ellison syndrome is a pathologic hypersecretory condition caused by adenomas of the gastrin-producing islet cells of the pancreas. Patients with this condition experience persistent ulcer pain and diarrhea. The drug of choice for this is considered to be omeprazole. *(11:474)*

15e. **(E)** Because cimetidine is a competitive antagonist of the hepatic cytochrome P-450 oxidase system, there will be a delay in the metabolism of many benzodiazepines. Others such as lorazepam, oxazepam, and temazepam, are not affected because they are metabolized by glucuronidation. *(1:1831; 11:472)*

15f. **(A)** Individual patients may have to be titrated to alleviate symptoms. Daily doses of 900 to 1200 mg will maintain plasma lithium levels of 0.6 to 0.8 mEq/L. To obtain plasma levels of 1 mEq/L, daily doses of 1500 to 2400 mg may be necessary. Toxic symptoms usually manifest themselves when plasma levels are greater than 1.5 mEq/L. Blood sampling is performed 10 to 12 h after the last dose. Usually, it is convenient to draw the blood just before the morning dose. *(11:1109)*

15g. **(A)** The reported symptoms are mild effects that probably relate to peaks in lithium levels. The first approach in correcting the problem is to spread the doses further apart. *(11:1110)*

15h. **(A)** Lithium is usually considered to be the drug of choice in the treatment of acute manic episodes. Symptoms of this condition include delusions, irritability, hallucinations, polyuria, and polydipsia. Some of the first signs that signal manic episodes are euphoric moods with hyperactivity, excessive energy, and perceived need for little sleep. Lithium has been used in treating schizophrenia, but it is not the drug of choice. *(11:1108)*

15i. **(B)** Nosocomial infections are those that have been acquired during hospital stays. *(27:1063)*

15j. **(C)** Fluoxetine is marketed under the tradename of Prozac by Lilly for the treatment of major depression. *(10)*

15k. **(B)** Prozac's antidepressive effects are believed to be due to the drug's ability to prevent the reuptake of serotonin. It appears to be more selective in its serotonin to norepinephrine reuptake inhibition than are the tricyclic antidepressants. *(9:434:11:1103–08)*

15l. **(C)** Prozac's side effect of causing anorexia is being explored as a method for weight loss. Insomnia is expected to occur in a number of patients, but the drug appears to decrease heart rate slightly, not increase it. *(11:1103)*

15m. **(C)** Prozac is available as both 10 and 20 mg capsules (Pulvules) and as an oral liquid (20 mg/5 mL), but no parenteral dosage form is marketed. *(1:1191; 3:264; 10)*

15n. **(C)** Olanzapine (Zyprexa) is intended for the management of manifestations of psychotic disorders. Although side effects are manageable, patients should be warned of possible orthostatic hypotension, especially when the drug is initiated. Titration up to the optimum dose is necessary. The drug is administered once daily either with or without food. *(10)*

15o. **(C)** The SSRIs offer many advantages over other classes of antidepressants including the first two listed answers. However, many patients require 6 to 12 months of therapy to treat a depressive episode. Stopping the drug too soon will cause relapses. *(11:1108)*

15p. **(C)** Because the incidence of insomnia with Zoloft (sertraline) is much lower than with Prozac (fluoxetine), it may be dosed either in the evening or morning. Zoloft's elimination half-life is approximately 26 hours versus 100 to 700 hours for Prozac. However, the therapeutic dose of Zoloft is 50 to 100 mg versus 20 mg for Prozac. This fact is evident when one reviews the commercial oral dosage form strengths available. *(11:1103)*

PROFILE NO. 16

16a. **(D)** Conventional therapy of urinary tract infections with ampicillin requires treatment for 7 to 14 days. Apparently, Ms. Johnson discontinued therapy after a few days, probably because the symptoms subsided. She should be encouraged to take a full dosage regimen to clear the infection. *(7:758)*

16b. **(D)** When bacterial counts reach greater than 1×10^5, the condition is considered to be bacteriuria even if it is asymptomatic. *(11:1319)*

16c. **(A)** Large single doses of drugs have been employed successfully in treatment of UTIs in nonpregnant patients. Amoxicillin (Amoxil) 3 g has been recommended. Sulfamethoxazole and trimethoprim combinations (Septra or Bactrim) have been administered in daily doses of 1600 mg sulfamethoxazole plus 320 mg trimethoprim for 3 days. However, Ms. Johnson is allergic to sulfa drugs. The suggested dose of Furadantin is too low for single-dose therapy. *(11:1315)*

16d. **(C)** Both ascorbic acid and ammonium chloride have been used to acidify the urine with varying degrees of success. The pharmacist must be aware of other drugs being consumed because the acidic urine may affect renal clearance. *(11:1321)*

16e. **(D)** The sympathomimetic agent phenylpropanolamine has been found to be safe and effective for short-term weight control. The stimulant caffeine, acting as a thermogenic agent, may be effective in increasing physical activity with a corresponding expenditure of energy. *(11:1170–72)*

16f. **(D)** There is evidence that the hypothalamus contains a "satiety" center. Normal-weight individuals appear to have internal cues such as hunger sensation and response to caloric density of foods that reduce the overeating habit. The genetic factor is also important. Statistically, the incidence of obesity is greater in children when either or both of the parents were obese. Because obesity is often associated with neurotic traits, overeating is commonly considered to be a behavioral defect. Either anxiety or depression may cause a tendency for some individuals to overindulge in eating. *(11:1165–66)*

16g. **(C)** Bulimia is characterized by uncontrolled rapid ingestion of large amounts of food followed by self-induced vomiting. The individual often has bouts of self-loathing and depression. Desipramine, a tricyclic antidepressant, and fluoxetine have been used to treat bulimia. *(11:1175; 27:218)*

16h. **(B)** Both bulimia and anorexia nervosa are eating disorders. The most common trait of the individual suffering from anorexia nervosa is the feeling of being overweight even when actually underweight. Usually, such individuals refuse to eat normal meals. Pharmacists should counsel clients, especially young females, who may be using enemas, appetite suppressants, or ipecac syrup for unrealistic weight control. *(11:1173)*

16i. **(D)** Several oral OTC products such as Pediacon DX, Triaminicin, and Robitussin CF contain phenylpropanolamine (PPA) as the nasal decongestant. However, most OTC oral decongestant products contain pseudoephedrine, rather than PPA, as the decongestant. *(2a:142; 2b:90,94,104)*

16j. **(E)** Insomnia and restlessness are more likely to be experienced by patients consuming phenylpropanolamine. *(19:84–86)*

16k. **(B)** Lubriderm is an O/W emulsion that is pourable from a bottle. The added ingredients would not increase its viscosity significantly. Thus the final product is most likely to be classified as a lotion. Obviously both "shake well" and "external use only" labels must be attached to the container. *(10)*

16l. **(C)** The designation "aa qs" translates as "of each a sufficient quantity to make 1%." Therefore, 0.5% each of menthol and camphor is needed. (120 mL × 0.5% = 0.6 g) *(23:40)*

16m. **(A)** Incorporating the two solids, menthol and camphor, into a lotion is best accomplished if a liquid is first formed. Simple mixing of the two chemicals will result in an eutectic liquid, which would mix readily with the alcoholic coal tar solution (LCD). Additional alcohol is not needed. It is not advisable to use alcohol as a solvent in ointment formulas because the alcohol may slowly migrate to the ointment surface, carrying dissolved drugs with it. There is no need to add polysorbate 80 to the product because it is already present in the LCD as a dispersing agent. *(1:874)*

16n. **(E)** Coal tar solution contains 20% coal tar in an alcoholic solvent. Coal tar, especially in combination with UV radiation, has been successful in the treatment of psoriasis. The combination is known as the Goeckerman regimen. *(2a:556)*

16o. **(C)** Coal tar is a photosensitizer. It increases a patient's tendency to sunburn for up to 24 h after application. The patient's medication record should also be reviewed for other photosensitizers such as the phenothiazines and tetracyclines. Coal tar is relatively safe when included in shampooing products partially because of the short contact period. There are several shampoos on the market, including Ionil T, Polytar, and Zetar. *(2a:556)*

PROFILE NO. 17

17a. **(E)** On reviewing the lab reports, the pharmacist concludes that none of the other conditions are present. The white blood count is within normal values (5000 to 10,000 cells/mm^3). The normal hemoglobin for males is 14 to 18 g/dL, and the hematocrit only slightly low (range of 40% to 54%). Diabetes is suspected when serum glucose levels are above 120 mg/dL. Both the BUN and serum creatinine values are normal. *(1:502,512–13)*

17b. **(B)** Clinical data suggest that administration of an antibiotic 1 to 2 h before surgery will reduce the incidence of postsurgical infections significantly. Usually one of the cephalosporins on formulary is prescribed. *(11:1453)*

17c. **(B)** Although an IV cephalosporin is indicated for most surgical procedures, it may be combined with neomycin for additional coverage. Another combination would be oral erythromycin and neomycin, 1 g of each, for a total of three doses before colorectal surgery. The dosage regimen greatly reduces the incidence of infection. *(11:1453)*

17d. **(C)** PEG/Electrolyte Lavage Solutions such as GoLYTELY are intended as a bowel evacuation and completely flush out the GI tract prior to surgery. The product is provided as a powder concentrate and reconstituted usually to a 4 L volume. The entire amount is to be consumed by the patient over a relatively short period of time—240 mL every 10 min. *(2a:237; 11:1404; 24:238)*

17e. **(C)** Both Aminosyn and FreAmine are standard formulas containing essential and nonessential amino acids. NephrAmine is a specially designed formula intended for use in renally impaired patients. It contains a mixture of the essential amino acids, but none of the nonessential amino acids except histidine. NephrAmine is significantly more expensive than are the other two products. *(3:36)*

17f. **(A)** TPN solutions are intended for slow parenteral infusion by either central administration through the subclavian vein or by peripheral administration through smaller veins. However, the TPN formula listed for this patient is very hypertonic, which precludes peripheral routes because the small veins may be damaged. Glucose concentrations of 10% or more should not be infused peripherally. *(11:183)*

17g. **(A)** The patient's chloride levels were 120 mEq/L, which is above the normal range of 98 to 109 mEq/L. Although it is possible to monitor blood pH, the pharmacist should suggest that potassium and sodium acetates be used in place of the respective chlorides. The "1 vial" designation for MVI refers to the standard 10 mL product. *(11:128,139)*

17h. **(A)** 500 mL amino acid solution × 8.5% = 42.5 g of amino acids. Because the average amount of nitrogen in amino acids is 16%, 42.5 g × 16% = 6.8 g of nitrogen. *(11:182)*

17i. **(A)** 500 mL dextrose × 40% = 200 g of dextrose.
200 g dextrose × 3.4 cal/g = 680 kcal.
(11:185)

17j. **(C)** TPN formulas should provide sufficient nonprotein calories to convert the amino acids present to lean body mass. A ratio of nonprotein calories to each gram of nitrogen (NPC:N) has been established. For most patients, a value of 150:1 is ideal, with a range of 125 to 175:1 acceptable. In stressed patients, such as burn victims, a 100 to 1 ratio may be used. When lower ratios are used, either other sources of calories must be employed (ie, body fats) or some of the amino acids will be used as calories. *(11:182)*

17k. **(C)** EFAD is a deficiency of essential fatty acids. Liposyn III is a parenteral fatty oil emulsion that will provide the linoleic acid needed in humans for cell membrane synthesis and stabilization. EFAD is characterized by scaly skin, alopecia, poor wound healing, and thrombocytopenia. *(11:185)*

17l. (C) Parenteral fatty oil emulsions are available in both 10% and 20% mixtures. Each milliliter of 10% emulsions gives 1.1 kcal, whereas each milliliter of 20% emulsions contributes 2 kcal. Therefore, 500 mL of 20% emulsion × 2 kcal/mL = 1000 kcal. If one did not know the exact calories present, the value could be estimated knowing that every gram of oil has approximately 9 calories. Thus: 500 mL × 20% = 100 g oil; 100 g oil × 9 kcal = 900 kcal. *(11:185)*

17m. (E) Patients experiencing delayed healing of wounds or burns have responded to therapeutic doses of zinc. *(22:276)*

17n. (D) Legionnaires' disease occurs mainly in the summer when the airborne gram-positive *Legionella pneumophilia* is present. Many victims are older males, especially smokers with chronic lung disease. *(11:1276)*

17o. (B) Aggressive treatment with erythromycin is usually necessary. An alternate choice is the tetracyclines or oral rifampin may be added to the therapy. *(11:1276)*

PROFILE NO. 18

18a. (D) Long-term therapy for treatment of Graves' disease includes either propylthiouracil or methimazole. The disease involves a hyperfunctional goiter, with clinical symptoms similar to that of thyrotoxicosis. Propylthiouracil is not used for this condition. *(11:1519)*

18b. (D) A regimen of chemotherapy known as MOPP is used in the treatment of Hodgkin's disease. Procarbazine (Matulane) and prednisone are given by the oral route on each day of the 14-day schedule. Mechlorethamine (Mustargen) and vincristine (Oncovin) are given intravenously on the first and eighth days of therapy. Experience has shown that combining drugs that have different mechanisms of action increases remission rates and lowers the incidence and severity of side effects. *(11:1625)*

18c. (A) Hepatocellular, bronchogenic, and pancreatic carcinomas have shown poor responses to presently used chemotherapeutic drugs. Ovarian and prostatic carcinomas are moderately responsive, with palliation and probable prolongation of life. Prolonged survival and probably some cures are expected in patients with testicular cancer and Hodgkin's disease. *(11:1552–54)*

18d. (B) Vincristine is available as a ready-to-use solution (1 mg/mL) in 1-, 2-, and 5-mL vials and 1- and 2-mL disposable syringes. It is intended for intravenous administration. It is never administered by the intramuscular, subcutaneous, or intrathecal routes. *(21:1091)*

18e. (B) Mechlorethamine is a potent vesicant. Serious localized damage may occur if the drug solution seeps into the area surrounding the infusion site. The thiosulfate ion will react with the nitrogen mustard. Cold compresses will relieve the burning sensation and slow the spread of mechlorethamine. Other solutions that have been infused are normal saline and sodium bicarbonate. *(19:91–12)*

18f. (A) A 1 molar solution of sodium thiosulfate will contain 248 g of chemical in 1 L of solution. A 1 normal strength will contain $\frac{248}{2}$ = 124 g. A one-sixth normal solution will contain $\frac{124}{6}$ = 21 g/L or 2.1 g/dL. *(1:1211)*

18g. (A) Although the official form of sodium thiosulfate contains five waters of hydration, the correct amount of active ingredient can be obtained by using the anhydrous form. Simply subtract 90 (weight of water in the molecule) from 248 to obtain 158 (the weight of anhydrous sodium thiosulfate), then follow the procedure outlined in Answer 18f. *(23:307)*

18h. (D) The dictionary defines nadir as the place or time of deepest depression. When discussing drug chemotherapy, the term usually refers to the length of time before maximum bone marrow depression occurs. Many oncologic drugs, especially the alkylating agents, cause a depression characterized by low leukocyte counts with increased susceptibility to infections. For example, the nadir for a given drug may be 7 to 10 days after the start of therapy, with bone marrow recovery in 14 to 18 days. *(6:1259)*

18i. **(E)** Bone marrow suppression is often the dose-limiting factor for toxicity during chemotherapy. Vincristine appears to have little effect on bone marrow. *(11:1621)*

18j. **(C)** Because neoplastic cells have properties similar to normal cells, it is virtually impossible to develop an antineoplastic agent that will not attack normal cells. Consequently, the antineoplastic drugs have very low therapeutic indexes, sometimes less than 1.0. *(7:29; 24:45)*

18k. **(C)** Cyanocobalamin injection (Redisol, Rubramin PC) is a pink-colored solution available in strengths of 30, 100, and 1000 µg/mL. It is administered by either IM or subcutaneous injection, but not IV. The injection route offers better bioavailability than oral administration. *(1:1125; 6:1331)*

18l. **(C)** Women that are on estrogen therapy for symptoms of menopause appear to have a lower incidence of osteoporosis. Doses of 0.625 mg are effective. It is well established that daily supplements of calcium, a minimum of 1500 mg, are also useful. Fibrous products such as psyllium may help maintain intestinal motility but do not prevent osteoporosis. *(11:1734; 19:46-29)*

18m. **(E)** Brompheniramine maleate is available as Dimetane tablets (4 mg). Chlorpheniramine is available as Chlor-Trimeton 4 mg tablets and Teldrin 4 mg tablets or prolonged release 12 mg capsules. Clemastine fumarate is now available OTC as Tavist liquid (0.5 mg/5 mL) and tablets (1.34 and 2.68 mg). *(2b:68,76,102)*

18n. **(C)** Advantages of dosing with astemizole (Hismanal 10 mg tablets) or terfenadine (Seldane 60 mg tablets) are that drowsiness or sedation are extremely rare. Seldane is avail-

able as 60 mg tablets given twice daily. Increasing the dose of Seldane does not increase its activity. A significant advantage of the drug is that it does not potentiate the action of alcohol, diazepam, or CNS depressants. *(11:886)*

18o. **(D)** Transdermal estradiol patches deliver 50 or 100 mg of estradiol, which is equivalent to 0.625 or 1.25 mg of Premarin in the prevention of postmenopausal symptoms and osteoporosis. Transdermal administration avoids early liver metabolism. The patches are replaced twice a week. *(19:46–31; 24:368)*

PROFILE NO. 19

19a. **(A)** Adria's Adriamycin is marketed in vials containing either 10 or 50 mg of powder for reconstitution. The drug is also available under the tradename of Rubex (Bristol). *(1:1249; 6:1265)*

19b. **(D)** Both doxorubicin and cyclophosphamide cause alopecia in a significant number of patients. *(5:2436)*

19c. **(E)** The nadir for the drug is approximately 10 to 15 days after administration. Recovery from the leukopenia occurs in about 20 days. Cardiomyopathy is a delayed, cumulative, dose-related adverse effect. *(1:1249; 5:2440)*

19d. **(B)** The patient weight is 140 lb

$$140 \text{ lb} \times \frac{1 \text{ kg}}{2.2 \text{ lb}} = 64 \text{ kg}$$

Because 700 mg of cyclophosphamide is being given, $\frac{700 \text{ mg}}{64 \text{ kg}} = 11 \text{ mg/kg}$. *(23:67)*

19e. **(A)** Almost all patients receiving cisplatin experience nausea and vomiting. Metoclopramide (Reglan) is administered in doses of 1 to 2 mg/kg approximately 30 min before cisplatin and every 2 h after cisplatin injection to control emesis. Reglan is also used orally to increase upper GI tract motility. Oral administration 30 min before meals will prevent gastroesophageal reflux. *(5:757–58)*

19f. **(B)** The elevated creatinine value (normal = 1 mg/dL) indicates renal damage. Cisplatin can cause proximal renal tubular damage that is not completely reversible. It is advisable to either discontinue the cisplatin or reduce the dosage while carefully monitoring the patient for acute renal failure. *(11:418)*

19g. **(B)** Bone marrow depression is the usual dose-limiting factor of cyclophosphamide therapy. High doses frequently result in sterile hemorrhagic cystitis. Patients should be counseled to maintain a high level of fluid intake and void frequently. Cytoxan is available as both tablets and injection forms. *(6:1239; 11:634)*

19h. **(D)** High serum levels of methotrexate will result in passive diffusion of the drug into normal cells. To avoid the resulting cytotoxic effects on normal cells, an injection of leucovorin is administered approximately 24 h after the methotrexate injection. Leucovorin is also used in treating megaloblastic anemia. It is administered by intramuscular injection. *(11:916)*

19i. **(C)** Methotrexate is sometimes given intrathecally because the drug does not normally enter the cerebrospinal fluid except if given at high levels (>1 g/m^2). Thiotepa is poorly absorbed from the GI tract. Because it is not a vesicant, it can be administered intravenously, by bladder irrigation, and intrathecal injection. *(1:1256)*

19j. **(A)** Progressive dose-related hepatotoxicity may occur in patients on long-term therapy with methotrexate. Oral weekly doses of methotrexate (7.5 mg) have been successful in reducing the symptoms of rheumatoid arthritis. The potential for toxicity has been reduced by giving leucovorin 1 day after the methotrexate dose. *(5:547)*

19k. **(D)** Vials of lyophilized powder are available as Folex (Adria). Both 2.5-mg tablets and a Solution for Injection (2.5 mg/mL) in 2-mL vials are available from Lederle. *(1:1256)*

19l. **(D)** Kytril as 1-mg tablet and injection (1 mg/mL) is administered at doses of 10 μg/kg prior to chemotherapy. Zofran as 4 and 8-mg tablet or injection (2 mg/mL) is dosed at 8 mg prior to surgery or chemo, then repeated 4 and 8 h after surgery then every 8 h for 1 or 2 days. Dronabinol, the active ingredient in marijuana, is only available in gelatin capsules (2.5, 5, and 10 mg). It is administered 1 to 3 h before chemotherapy, then every 2 to 4 h for a total of 4 to 6 doses per day. It has also been found effective as an appetite stimulant. *(3:259)*

19m. **(E)** All the listed drugs are appropriate. Another drug used for breast cancer is the anti-estrogen Tamoxifen. It is important to reduce doses of mercaptopurine to 25% of normal when allopurinol is being used. *(1:1255,1831; 6:1252,1260–62)*

19n. **(A)** The antihypertensive enalapril maleate (Merck's Vasotec) is available as 5-, 10-, and 20-mg tablets, with usual maintenance dosing of 10 to 40 mg daily. *(11:708)*

19o. **(C)** Vasotec is an angiotensin-converting enzyme (ACE) inhibitor. *(11:708)*

19p. **(C)** Several of the ACE inhibitors cause the unusual side effect of an occasional dry and nonproductive cough. Patients should also be warned of incidences of hypotension, especially during the first few days of therapy. The drugs also appear to increase alertness and produce mood elevation. Vasotec does not cause reflex tachycardia. *(10; 11:715)*

PROFILE NO. 20

20a. **(E)** The 30-day supply of HCTZ appears to have been dispensed only once with tablets depleted by April 1. Either Mr. Tralor has had the prescription filled elsewhere or is not complying with the once-daily dosing. This may explain why Dr. Lange has issued a new prescription for the stronger acting verapamil. Mevacor is available in several strengths (10-, 20-, and 40-mg tablets). Verapamil may increase digoxin levels by 50% to 70% during the first week of therapy. Monitoring of the patient may be necessary. *(1:1833; 14:481; 19:1315)*

20b. **(B)** Verapamil is a calcium entry or calcium channel blocker used as an antihypertensive agent, antianginal, and antiarrhythmic. It is available as both regular tablets and controlled release dosage forms. The products may be given with food. *(1:966)*

20c. **(B)** The term circadian relates to a biologic variation or rhythm with a cycle of 24 h. Searle's Covera-HS capsules provide a controlled onset of action coupled with extended release of drug. The 180- or 240-mg tablet is taken at bedtime with a significant amount of drug released in the morning when the highest blood level is desired because at this time the patient is at greatest risk. Additional amounts of drug are released over the next 24 h. *(10; 27:309)*

20d. **(A)** When drugs such as verapamil have significant differences between the oral and parenteral doses administered, there are several explanations. One is poor absorption from the GI tract. Another is that the drug undergoes significant first-pass effect, usually due to rapid metabolism by the liver. Because this occurs before the drug reaches sites of activity, the oral dose must be relatively high as compared to the intravenous dose, which avoids the first-pass effect. Another drug example is propranolol, which has an IV dose of 4 mg compared to the oral dose of 40 to 80 mg. *(1:966; 19:13–17)*

20e. **(E)** Taking Mevacor with the evening meal appears to maximize the GI absorption of the drug. *(19:9–16)*

20f. **(C)** A fast disintegration time for tablets indicates that the tablet has broken into smaller pieces, which allows the dissolution process

to occur. The fastest disintegration occurred with brand D, followed by brand C. However, brand C dissolved faster than brand D. Because dissolution is critical for drug absorption and is usually the rate-limiting step, brand C probably has the greatest bioavailability. *(1:594)*

20g. **(E)** Niacin is one of the most economical drugs in attempting to reduce blood triglycerides and cholesterol. It causes the catabolism of low-density lipoproteins (LDL). Pyridoxine is used to treat peripheral neuritis. *(11:399; 19:9–14)*

20h. **(D)** The vasodilation effect of niacin causes peripheral flushing that may last up to 1 h after administration. The drug may also irritate the stomach, causing abdominal discomfort. The flushing and pruritus can be prevented by administration of 325 mg of aspirin 30 min before the niacin. *(11:399)*

20i. **(B)** Screening is usually based on total cholesterol, with a targeted goal of less than 200 mg/dL (5.17 mM/L in the nonfasting adult). People with higher cholesterol levels should have their LDL value calculated by determining their triglyceride and high-density lipoprotein (HDL) while in the fasting state. Hyperlipidemia is closely associated with increase incidences of CHD (coronary heart disease). *(11:387,392)*

20j. **(D)** High levels of LDL and VLDL (very low–density lipoproteins) indicate a high atherosclerotic risk. Patients with LDL values greater than 130 mg/dL should consider both dietary changes and possible drug therapy. For example, patients should limit their intake of meats (up to 6 oz per day of lean red meat or chicken with the skin removed is permissible). HDL appears to be a scavenger of cholesterol and protects arteries from deposition of cholesterol. Generally, a LDL-/HDL ratio of less than 3.0 is ideal. *(11:392)*

20k. **(E)** When comparing the dosing regimen of the listed drugs, simvastatin (Zocor) has the lowest dosing regimen—5 to 40 mg daily—which is reflected in the tablet strengths available (5-, 10-, 20-, and 40-mg). Lovastatin (Mevacor) has the next lowest dose—20 mg daily—with 10-, 20-, and 40-mg tablets marketed. The remaining drugs were cholestyramine (Questran)—4 g t.i.d.; colestipol (Colestid)—15 g daily; and gemfibrozil (Lopid)—300 mg b.i.d. *(3:171; 11:398)*

20l. **(C)** Weak acidic compounds such as warfarin, digoxin, and penicillin will bind to cholestyramine and colestipol. Bile acids also bind. This is the mechanism by which the resins exert their activity. *(11:339)*

20m. **(C)** Although the depressant effects of alcohol may occur at lower blood levels, mental impairment and loss of motor coordination is obvious in most individuals once blood alcohol levels exceed 0.1%. The major problem with alcohol metabolism is the limited supply of enzymes for the oxidation procedure. Therefore, alcohol may be described as mainly following zero-order kinetics with limited amounts metabolized each hour. *(11:1180)*

20n. **(C)** Deficiencies in thiamine (vitamin B_1) may result in Wernicke's syndrome or Korsakoff's syndrome characterized by peripheral neuropathy and confusion. Depletion of folic acid leads to moderate or severe anemia. Folic acid has been a valuable supplement for pregnant women in the prevention of fetal spina bifida. *(1:1118; 11:1191)*

PROFILE NO. 21

21a. **(A)** Hypothyroidism (myxedema) is characterized by the slowing of body processes because of a deficiency of thyroid hormone. The classic treatment was thyroid tablets. Today, this drug has been replaced with L-thyroxine (T_4), L-thyronine (T_3), and liotrix (a mixture of T_4 and T_3). Synthroid is levothyroxine sodium (L-thyroxine). Graves' disease is a form of hyperthyroidism (thyrotoxicosis). *(11:333)*

21b. **(E)** Omission of a single dose of Synthroid will not have significant effects on the disease state. *(10)*

21c. **(B)** Acesulfam, aspartame, and saccharin are artificial sweeteners that are 200, 180, and 400 times sweeter, respectively, than sucrose. The agents are used in many dietary foods and in some pharmaceuticals. The use of saccharin in place of 1 teaspoonful of sugar saves the consumer 33 calories. Because of a weak relationship between saccharin and cancer in animals, a warning label is required in stores selling foods or beverages containing saccharin. Similar relationships between acesulfam and aspartame have not been established. *(2a:335; 24:128–30)*

21d. **(C)** The tannins in teas may react with iron to form insoluble iron tannates. It is well established that many antacids combine with iron, thereby reducing the absorption of iron. *(11:201)*

21e. **(D)** Amantadine is a selective antiviral agent for prophylactic action (200 mg daily) against influenza **A**, but **not B**. It is also useful in reducing the signs and symptoms of Parkinson's disease, in which it augments dopamine release. Amantadine can be used as the sole agent or with levodopa. Amantadine is available in both 100-mg capsules and syrup (50 mg/5 mL) under the tradename of Symmetrel. *(1:1034; 3:290)*

21f. **(C)** Although there is some patient-to-patient variation, one of the earliest signs of Alzheimer's disease is the forgetfulness of current events; for example, what one has eaten for lunch. Although gradual, this memory loss becomes progressively worse. *(11:1804)*

21g. **(D)** Ergoloid mesylates (Hydergine), an ergot drug, has been used for several years in attempts to improve patients' memories and increase the feeling of well being. Tacrine (Cognex) is a cholinesterase inhibitor that has reduced the clinical symptoms of Alzheimer's. Selegiline is available as Eldepryl and is used in the treatment of parkinsonism. *(1:1007,1038; 11:1802–04)*

21h. **(D)** Tacrine is usually dosed at 10 mg four times a day and increased to 20 mg if necessary. The pharmacist should inform the patient to take the drug on an empty stomach because food decreases the drug's absorption significantly. The most serious side effect of tacrine is abnormal liver function as reflected in elevated transaminase. Fortunately, the condition is usually reversible. *(1:1828; 11:1802; 19:102–6)*

21i. **(D)** Normally, the patient would be counseled to take digoxin in the morning to assure compliance. However, she is taking an antacid in the morning and at night that may interfere with digoxin absorption. Suggest that the digoxin be taken either at noon or in the morning, separated by 2 hours from the antacid. *(19:23–9)*

21j. **(C)** Women, especially postmenopausal women, should increase their intake of calcium to avoid osteoporosis. Tums is available as 500-mg of calcium carbonate per chewable tablet, 750-mg chewable tablets (Tums E-X) and 1000-mg chewable tablets (Tums Ultra). Although calcium carbonate can be used in the prevention of gastroesophageal reflux (GERD), there are better products on the market and the dosing regimen would be after each meal as well as at bedtime. *(2b:256; 3:293)*

21k. **(A)** Many of the elderly have an increase in the relative amount of fat in their bodies, partially because of dehydration and less activity. The corresponding volume of distribution for lipophilic drugs may increase. Renal clearance rates are often lower in the elderly because of impaired kidney function. The plasma albumin levels are sometimes lower than normal, thereby effecting the amount of protein binding. *(6:50)*

21l. **(C)** If both dosage forms had 100% bioavailability (F value of 1.0), the answer would be 5 mL.

$$\frac{0.05 \text{ mg}}{1 \text{ mL}} = \frac{0.25 \text{ mg}}{x \text{ mL}}$$

$$x = 5 \text{ mL of elixir}$$

However, not all of the drug is available as reflected in the "F" values of 0.6 for the tablet and 0.75 for the elixir. Therefore,

$$[Q_1] [C_1] = [Q_2] [C_2]$$

$$[0.25 \text{ mg}] [0.6] = [x \text{ mg}] [.75]$$

$$x = 0.2 \text{ mg of digoxin needed}$$

Since the elixir contains 0.05 mg per mL

$$\frac{0.05 \text{ mg}}{1 \text{ mL}} = \frac{0.2 \text{ mg}}{x \text{ mL}}$$

$$x = 4 \text{ mL of elixir}$$

(23:201)

21m. **(A)** Many of the elderly exhibit digoxin toxicity by experiencing a hazy vision rather than the more classic halo and color vision changes that occur in the younger population. Rather than having an increase in appetite, anorexia often occurs. *(11:744)*

21n. **(E)** All of the choices decrease digoxin's volume of distribution and renal clearance rate. It is usually necessary to reduce the digoxin by 50%. *(6:817; 11:743)*

PROFILE NO. 22

22a. **(C)** The term tocolytic refers to a drug that will reduce uterine contractility, thereby preventing premature birthing. *(19:44–23)*

22b. **(B)** Terbutaline is available under the trade names of Brethine (Geigy) and Bricanyl. To inhibit preterm labor, it is administered orally, SC, or IV. However, its greatest market is as a bronchodilator. A second agent that has been very successful for tocolytic therapy is ritodrine (Yutopar) which can be given either orally or IV. *(1:998; 19:44–23)*

22c. **(D)** The medication order calls for 25 μg of drug per minute. The pharmacist added 2 mL (2 mg or 2000 μg) to 250 mL of diluent.

$$\frac{2000\ \mu g}{250\ mL} = \frac{25\ \mu g}{x\ mL}$$

$$x = 3.125\ mL$$

$$\frac{15\ gtt}{1\ mL} = \frac{x\ gtt}{3.125\ mL}$$

$$x = 46.8\ \text{drops per minute}$$

(23:180)

22d. **(B)** The total amount of drug present is 2000 μg. It is being administered at a rate of 25 μg/min.

$$\frac{250\ mL}{x\ min} = \frac{3.125\ mL}{1\ min}$$
$$x = 80\ min$$

(23:182)

22e. **(E)** Elastomeric containers contain an elastic balloon that is filled with sterile solution. They slowly but constantly collapse, thus providing a steady volume of drug at zero-order kinetics solution through a small diameter infusion line. Syringe pumps are used in many institutions in place of standard infusion pumps. The pharmacist simply fills syringes instead of infusion bags. PCA stands for "patient-controlled analgesia." Although originally designed for slow infusion of analgesic solutions, it is currently used for many other infusion solutions. *(13:171,483)*

22f. **(C)** Barium sulfate is used to render the intestinal tract opaque for x-rays. A dose of 60 to 250 g is administered as a suspension. *(1:1370)*

22g. **(E)** Barium sulfate is practically insoluble in water; thus, there is little danger of toxicity from systemic absorption of the chemical. It is administered either orally or rectally, depending on the portion of the GI tract to be x-rayed. *(1:1370)*

22h. **(B)** Atropine is classified as an antimuscarinic/antispasmodic agent used to inhibit salivation and other excessive secretions during surgery. It may also prevent cholinergic effects such as cardiac arrhythmias, hypotension, and bradycardia during surgery. An al-

ternative drug is glycopyrrolate (Robinul) which may be administered 30 min prior to surgery for action similar to that of atropine. It is also available as oral tablets (1 and 2 mg) to suppress gastric secretions for the treatment of peptic ulcers. *(1:1020,1025)*

22i. **(B)** The usual adult dose of atropine is 0.4 mg SC, IM, or even IV. Atropine sulfate and chlorpromazine HCl (Thorazine) will be compatible in a syringe. The purpose of chlorpromazine is to relieve presurgical apprehension and control nausea and vomiting during surgery. *(1:1021,1182)*

22j. **(A)** Because of their sizing and use, urinary catheters bear a federal warning concerning dispensing without a prescription. Ostomy pouches are available in several sizes and designs, but the consumer may purchase them, as well as bandages and dressings, without a prescription. *(1:1863–66)*

22k. **(B)** The active ingredient in Metamucil is the bulk former psyllium. Some psyllium-containing products contain sucrose for sweetening. A pharmacist may wish to counsel diabetics away from this type of product to one that contains an artificial sweetener such as aspartame; for example, Orange Flavor Metamucil Instant Mix. *(1:899; 2b:149)*

22l. **(A)** Bulking agents such as Metamucil should be dispersed in water or a flavored vehicle such as orange juice, stirred quickly, then drunk immediately. Otherwise the powder will swell, forming a gel that would be difficult to swallow. *(2a:232)*

22m. **(B)** Both Slo-Bid and Theo-Dur contain anhydrous theophylline for the prevention of asthma. Slo-Bid consists of timed-release capsules (50, 100, 200, and 300 mg), whereas Theo-Dur is available as sustained-action tablets and sustained-action capsules. *(10)*

22n. **(D)** The centrally acting beta-2 agonist methyldopa (Aldomet) is the most commonly used antihypertensive during pregnancy. Other alternatives include labetalol (Normodyne or Trandate) or hydralazine (Apresoline). *(19:44–17)*

PROFILE NO. 23

23a. **(B)** The active ingredient in Monistat-7 is miconazole, an antifungal agent effective against numerous species, including *Candida albicans* and *Trichophyton mentagrophytes*, which infect the vagina and the foot, respectively. Monistat-7 consists of suppositories for vaginal insertion. Many products containing miconazole are now OTC as 2% creams, powders, and sprays. *(2a:95–96)*

23b. **(B)** With the successful treatment of gonorrhea with either penicillin or tetracyclines, other causes of sexually transmitted urethritis have emerged. More than 50% of cases of nongonorrheal urethritis are caused by the obligate intracellular parasite *Chlamydia*. *(11:1392)*

23c. **(D)** Syphilis is usually transmitted by direct contact with an active lesion containing spirochetes. Although there are several stages and types of syphilis, the drug of choice is still parenteral penicillin, such as 2.4 million units of benzathine penicillin G. For patients allergic to penicillin, tetracycline is used. *(11:1396)*

23d. **(C)** Chlamydia is usually asymptomatic in females, whereas males experience dysuria. Primary treatment will be either doxycycline 100 mg twice a day for 7 days or azithromycin as a single 1000-mg dose. Alternatives include erythromycin or ofloxacin 400 mg b.i.d. Ciprofloxacin has been used but is not as successful as doxycycline. *(11:1393)*

23e. **(C)** Oral contraceptives appear to be the best method to avoid conception, followed by intrauterine devices (IUDs). *(2a:117; 19:43–4, 43–28)*

23f. **(C)** White Vaseline or any petrolatum product is not acceptable as a lubricant for either condoms or diaphragms, because small openings will develop due to the solvent characteristics of petrolatum toward rubber. *(2a:120)*

23g. **(C)** Skin implants such as Norplant offer long-term contraceptive protection. Six capsules are implanted subcutaneously into the upper arm. A constant rate release of 20 to 30 µg of levonorgestrel occurs daily. The implants appear to be even more effective than are oral contraceptives. *(2a:118; 19:43-19; 24:223)*

23h. **(A)** The testicular hormone danazol (Sanofi Winthrop's Danocrine) is given orally in 100- to 200-mg doses to treat endometriosis, a condition characterized by menstrual-like bleeding and localized inflammation and pain, usually within the pelvis. A second drug successful in the treatment of endometriosis is Nafarelin acetate (Synarel), which is available as an intranasal spray. *(1:1102)*

23i. **(B)** Obsessive–compulsive disorder (OCD) is an anxiety disorder characterized by compulsions such as a fear of dirt or microorganisms, recurrent fear that a stove has not been shut off, constant checking to see if lights have been turned off, or having persistent thoughts that one might injure a loved one. *(11:1076)*

23j. **(A)** The antiobsessional drug clomipramine (Ciba's Anafranil), is a tricyclic antidepressant related to imipramine (Tofranil). Its mode of action in the treatment of OCDs is believed to be that it inhibits reuptake of serotonin. Dosing has to be carefully adjusted to avoid adverse effects, especially seizures. *(11:1079)*

23k. **(C)** Methylphenidate (Ritalin) is classified as a centrally acting sympathomimetic. It is used in the therapy of attention deficit hyperactivity disorder. *(11:1077–79)*

23l. **(E)** The benzodiazepines exert their antianxiety effects by potentiation of the inhibitory neurotransmitter GABA. *(11:1077)*

23m. **(E)** Therapy with clozapine should be reserved for severely ill schizophrenic patients. Although the drug has many valuable attributes, blood monitoring is necessary. One serious side effect is the development of agranulocytosis. *(11:1128)*

23n. **(D)** The incidence of extrapyramidal effects (EPS), including tardive dyskinesia, is minimal with clozapine, especially when compared with other psychiatric drugs. *(11:1128)*

23o. **(D)** Risperidone (Risperdal) is an antipsychotic drug used for many of the same conditions as clozapine. Although there is a lower incidence of agranulocytosis, there is an increase in EPS. Clonazepam is used to treat petit mal, and the other choices are antidepressants. *(3:267; 11:1078)*

PROFILE NO. 24

24a. **(D)** These two microorganisms are major causes of both ear infections and sinusitis. A third microorganism often implicated is *Moraxella catarrhalis*. *(11:953)*

24b. **(D)** Other appropriate antibiotics include erythromycin + sulfisoxazole, loracarbef (Lorabid), and amoxicillin + potassium clavulanate (Augmentin). *(11:953)*

24c. **(B)** All three drugs possess antipyretic activity. However, Jason is sensitive to salicylates and neither aspirin nor ibuprofen (to which he may also be sensitive) should be dispensed. The newer OTC agents such as naproxen and ketoprofen carry label warning that they should not be used in young children unless under a physician's supervision. *(2a:60,67–68)*

24d. **(C)** Ibuprofen is 2 (p-isobutylphenyl) propionic acid. *(1:1223)*

24e. **(A)** Fever may be the sign of a serious systemic infection. If the fever is masked by the use of an antipyretic, prompt treatment may be delayed. *(2a:56)*

24f. **(A)** Amount of cromolyn needed for Rx is 30 mL × 2.5% = 0.75 g. The amount of the available 4% solution to use:

$$\frac{4\,g}{100\,mL} = \frac{0.75\,g}{x\,mL}$$

$$x = 19\,mL \text{ (which is already isotonic)}$$

Therefore, the pharmacist must make only the remaining 11 mL isotonic.

11 mL × 0.9% NaCl = 0.099 g, or 99 mg
(23:149; 24:398–401)

24g. **(A)** Removal of bacteria and fungi from extemporaneously prepared solutions may be accomplished by passage through a 0.20- or 0.22-micron filter into a sterile container. *(1:1478; 24:296)*

24h. **(C)** "OS" or "sinister eye" translates as left eye. *(23:40)*

24i. **(B)** Ophthalmic solutions containing cromolyn sodium have been effective in treatment of allergic conjunctivitis. Chronic allergic conjunctivitis patients should also avoid using OTC sympathomimetic decongestants, which may cause rebound vasodilation. A second agent that offers more rapid relief is Iodoxamide 0.1% ophthalmic solution. *(1:1229; 11:946)*

24j. **(C)** Tofranil in doses of 25 mg 1 h before bedtime reduces the incidence of childhood enuresis. If unsuccessful, the dose may be increased up to 75 mg. *(1:1191)*

24k. **(B)** Diphenhydramine (Benadryl) is a well-known antihistamine exhibiting drowsiness as a major side effect. It is sometimes prescribed as a sleep aid and is available in several commercial OTC sleep aid products including Compoz, Sominex, and Unisom. *(2b:125–127)*

24l. **(D)** Because of the limited capacity of the eye surface, separating the 2 drops by a few minutes will increase the amount of solution that actually enters and remains in the eye. Blocking the passageway between the eye and nose will reduce the amount of drug lost interiorly through the tear duct. *(24:396,409)*

24m. (C) The tympanic thermometer is a device, the tip of which is placed gently in the ear and a sensor receives infrared emission from the tympanic membrane. A digital readout of temperature occurs in approximately 3 sec. TENS refers to transcutaneous electrical nerve stimulation. TENS devices are worn on the body, usually to relieve pain. *(1:1861–62; 2a:54)*

24n. (A) Debrox drops contain carbamide peroxide, which will soften ear wax, easing its removal. S.T. 37 is a mouthwash and topical anti-infectant with hexylresorcinol as the active ingredient. Anbesol is used in the treatment of cold sores and contains both benzocaine and phenol. *(2b:302–03,368)*

24o. (E) Tartrazine (F.D. & C. Yellow #5) is included in both solid and liquid products. A percentage of the general population is sensitive to the dye and may respond with typical allergic responses. There appears to be a high incidence of cross allergies in individuals sensitive to aspirin and to tartrazine. *(2a:60; 24:132)*

PROFILE NO. 25

25a. (A) Gout is a chronic metabolic disease characterized by hyperuricemia. The uric acid is an end product of protein catabolism. Either uric acid production has increased or impaired renal clearance is slowing the removal. The immediate concern during an acute attack is to relieve pain. Only after this relief should longer term therapy be initiated. *(11:611; 19:40–2)*

25b. (D) To relieve an acute attack, an anti-inflammatory drug (NSAID) or colchicine is administered. Colchicine is most effective if given within the first 12 to 36 h of the acute attack.

Allopurinol is reserved for patients who appear to be refractory to colchicine or the NSAIDs. *(11:611; 19:40–4)*

25c. (A) Allopurinol (Zyloprim) is the most commonly used agent for long-term control of chronic gout and is the drug of choice for patients that are overproducers of uric acid. Not only does allopurinol inhibit xanthine oxidase, which converts xanthine to uric acid, but allopurinol's metabolite, oxypurinol, also inhibits xanthine oxidase. *(1:1219; 11:617)*

25d. (C) Sufficient liquid intake of at least 2 L daily is necessary to prevent formation of xanthine calculi. Acute attacks of gout may occur on initial therapy; therefore, colchicine therapy should be continued for a few days. Because of possible stomach irritation, it is best to take allopurinol with food. *(1:1220; 10; 11:611)*

25e. (A) Antacids appear to increase the absorption of levodopa. Because levodopa dosing for Parkinson's is usually by titration, either the addition or discontinuation of concurrent antacids may change plasma levels of levodopa significantly. Most drugs decrease the effectiveness of levodopa, the classic being pyridoxine (B6), which speeds the transformation of levodopa to dopamine before it can cross the blood–brain barrier. There is evidence that combination products such as Sinemet are less affected by pyridoxine than is pure levodopa. *(2a:211; 19:40–4)*

25f. (C) Combinations of aluminum and magnesium hydroxides are very effective antacids. The combination also reduces the constipation effect of aluminum and the laxative effect of magnesium. The greatest risk is in renally impaired patients who may not be able to excrete magnesium ions readily. *(2a:207; 2b:137)*

25g. (E) Minoxidil was originally marketed as Loniten, an antihypertensive agent. However, one side effect was stimulation of hair growth. The drug was further developed for the treatment of alopecia. Its greatest success is with males younger than 40 years of age who have had thin hair or baldness for less than 10 years. *(1:947; 6:1612)*

25h. **(C)** Loniten is available as 2.5- and 10-mg tablets. A topical 2% solution is marketed as Rogaine. *(1:947)*

25i. **(D)** The prescribed dose was 0.6 mg/kg/h. Because the patient weighs 160 lb:

Step 1. $160 \text{ lb} \times 1 \text{ kg}/2.2 \text{ lb} = 77 \text{ kg}$

Step 2. $77 \text{ kg} \times 0.6 \text{ mg/kg} = 46.2 \text{ mg/h}$

Step 3. $\dfrac{500 \text{ mg}}{1000 \text{ mL}} = \dfrac{46.2 \text{ mg}}{x \text{ mL}}$

$x = 92.4 \text{ mL/h}$
or 1.5 mL/min

Step 4. $\dfrac{15 \text{ gtt}}{1 \text{ mL}} = \dfrac{x \text{ gtt}}{1.5 \text{ mL}}$

$x = 22.5 \text{ gtt}$

(23:180)

25j. **(A)** The half-life of theophylline in smokers is 4 to 5 h, as compared to 7 to 9 h in non-smokers. Infusion rates of 0.7 mg/kg/h are needed, as compared to 0.4 mg/kg/h in non-smokers. Aminophylline is the ethylenediamine salt of theophylline, and therefore has only 85% of the potency. The desired serum levels of theophylline are between 10 and 20 μg/mL. *(1:973; 11:663)*

25k. **(E)** Because ranitidine does not interact with hepatic cytochrome P-450, it has minimal effect on the pharmacokinetics of theophylline. All of the other choices inhibit the metabolism of theophylline, thereby increasing its half-life. *(11:662–665)*

25l. **(C)** If the rate of initial distribution is not greater than the rate of elimination, two slopes will not be evident when the plasma drug levels are plotted on graph paper. Half-lives of drugs are not directly related to whether a one- or two-compartment model is present. The half-life relates to the clearance of the drug. *(17:72)*

25m. **(E)** A faster heartbeat is a fairly early sign of theophylline overdosing. It is actually more reliable than are nausea and anorexia, which do not occur in all patients. *(1:973; 11:662)*

25n. **(C)** Phenytoin will increase the clearance of theophylline resulting in an approximate 40% drop in expected serum levels. Interferon decreases theophylline clearance significantly, resulting in a 100% increase in activity. Allopurinol and alcohol decrease clearance by approximately 25%. Propranolol and cimetidine inhibit cytochrome P-450, requiring that theophylline dosing be reduced. *(7:993; 11:664; 14:568)*

25o. **(E)** Rifampin (Rifadin or Rimactane) discolors urine, sweat, and tears. The drug's major use is in the treatment of tuberculosis, usually in combination with isoniazid or pyrazinamide. *(1:1316; 11:1291)*

PROFILE NO. 26

26a. **(B)** Both amitriptyline (Elavil) and nortriptyline (Pamelor) are tricyclic antidepressants. Compazine is a phenothiazine, Nardil is a monoamine oxidase inhibitor, and Clozaril and Loxitane are antipsychotic agents. *(7:455)*

26b. **(E)** Hirsutism, or abnormal growth of hair, has not been reported as a significant adverse effect of Elavil. *(19:76–12; 10)*

26c. **(C)** Patients using Lithobid should be advised to consume 8 to 12 glasses of water daily. This will stabilize lithium levels in the blood and prevent lithium toxicity. *(3:268; 10)*

26d. **(A)** Adverse reactions to lithium rarely occur when serum lithium levels are below 1.5 mEq/L. Mild to moderate toxic reactions may occur at a level of 1.5 to 2.5 mEq/L, and severe toxicity is seen above these levels. *(11:1110; 14:502)*

26e. **(A)** The addition of HydroDIURIL to this patient's regimen is likely to increase serum lithium levels because when sodium is depleted from the body, the body will conserve lithium, thereby resulting in lithium accumulation. *(11:1111; 14:507)*

26f. **(C)** Blood samples are drawn just prior to taking a dose, because lithium levels will be steady at that time and will represent the trough value for lithium. *(14:503)*

26g. **(B)**

$$300 \text{ mg} = \frac{(x \text{ mEq}) (74)}{2}$$

$$x = 8 \text{ mEq}$$

(23:157)

26h. **(E)** Hydrochlorothiazide (HydroDIURIL) is an example of a thiazide diuretic. *(1:1045)*

26i. **(E)** Triazolam (Halcion) is an ultrashort hypnotic with a half-life of 2 to 3 h. It is the least likely of any of the benzodiazepines to produce a morning hangover; however, it does produce short-term amnesia in some patients. *(19:74–6)*

26j. **(E)** Ambien and Halcion both have an onset of action of less than 30 min and half-lives of 2 to 5 h. Thus, a patient will fall asleep quickly, and the drug wears off before waking. Prosom and Restoril have an onset of 1 to 2 h with half-lives of 10 to 20 h. *(19:74–8)*

26k. **(D)** Azulfidine (sulfasalazine) is used in the treatment of ulcerative colitis. Usually 1 to 2 g of drug is needed daily. *(1:1277)*

26l. **(C)** Sulfasalazine (Azulfidine) is usually administered for ulcerative colitis in doses of 500 mg q.i.d. A second drug, olsalazine (Dipentum), may also be used. It is a topical anti-inflammatory agent that forms 5 aminosalicylic acid in the intestines. *(1:1277; 10)*

26m. **(A)** Amiloride blocks reuptake of lithium into cells of the distal tubules and collection ducts. Other drug classes such as the ACE inhibitors significantly increase lithium levels by 100% to 200%. *(11:1111–12)*

26n. **(B)** Anticholinergic action such as that caused by diphenhydramine or doxylamine

include constipation. A major symptom of prostatitis is restricted urinary flow. *(2a:183)*

26o. **(E)** PSA refers to the prostate-specific antigen, which as a glycoprotein product is almost exclusively produced by prostate epithelial cells. Routine determination of PSA allows comparison of newer values to the individual's baseline value. Increases indicate the possibility of prostate cancer. *(19:4–12)*

26p. **(D)** Mitrolan tablets contain calcium polycarbophil, which possesses both laxative and antidiarrheal properties. It quickly binds water in the GI tract, thus reducing fluidity by forming a bulk. *(2:325,350)*

PROFILE NO. 27

27a. **(A)** All of the choices are nonsteroidal anti-inflammatory drugs (NSAIDS). *(3:251)*

27b. **(E)** NSAIDS have analgesic and antipyretic action, which is believed to be related to their ability to inhibit cyclooxygenase activity and prostaglandin synthesis. *(3:251)*

27c. **(C)** Advil is a nonprescription brand of ibuprofen. Ibuprofen is usually administered three to four times daily, although more frequent administration may be required in some cases. Antacids may be taken with ibuprofen to increase its GI tolerance. *(2a:66)*

27d. **(D)** Mylanta is an antacid containing aluminium hydroxide, magnesium hydroxide, and simethicone. Simethicone is included in the formulation to dispel gas, which may otherwise accumulate in the stomach. *(3:296)*

27e. **(C)** Piroxicam is available as the brand Feldene. *(3:251m)*

27f. **(E)** Piroxicam (Feldene) is a relatively long-acting NSAID that requires only a single daily 20-mg dose for most patients. *(3:251m)*

27g. (D) Auranofin (Ridaura) is an oral gold product used to treat rheumatoid arthritis that cannot be managed effectively or safely by NSAIDS and other more conservative forms of therapy. *(3:254c)*

27h. (C) Misoprostol is a synthetic prostaglandin analog that has both antisecretory activity and mucosal protective properties. It is employed primarily in preventing NSAID-induced gastric ulcers. *(3:305h)*

27i. (A) Misoprostol is contraindicated for use during pregnancy and is classified as a pregnancy category X drug by the US Food and Drug Administration. *(3:305h)*

27j. (D) Anacin is an OTC analgesic product containing 400 mg of aspirin and 32 mg of caffeine in each tablet. *(2b:33)*

PROFILE NO. 28

28a. (C) Digoxin is a cardiac glycoside that produces a negative chronotropic effect (slowed heart rate), a positive inotropic effect (greater force of contraction), and a vagomimetic effect on the heart. *(5:242)*

28b. (D) Most patients using digoxin will experience a slowed heart rate (negative chronotropic effect). *(5:242)*

28c. (E) Amrinone (Inocor), although not a digitalis glycoside, is a positive inotropic agent. *(5:232)*

28d. (D) Digitoxin is a cardiac glycoside suitable for use in patients with renal impairment because most digitoxin is cleared by the liver. The other cardiac glycosides currently available are cleared primarily by the kidneys. *(5:243)*

28e. (C) Lanoxicaps are liquid-filled capsules that contain a solution of digoxin in polyethylene glycol. Because the digoxin is already in solution, the Lanoxicap dosage form provides greater bioavailability of digoxin than is

achieved from digoxin tablets. A dose of 0.25 mg (250 µg) of digoxin from a tablet dosage form is equivalent to 0.2 mg (200 µg) from the Lanoxicap dosage form. *(3:142b)*

28f. (C) Digoxin toxicity is characterized by nausea and vomiting, diarrhea, disorientation, and ventricular tachycardia. *(5:245)*

28g. (B) If amiloride (Midamor) is substituted for Lasix in this patient's regimen, the patient should no longer receive the potassium supplement Klorvess because amiloride is a potassium-sparing diuretic and the administration of the combined agents will result in hyperkalemia. *(3:138f)*

28h. (E) Klorvess is a potassium supplement available in a variety of different dosage forms, including effervescent granules and tablets as well as a solution. *(3:16)*

28i. (A) Torsemide (Demadex) and furosemide (Lasix) are both loop diuretics. Midamor and Dyrenium are potassium-sparing diuretics, and Diamox is a carbonic anhydrase inhibitor. *(3:138c)*

28j. (B) The patient appears to be noncompliant because he received a month's supply of digoxin but did not get a refill until about 1 1/2 months later. *(10)*

PROFILE NO. 29

29a. (E) Diphenhydramine (Benadryl) is an ethanolamine antihistamine with both sedative and antipruritic properties. *(2a:140)*

29b. (B) Pyrethrins, one of the active ingredients in RID, is a parasite neurotoxin that is used for the treatment of human lice and scabies. *(2a:585)*

29c. (B) When RID Shampoo is used, it is essential that the product not come in contact with the eyes because it can cause significant irritation. RID should not be used on the face or on open cuts or excoriated areas of the body. *(3:585)*

29d. **(D)** The term "pediculus" refers to lice. *Pediculus capitis* refers to head lice, whereas *Pediculus pubis* refers to pubic lice. *Sarcoptes scabiei* is the organism that causes scabies. The term "tinea" refers to a type of fungal organism. *(27:1153)*

29e. **(E)** RID Shampoo is generally administered once. After working it thoroughly into the shampood and dried hair, it remains in place for 10 minutes and is then worked into a lather with water. It is then rinsed well from the hair, and the hair is towel-dried and combed to ensure the removal of any remaining nit shells. Retreatment may occur after 7 days if there is still evidence of living lice at that time. *(3:585a)*

29f. **(E)** Diprosone Cream contains 0.05% betamethasone dipropionate in a hydrophilic emollient base. *(3:590a)*

29g. **(E)** Diprosone Cream or any other potent corticosteroid topical product should not be used on areas of the skin that are infected by bacteria, fungi, or a virus because the corticosteroid will inhibit the body's defense mechanisms and potentially cause spreading of the infection. *(3:590a)*

29h. **(C)** Both Nix (permethrin) and A-200 Pyrinate (pyrethrins, piperonyl butoxide, and petroleum distillate) are available for OTC use. Eurax (crotamiton) is available only by prescription. *(3:585a)*

29i. **(A)** Pyrethrin-containing products should be avoided by people with ragweed allergy because pyrethrins are plant derivatives that may precipitate a hypersensitivity reaction in such patients. *(2a:658)*

29j. **(B)** Scabies is a skin condition caused by the mite *Sarcoptes scabiei*. The mite burrows into the skin and causes severe itching and excori-

ation of the affected area. Lindane and crotamiton are effective drugs for the treatment of scabies. *(2a:659)*

PROFILE NO. 30

30a. **(C)** Naloxone is a pure narcotic antagonist that, when administered parenterally, rapidly reverses the effects of opioid narcotic agents such as heroin. Because it has no agonist action of its own, there is no danger in administering this agent to an unconscious patient even if the source of drug toxicity is unknown. *(3:709a)*

30b. **(E)** Heroin is diacetylmorphine. Codeine is methylmorphine, whereas dionin is ethylmorphine. *(6:527)*

30c. **(C)** Pneumocystis carinii pneumonia (PCP) is a condition seen commonly in AIDS patients. It is an opportunistic infection that emerges when the immune system of a patient is suppressed by disease or drugs. *(5:2368)*

30d. **(D)** Zidovudine or azidothymidine (AZT) is an antiviral agent commonly used in the management of patients with HIV infection who have evidence of impaired immunity. The drug is available by the brand name Retrovir. *(5:2361)*

30e. **(D)** Patients on Retrovir are at risk of developing granulocytopenia or anemia that may require discontinuation of the medication or blood transfusions. It is therefore important to monitor the patient's hematologic status closely while on Retrovir therapy. *(3:873)*

30f. **(E)** Retrovir capsules are administered every 4 hours around the clock, even though it may interrupt normal sleep. This is necessary because of the rapid absorption and rapid clearance of the drug from the body. *(3:873)*

30g. (C) Acetaminophen use may competitively inhibit the glucuronidation of zidovudine (Retrovir). This may increase the likelihood of granulocytopenia developing with the use of Retrovir. *(6:1206)*

30h. (C) Pentamidine isethionate (Pentam 300, NebuPent) is an agent that is useful in the treatment of Pneumocystis carinii pneumonia. It is available as an injectable product that may be administered intravenously or intramuscularly and as an aerosol solution administered by inhalation using a nebulizer. *(3:411b)*

30i. (E) Patients receiving pentamidine must be monitored for a variety of serious adverse effects, including sudden, severe hypotension that may occur after a single parenteral dose. Other adverse effects include hypoglycemia, bronchospasm, and cough. *(3:411b)*

30j. (D) Robitussin DM is an OTC product used for the treatment of cough. It contains guaifenesin, an expectorant, and dextromethorphan HBr, a cough suppressant. *(2b:94)*

--- **CHAPTER 8** ---

Practice Test

You have come a long way to get here. You have completed hundreds of test items and have studied 30 medication profiles and records. This practice test should confirm what you may already feel— that is, confidence that your time and effort have been well spent. You should set aside about 2 hours of uninterrupted time to take this test. You should be able to answer 80 or more Practice Test questions without guessing, because most test the same competencies that you mastered in previous chapters.

Of course, the Practice Test is also a learning and self-assessment experience. Correct answers will build your confidence in the knowledge base that you have developed. Incorrect answers will enable you to focus on specific areas that may require more time for you to master. Good luck!

Questions

DIRECTIONS (Questions 1 through 100): Each of the numbered items or incomplete statements in this section is followed by answers or by completions of the statement. Select the ONE lettered answer or completion that is BEST in each case.

1. One course of fluorouracil therapy is 6 mg/kg twice a day for 4 days. How many mg will be given daily to a 140-lb patient?

   (A) 380 mg
   (B) 48 mg
   (C) 3040 mg
   (D) 1500 mg
   (E) 760 mg

2. According to the National Bureau of Standards (NBS), the initial calibration mark on a 250-mL graduate should be

   (A) 10 mL
   (B) 25 mL
   (C) 50 mL
   (D) 75 mL
   (E) 100 mL

3. The most common type of drug transport in humans is

   (A) active transport
   (B) Newtonian transport
   (C) facilitated transport
   (D) passive transport
   (E) pinocytosis

4. Which of the following agents may be classified as an angiotensin-II antagonist?

   (A) Lisinopril
   (B) Minoxidil
   (C) Guanadrel
   (D) Losartan
   (E) Gemfibrozil

5. Which of the following is NOT a common adverse effect associated with the use of tricyclic antidepressants?

   (A) Urinary retention
   (B) Sedation
   (C) Orthostatic hypotension
   (D) Dry mouth
   (E) Hirsutism

6. An elixir contains 100 µg of drug per teaspoon dose. How many mg are present in each mL?

   (A) 0.02 mg
   (B) 0.025 mg
   (C) 0.1 mg
   (D) 2.0 mg
   (E) 20 mg

7. Patients with phenylketonuria (PKU) should avoid food products containing

   (A) aspartame
   (B) medium-chain triglycerides
   (C) soy protein
   (D) sodium chloride
   (E) unsaturated fats

8. Generic product A has a greater AUC than generic product B, containing the same quantity of drug per dose. One can conclude that

(A) product B is more bioavailable than is product A

(B) product A is more bioavailable than is product B

(C) product A has a shorter half-life than is product B

(D) product B has a shorter half-life than is product A

(E) product A is more readily excreted in the urine than is product B

9. Which one of the following drugs will NOT cause miosis of the pupil when instilled in the eye?

(A) Echothiophate

(B) Carbachol

(C) Physostigmine

(D) Pilocarpine

(E) Homatropine

10. Misoprostol (Cytotec) can best be described as a(an)

(A) ulcer-adherent complex

(B) anticholinergic

(C) H_2-receptor antagonist

(D) synthetic prostaglandin analog

(E) abortifacient

11. A hospital pharmacist adds 100 mL of alcohol USP (95% V/V ethanol) to 1 L of cough syrup that contains 8% V/V ethanol. What is the new percentage of ethanol present in the mixture?

(A) 10%

(B) 12%

(C) 14%

(D) 16%

(E) 18%

12. Which of the following needles is most suited for the administration of insulin products?

(A) 16G $^5/_8''$

(B) 21G $^1/_2''$

(C) 21G $^5/_8''$

(D) 25G 1''

(E) 25G $^5/_8''$

13. Assuming first-order kinetics, the characteristic that readily allows the calculation of time to reach plasma steady-state is the drug's

(A) AUC

(B) half-life

(C) absorption constant

(D) elimination constant

(E) F value

14. Midamor is most similar in action to

(A) Demadex

(B) HydroDIURIL

(C) Midazolam

(D) Dyrenium

(E) Lasix

15. A patient with an abnormally elevated number of erythrocytes is said to have

(A) macrocytic anemia

(B) polycythemia

(C) sickle cell anemia

(D) aplastic anemia

(E) microcytic anemia

16. A dietician adds 5 g of potassium chloride to 500 mL of an enteral formula. How many milliequivalents of potassium are present? (K = 39; Cl = 35.5; KCl = 74.5)

(A) 25 mEq

(B) 45 mEq

(C) 67 mEq

(D) 128 mEq

(E) 134 mEq

17. The agent most likely to precipitate when added to D5W or NS is

(A) tetracycline HCl (Achromycin V)

(B) ethacrynic acid (Edecrin)

(C) tobramycin sulfate (Nebcin)

(D) phenytoin sodium (Dilantin)

(E) ascorbic acid

18. Sodium bicarbonate is likely to increase the rate of urinary elimination of

    I. phenobarbital sodium
    II. penicillin G potassium
    III. cocaine HCl

    (A) I only
    (B) III only
    (C) I and II only
    (D) II and III only
    (E) I, II, and III

19. Which one of the following cephalosporins has the greatest activity against gram-negative microorganisms?

    (A) Cefaclor (Ceclor)
    (B) Ceftizoxime (Zefizox)
    (C) Cefonicid (Monocid)
    (D) Cefazolin (Ancef, Kefzol)
    (E) Cephalexin (Keflex)

20. Peripheral veins are SELDOM used for the administration of

    (A) electrolyte infusions
    (B) cephalosporins
    (C) vitamin infusions
    (D) heparin
    (E) TPN solutions

21. How many mL of glycerin would be needed to prepare 1 lb of an ointment containing 8.5% (W/W) glycerin? The density of glycerin is 1.25 g/mL.

    (A) 10.6
    (B) 18.5
    (C) 30.9
    (D) 32.6
    (E) 48.2

Questions 22 through 25

Questions 22 through 25 are based on the following order received from a hospital outpatient clinic:

> For: Happy Hospital Ophthalmology Clinic
>
> **Rx**
> Atropine sulfate   0.25%
> Boric acid   1.0%
> Pur. Water qs   60 mL
>
> Please make isotonic and sterilize. Label as "Atropine sulfate 0.25% ophthalmic solution."

22. Boric acid is present in the formula as a (an)

    I. chelating agent
    II. viscosity builder
    III. antimicrobial preservative

    (A) I only
    (B) III only
    (C) I and II only
    (D) II and III only
    (E) I, II, and III

23. How many milligrams of sodium chloride are required to adjust the tonicity of the formula? (The following "E" values are available: atropine sulfate = 0.20; boric acid = 0.50.)

    (A) 210 mg
    (B) 330 mg
    (C) 425 mg
    (D) 540 mg
    (E) 900 mg

24. The most practical method for sterilizing this ophthalmic solution is

    (A) autoclaving for 15 min
    (B) autoclaving for 30 min
    (C) membrane filtration through an 5-μ filter
    (D) membrane filtration through a 0.2-μ filter
    (E) the use of ethylene oxide gas

25. Kwell Lotion is indicated for the treatment of conditions caused by

    I. tinea versicolor
    II. *Pediculus capitis*

III. *Sarcoptes scabiei*

(A) I only
(B) III only
(C) I and II only
(D) II and III only
(E) I, II, and III

26. An administration set delivers 50 drops to the mL. How many drops per minute are needed to obtain 12 units of heparin per minute if the IV admixture contains 10,000 units of heparin per 500 mL of normal saline?

(A) 40
(B) 60
(C) 20
(D) 600
(E) 30

27. Which one of the following would be likely to render benzalkonium chloride solution inactive?

(A) Acetic acid
(B) *Pseudomonas aeruginosa*
(C) Ethanol
(D) Sodium chloride
(E) Sodium stearate

28. Fick's law is related to

(A) diffusion
(B) viscosity
(C) pediatric dosage
(D) adsorption
(E) buffers

29. The naturally occurring enkephalins, endorphins, and dynorphins are chemically classified as

(A) alkaloids
(B) peptides
(C) phospholipids
(D) polysaccharides
(E) prostaglandins

30. A drug approved by the FDA for the treatment of enuresis is

(A) furosemide (Lasix)
(B) imipramine (Tofranil)
(C) nitrofurantoin (Macrodantin)
(D) nadolol (Corgard)
(E) hydroxyurea (Hydrea)

31. How many milliliters of a 1:150 stock solution of atropine sulfate would be needed to prepare the following prescription?

Rx	
Atropine sulfate	0.5%
Normal saline	qs. 30.0 mL

(A) 45.0 mL
(B) 15.0 mL
(C) 22.5 mL
(D) 66.7 mL
(E) 17.8 mL

32. The Henderson–Hasselbalch equation can be used to determine the pH of a

I. mixture of lactic acid and sodium lactate
II. 0.15 mole/L hydrochloric acid
III. 2% morphine sulfate solution

(A) I only
(B) III only
(C) I and II only
(D) II and III only
(E) I, II, and III

33. A high F value for a drug indicates that the drug is

(A) chemically unstable
(B) very soluble in water
(C) very bioavailable
(D) susceptible to hepatic first-pass metabolism
(E) renally eliminated

34. The product Sinemet 25/100 contains

(A) carbidopa 25 mg + levodopa 100 mg
(B) carbidopa 100 mg + levodopa 25 mg
(C) HCTZ 25 mg + propranolol 100 mg
(D) HCTZ 25 mg + triamterene 100 mg
(E) HCTZ 100 mg + triamterene 25 mg

35. A drug commonly employed in the treatment of acute morphine overdose is

(A) physostigmine
(B) EDTA
(C) chlordiazepoxide
(D) naloxone
(E) disulfiram

36. How many grams of hydrocortisone powder must be added to 2 lb of 1% W/W hydrocortisone cream to obtain a 4% W/W cream?

(A) 20 g
(B) 23 g
(C) 27 g
(D) 28 g
(E) 38 g

Questions 37 through 39

Answer questions 37 through 39 based on the following prescription:

> **Rx**
> | Phenylephrine HCl | 0.5% |
> | Menthol | |
> | Thymol | aa 2.0% |
> | Methyl salicylate | 0.5% |
> | Mineral oil | qs 30 mL |
>
> Sig: gtt ii both sides t.i.d.

37. Which of the following ingredients will NOT dissolve in the prescribed solvent?

I. Phenylephrine HCl
II. Methyl salicylate
III. Menthol

(A) I only

(B) III only
(C) I and II only
(D) II and III only
(E) I, II, and III

38. This prescription is intended for use in the

(A) eyes
(B) lungs
(C) ears
(D) nose
(E) buccal cavity

39. In compounding this prescription, which of the following would be useful to employ?

(A) Fusion
(B) Levigation
(C) Eutexia
(D) Trituration by intervention
(E) Emulsification

40. An order for a TPN formula requests 500 mL of D30W. How many milliliters of D50W may be used if D30W is not available?

(A) 200 mL
(B) 300 mL
(C) 400 mL
(D) 500 mL
(E) 600 mL

41. The decay constant of a radioisotope is 0.69/h. The half-life of the radioisotope is

(A) 100 h
(B) 14 h
(C) 10 h
(D) 1 h
(E) 69 h

42. Which of the following is true of active transport systems?

I. They do not consume energy.
II. They never become saturated.
III. They do not reach equilibrium.

(A) I only
(B) III only

(C) I and II only
(D) II and III only
(E) I, II, and III

43. Which of the following agents are useful in the treatment of patients who are HIV positive and show signs of immunological deficiency?

   I. Acyclovir
   II. Zidovudine
   III. Pentamidine isethionate

   (A) I only
   (B) III only
   (C) I and II only
   (D) II and III only
   (E) I, II, and III

44. Patients with gluten intolerance should avoid foods containing

   (A) eggs
   (B) wheat
   (C) tyramine
   (D) milk
   (E) fats

45. A pharmacist has 80 mL of a 1.5% benzalkonium chloride solution. What will be the final ratio strength if this solution is diluted to 1500 mL with purified water?

   (A) 1:125
   (B) 1:1250
   (C) 1:100
   (D) 1:1875
   (E) 1:2250

46. Which of the following are mixtures containing both aluminum hydroxide and magnesium hydroxide?

   I. Maalox Suspension
   II. Mylanta Suspension
   III. Tums Chewable Tablets

   (A) I only
   (B) III only
   (C) I and II only

(D) II and III only
(E) I, II, and III

47. The peak of the serum concentration vs. time curve approximates the time when

   (A) the maximum pharmacologic effect occurs
   (B) all of the drug has been absorbed from the GI tract
   (C) absorption and elimination of the drug has equalized
   (D) saturation of metabolizing enzymes has occurred
   (E) renal elimination of the drug begins

48. The pharmacist should advise a patient who has just received a prescription for prazosin 2 mg t.i.d. to take the initial dose

   (A) at noon
   (B) at bedtime
   (C) in the morning before breakfast
   (D) in the morning after breakfast
   (E) 1 hour before the evening meal

49. A disease characterized by inflammation of layers of the intestinal tract is

   (A) Bright's disease
   (B) Goeckerman's disease
   (C) Graves' disease
   (D) Crohn's disease
   (E) Cushing's disease

50. Which one of the following pharmaceutical adjuvants is most likely to cause asthma-like reactions?

   (A) Benzalkonium chloride
   (B) Benzyl alcohol
   (C) Edetate
   (D) Sodium bisulfite
   (E) Methylparaben

51. A drug is said to have a biologic half-life of 2 hours. At the end of 8 hours, what percentage of the drug's original activity will remain?

    (A) 6.25%
    (B) 12.5%
    (C) 25%
    (D) 50%
    (E) 2.5%

52. Bupropion is used as an

    (A) anticholinergic
    (B) immunosuppressant
    (C) antidepressant
    (D) antipsychotic
    (E) anti-inflammatory agent

Questions 53 through 56

Questions 53 through 56 refer to the following prescription:

For: David Harris	Age: 14
Rx	
Codeine phosphate	90 mg
Diphenhydramine	900 mg
NAPAP	2500 mg
Ft. Cap. #12	
Sig: 1 q.i.d. p.r.n. pain	

Note: The pharmacist has 50-mg diphenhydramine capsules, each containing 130 mg of powdered contents, as well as $\frac{1}{4}$-grain codeine phosphate tablets, each weighing 90 mg. The NAPAP is available as a pure powder.

53. Which of the following statements concerning this prescription is (are) true?

    I. The amount of codeine being consumed per dose is an overdose.
    II. There is a chemical incompatibility between diphenhydramine and codeine phosphate.

    III. The patient should be cautioned about the possibility of drowsiness from the capsules.

    (A) I only
    (B) III only
    (C) I and II only
    (D) II and III only
    (E) I, II, and III

54. The final weight of each capsule will be approximately

    (A) 270 mg
    (B) 410 mg
    (C) 340 mg
    (D) 180 mg
    (E) 450 mg

55. Aminophylline injection is likely to be compatible with which of the following parenteral solutions?

    I. Heparin
    II. Verapamil
    III. Dopamine

    (A) I only
    (B) III only
    (C) I and II only
    (D) II and III only
    (E) I, II, and III

56. Which of the following stimulate red blood cell production?

    I. Neupogen
    II. Leukine
    III. Procrit

    (A) I only
    (B) III only
    (C) I and II only
    (D) II and III only
    (E) I, II, and III

57. A tine test is employed in identifying patients who have been exposed to

(A) acquired immunodeficiency syndrome (AIDS)

(B) influenza

(C) tuberculosis

(D) hepatitis virus

(E) herpes simplex

58. Nifedipine is classified as a (an)

(A) narcotic antagonist

(B) antihistamine

(C) narcotic agonist

(D) beta-adrenergic receptor blocker

(E) calcium entry blocker

59. A patient is using hydrochlorothiazide (HydroDIURIL) and guanethidine (Ismelin) for the treatment of hypertension. This patient should not receive

(A) potassium supplementation

(B) antihistamines

(C) aluminum-containing antacids

(D) folic acid supplementation

(E) tricyclic antidepressants

60. Which one of the following is an example of an absorption base?

(A) Polyethylene glycol ointment

(B) Cold cream

(C) Jelene

(D) Eucerin

(E) White petrolatum

Questions 61 through 66

Answer questions 61 through 66 based on the following prescription:

```
Rx
  Burow's solution          10 mL
  Salicylic acid            4%
  Phenol                    1%
  White petrolatum          qs 60 g

  Sig: apply to affected area t.i.d.
```

61. The active ingredient in Burow's solution is

(A) aluminum hydroxide

(B) acetic acid

(C) aluminum chloride

(D) calcium hydroxide

(E) none of the above

62. When preparing this prescription the pharmacist may wish to include

I. alcohol

II. polysorbate 80

III. Aquaphor

(A) I only

(B) III only

(C) I and II only

(D) II and III only

(E) I, II, and III

63. The most appropriate way to incorporate salicylic acid into this product is by

(A) levigation

(B) fusion

(C) dissolution in alcohol

(D) trituration

(E) attrition

64. The concentration (% W/W) of Burow's solution in the final preparation will be

(A) 10

(B) 16.7

(C) 22.5

(D) 20.0

(E) 13.4

65. Which of the following may be employed as one of the ingredients of this prescription?

(A) Carbolic acid

(B) Aspirin

(C) Thymol

(D) Salicylamide

(E) Lactic acid

66. The function of salicylic acid in this product is as a (an)

    (A) preservative
    (B) local anesthetic
    (C) keratolytic
    (D) analgesic
    (E) abrasive

67. Which one of the following may be considered a viral disease?

    (A) Pertussis
    (B) Tuberculosis
    (C) Hepatitis
    (D) Cholera
    (E) Typhoid fever

68. Retinoic acid is used therapeutically

    (A) by the oral route only
    (B) to accelerate the production of epithelial cells in the skin
    (C) to reverse the symptoms of psoriasis
    (D) to promote healing of actinic keratoses
    (E) to treat malignant melanoma

69. Which of the following drugs is (are) indicated for the treatment of gout?

    I. Lamotrigine (Lamictal)
    II. Probenecid (Benemid)
    III. Sulfinpyrazone (Anturane)

    (A) I only
    (B) III only
    (C) I and II only
    (D) II and III only
    (E) I, II, and III

70. Oxidation will cause solutions of which of the following to turn pink?

    I. Epinephrine
    II. Milrinone acetate
    III. Streptokinase

    (A) I only
    (B) III only
    (C) I and II only

    (D) I and III only
    (E) I, II, and III

71. Which one of the following is true of cholestyramine resin?

    (A) It is not absorbed from the GI tract.
    (B) It is a cationic exchange resin.
    (C) It increases the synthesis of cholesterol.
    (D) It is commercially available as a viscous syrup.
    (E) It will solubilize gallstones.

72. In addition to being used as an anticonvulsant, phenytoin (Dilantin) is also used in treating

    (A) tuberculosis
    (B) cardiac arrhythmias
    (C) systemic lupus erythematosus (SLE)
    (D) Parkinson's disease
    (E) cataracts

73. The HLB system is used to classify

    (A) the danger of drugs in pregnant patients
    (B) droplet size of aerosols
    (C) pharmaceutical dyes
    (D) drug solubility
    (E) surfactants

74. Terfenadine (Seldane) can best be classified pharmacologically as an

    (A) antidepressant
    (B) H_2-receptor antagonist
    (C) antihypertensive agent
    (D) antipsychotic
    (E) H_1-receptor antagonist

75. A nurse informs you that a patient has polydipsia. This refers to

    (A) excessive urination
    (B) excessive craving for food
    (C) excessive thirst
    (D) diarrhea
    (E) double vision

76. Which one of the following body areas usually has the lowest (most acidic) pH?

    (A) Blood
    (B) Lacrimal fluid
    (C) Oral cavity
    (D) Intestinal fluid
    (E) Vagina

77. Lotensin is most similar in action to

    (A) Dyrenium
    (B) Calan
    (C) Minipress
    (D) Lotrisone
    (E) Capoten

78. A drug interaction is likely to occur when 6-mercaptopurine (Purinethol) is used with

    (A) aspirin
    (B) pyridoxine
    (C) allopurinol (Zyloprim)
    (D) streptokinase (Streptase)
    (E) iron products

79. Simethicone is employed in pharmaceutical products as a (an)

    (A) buffer
    (B) laxative
    (C) chelating agent
    (D) viscosity builder
    (E) antifoaming agent

80. Acetylcysteine (Mucomyst) exerts its mucolytic effect by

    (A) complexing with mucus protein
    (B) altering the normal synthesis order of DNA
    (C) altering the cellular synthesis of mucoproteins
    (D) breaking chemical bonds of mucoproteins
    (E) increasing the secretion of low viscosity mucus from the walls of the respiratory tract

81. A patient's chart reveals a hypersensitivity to penicillin. The patient should be suspected of exhibiting a similar reaction to

    (A) nystatin (Mycostatin)
    (B) erythromycin
    (C) vancomycin (Vancocin)
    (D) cefixime (Suprax)
    (E) phenazopyridine (Pyridium)

82. An antacid that is most likely to induce gastric hypersecretion is

    (A) calcium carbonate
    (B) magaldrate
    (C) aluminum hydroxide
    (D) magnesium hydroxide
    (E) glycine

83. Which of the following is utilized in the treatment of viral infections?

    (A) Pentoxifylline
    (B) Ergonovine
    (C) Misoprostol
    (D) Amantadine
    (E) Moricizine

84. A patient's blood test reveals an excessively high level of amylase. This may indicate a disease of the

    (A) liver
    (B) heart
    (C) kidney
    (D) lung
    (E) pancreas

85. Basal thermometers and rectal thermometers are similar in that both

    I. have the same degree of accuracy
    II. can be used to determine ovulation
    III. can be used orally

    (A) I only
    (B) III only
    (C) I and II only
    (D) II and III only
    (E) I, II, and III

86. Patients with estrogen-dependent neoplasms often benefit from the use of

    (A) oral contraceptives
    (B) methotrexate
    (C) cyanocobalamin
    (D) tamoxifen
    (E) cisplatin

87. Another name for diacetylmorphine is

    (A) meperidine
    (B) heroin
    (C) dionin
    (D) cocaine
    (E) methadone

88. A patient receiving isocarboxazid (Parnate) should be advised to

    (A) avoid foods high in potassium
    (B) avoid foods high in tyramine
    (C) avoid foods high in sodium
    (D) avoid foods high in vitamin K
    (E) consume a low-fat diet

89. Dextranomer (Debrisan) is employed pharmaceutically as a (an)

    (A) topical corticosteroid
    (B) plasma expander
    (C) antipsoriatic agent
    (D) abrasive cleanser for the skin
    (E) absorbant for secreting wounds

90. The antidiarrheal Mitrolan contains

    (A) attapulgite

    (B) bismuth subsalicylate
    (C) polycarbophil
    (D) gelatin
    (E) kaolin

91. A drug of choice for the treatment of typhoid fever is

    (A) nafcillin (Unipen)
    (B) vancomycin (Vancocin)
    (C) sulfasalazine (Azulfidine)
    (D) chloramphenicol (Chloromycetin)
    (E) ganciclovir (Cytovene)

92. Polyvinyl alcohol is commonly employed in pharmaceutical systems as a

    (A) solvent
    (B) preservative
    (C) buffer
    (D) lubricant
    (E) viscosity builder

93. Which of the following drugs exhibits H_2-receptor antagonist activity?

    I. Sucralfate
    II. Tagamet
    III. Axid

    (A) I only
    (B) III only
    (C) I and II only
    (D) II and III only
    (E) I, II, and III

94. The hub of a needle is

    (A) the portion that fits onto the syringe
    (B) the needle shaft
    (C) the portion of the needle that is ground for sharpness
    (D) the needle hole
    (E) the needle bevel

95. The use of which of the following drugs is associated with the development of a SLE-like syndrome?

    (A) probenecid (Benemid)

Questions: 85–100   333

(B) hydralazine (Apresoline)

(C) nitrofurantoin (Macrodantin)

(D) diazepam (Valium)

(E) phenytoin (Dilantin)

96. Which of the following drugs is least likely to interact with cholestyramine (Questran)?

(A) Phenobarbital

(B) Warfarin

(C) Atropine

(D) Chlorothiazide

(E) Penicillin

97. Pyridoxine supplementation should be provided to patients chronically using

(A) phenytoin (Dilantin)

(B) propranolol (Inderal)

(C) levodopa (Larodopa)

(D) sulindac (Clinoril)

(E) isoniazid

98. Vasopressin is a hormone elaborated by the

(A) anterior pituitary gland

(B) posterior pituitary gland

(C) adrenal gland

(D) pancreas

(E) kidney

99. An inverse relationship exists between the concentration of calcium in the blood and the blood concentration of

(A) magnesium

(B) thyroid hormone

(C) testosterone

(D) sodium

(E) phosphorus

100. Drug metabolites are generally

(A) more lipid soluble than their parent compound

(B) referred to as "prodrugs"

(C) eliminated more slowly from the body than is their parent compound

(D) more water soluble than their parent compound

(E) incapable of producing pharmacologic effects

Answers

1. (E)
2. (C)
3. (D)
4. (D)
5. (E)
6. (A)
7. (A)
8. (B)
9. (E)
10. (D)
11. (D)
12. (E)
13. (B)
14. (D)
15. (B)
16. (C)
17. (D)
18. (C)
19. (B)
20. (E)

21. (C)
22. (B)
23. (A)
24. (D)
25. (D)
26. (E)
27. (E)
28. (A)
29. (B)
30. (B)
31. (C)
32. (E)
33. (C)
34. (A)
35. (D)
36. (D)
37. (A)
38. (D)
39. (C)
40. (B)

41. (D)	67. (C)
42. (B)	68. (B)
43. (D)	69. (D)
44. (B)	70. (A)
45. (B)	71. (A)
46. (C)	72. (B)
47. (C)	73. (E)
48. (B)	74. (E)
49. (D)	75. (C)
50. (D)	76. (E)
51. (A)	77. (E)
52. (C)	78. (C)
53. (B)	79. (E)
54. (E)	80. (D)
55. (A)	81. (D)
56. (E)	82. (A)
57. (C)	83. (D)
58. (E)	84. (E)
59. (E)	85. (D)
60. (D)	86. (D)
61. (E)	87. (B)
62. (B)	88. (B)
63. (A)	89. (E)
64. (B)	90. (C)
65. (A)	91. (D)
66. (C)	92. (E)

93. **(D)**

94. **(A)**

95. **(B)**

96. **(C)**

97. **(E)**

98. **(B)**

99. **(E)**

100. **(D)**

Frequently Dispensed Drugs

The practicing pharmacist should be familiar with commonly prescribed pharmaceutical products. If given the generic name, he or she should be able to match the following information with the drug:

1. brand or tradename
2. general pharmacologic category or use
3. commonly available dosage forms
4. available strengths
5. names of other products with identical or similar ingredients

The table contains the following abbreviations:

COMPANIES

G-W   Glaxo-Wellcome
M-J   Mead Johnson
MSD   Merck Sharp & Dohme
P-D   Parke-Davis
R-PR   Rhone-Poulenc Rorer
SK-B   SmithKline-Beecham
W-A   Wyeth-Ayerst
W-C   Warner Chilcott
ESI   Elkins-Sinn Inc.
B-W   Burroughs Wellcome

DRUGS

ASA   aspirin
APAP   acetaminophen
HCTZ   hydrochlorthiazide
NSAID   nonsteroidal anti-inflammatory drug
PE   phenylephrine
PPA   phenylpropanolamine

TABLE OF FREQUENTLY DISPENSED DRUGS

Generic Name	Tradename & Company	Category or Use	Dosage Forms and Strength
Acetaminophen + Codeine	Tylenol with Codeine (McNeil) Empracet with Codeine (G-W)	analgesic	300 mg APAP with 7.5, 15, 30, or 60 mg Cod.
Acyclovir sodium	Zovirax (B-W)	treatment of herpes	injection vial (600 mg); cap 200 mg; oint 5%; susp
Albuterol	Proventil (Schering) Ventolin (Glaxo) Volmax (Muro)	bronchodilator	tab (2 & 4 mg); syrup; inhalation nebulizer solution; extended-release tab (4 & 8 mg)
Allopurinol	Zyloprim (B-W)	treatment of hyperuricemia (gout, etc.)	tab (100 & 300 mg)
Alprazolam	Xanax (Upjohn)	treatment of anxiety	tab (0.25, 0.5, & 1 mg)
Amitriptyline HCl	Elavil (MSD)	antidepressant	tab (10, 25, 50, 75, 100, & 150 mg); injection
Amlodipine	Norvasc (Pfizer)	antihypertensive (calcium channel blocker)	tab (2.5, 5, & 10 mg)
Amoxicillin	Amoxil (SK-B) Polymox (Apothecon) Trimox (Apothecon) Wymox (Wyeth)	broad-spectrum antibiotic	cap (250 & 500 mg); susp
Amoxicillin + clavulanate K	Augmentin (SK-B)	broad-spectrum antibiotic	tab (250, 500, & 875 mg); chewable tab (125 & 250 mg); susp
Ampicillin	Omnipen (Wyeth) Principen (Squibb) Polycillin (Bristol) Totacillin (Beecham)	same as above	cap and susp (250 & 500 mg)
Aspirin with codeine	Empirin with codeine (B-W)	analgesic; antitussive	tab—No. 1 (1/8 gr), No. 2 (1/4 gr), No. 3 (1/2 gr), No. 4 (1 gr)
Astemizole	Hismanal (Janssen)	antihistamine (H_1-receptor antagonist)	tab (10 mg)
Atenolol	Tenormin (ICI Pharma)	antihypertensive (beta-adrenergic blocking agent)	tab (50 & 100 mg)
Atenolol + chlorthalidone	Tenoretic (ICI Pharma)	same	tab 50 = 50 mg + 25 mg tab 100 = 100 mg + 25 mg
Azithromycin	Zithromax (Pfizer)	antibiotic (macrolide)	cap (250 mg)
Beclomethasone dipropionate	Vanceril, Vancenase AQ (both Schering) Beconase AQ (Allen & Hanburys)	bronchodilator to treat rhinitis	inhalation aerosol; aerosol nasal inhaler
Benazepril HCl	Lotensin (Ciba)	antihypertensive (ACE inhibitor)	tab (5, 10, 20, & 40 mg)
Buspirone HCl	Buspar (M-J)	antianxiety	tab (5 & 10 mg)
Butalbital + ASA + caffeine	Fiorinal (Sandoz)	sedative; analgesic	tab; cap
Butalbital, ASA, caffeine, + codeine	Fiorinal with codeine (Sandoz)	same	same

(continued)

Generic Name	Tradename & Company	Category or Use	Dosage Forms and Strength
Butalbital, APAP, caffeine	Fioricet (Sandoz)	same	tab
Carbamazepine	Tegretol (Cibageneva)	anticonvulsant	tab (200 mg); chewable tab (100 mg)
Carbidopa + levodopa	Sinemet (MSD)	antiparkinson agent	tab 10/100 (10 mg + 100 mg); 25/250 (25 mg + 250 mg)
Carisoprodol	generic Soma (Wallace)	skeletal muscle relaxant	tab (350 mg)
Cefaclor	Ceclor (Lilly)	antibiotic	cap (250 & 500 mg); susp
Cefadroxil	Duricef (M-J)	antibiotic	tab (1 g); cap (500 mg); susp (125, 250, & 500 mg)
Cefixime	Suprax (Lederle)	antibiotic	tab (200 & 400 mg); pwd for suspension
Cefuroxime	Ceftin (Allen & Hanburys) Kefurox (Lilly) Zinacef (Glaxo)	antibiotic	tab (125, 250, & 500 mg) pwd for injection same
Cephalexin HCl monohydrate	Keftab (Dista)	antibiotic	tab (250 & 500 mg)
Chlorhexidine gluconate	Peridex (Procter & Gamble)	microbicide	0.12% oral rinse
Chlorpropamide	Diabinese (Pfizer)	oral hypoglycemic	tab (100 & 250 mg)
Chlorthalidone	Hygroton (Rorer)	antihypertensive	tab (25, 50, & 100 mg)
Cholestyramine	Questran (Bristol)	antihyperlipidemic	pwd
Cimetidine	Tagamet (SK-B)	prevent and treat peptic ulcers	tab (200, 400, & 800 mg); liq; injection
Ciprofloxacin	Cipro (Miles)	broad-spectrum antibiotic (a fluoroquinolone)	tab (250, 500, & 750 mg); injection sol
Cisapride	Propulsid (Janssen)	treat gastroesophageal reflux	tab (10 & 20 mg)
Clindamycin	Cleocin (Upjohn)	antibiotic	cap (75, 150, & 300 mg)
Clindamycin topical	Cleocin T (Upjohn)	treatment of acne	gel; sol; lotion (all 10 mg/mL)
Clonidine HCl	Catapres (Boehringer)	antihypertensive	tab (0.1, 0.2, & 0.3 mg); trans-dermal patches
Clonazepam	Klonopin (Roche)	treatment of petit mal seizures	tab (0.5, 1, & 2 mg)
Clotrimazole	Gyne-Lotrimin (Schering) Lotrimin (Schering) Lotrimin AF (Schering) Mycelex-G (Miles)	broad-spectrum antifungal	vag. cream (1%); vag. tab (100 mg) cream; lotion; sol (all 1%) AF = antifungal; same topical conc. as above but OTC tab; cream
Clotrimazole + betamethasone	Lotrisone (Schering)	antifungal and anti-inflammatory	cream
Cromolyn sodium	Intal (Fisons) Nasalcrom (Fisons)	management of asthma & rhinitis	aerosol spray; sol for nebulizer nasal sol

(continued)

Generic Name	Tradename & Company	Category or Use	Dosage Forms and Strength
Cyclobenzaprine	Flexeril (MSD)	skeletal muscle relaxant	tab (10 mg)
Diazepam	Valium (Roche) Valrelease (Roche)	antianxiety	tab (2, 5, & 10 mg); cap (15 mg)
Diclofenac	Voltaren (Geigy)	NSAID	tab (25, 50, & 75 mg)
Dicyclomine	generic Bentyl	GI anticholingeric & antispasmodic	cap (10 & 20 mg); tab (10 mg); syrup; injection
Digoxin	Lanoxin (B-W) Lanoxicaps	cardiovascular agent	tab (0.125, 0.25, & 0.5 mg); pediatric elix.; injection cap (50, 100, & 200 µg)
Diltiazem	Cardizem (Marion) Dilacor XR (R-PR) Tiazac (Forest)	antianginal agent	tab (30, 60, 90, & 120 mg); SR cap (60, 90, & 120 mg) for hypertension
Diphenoxylate HCl + atropine	Lomotil (Searle)	antidiarrheal	tab (2.5 mg); liq
Dipyridamole	Persantine (Boehringer)	antianginal agent	tab (25, 50, & 75 mg)
Doxazosin	Cardura (Roerig)	antihypertensive	tab (1, 2, 4, & 8 mg)
Doxycycline	Vibramycin, Vibra-Tab (Pfizer)	broad-spectrum antibiotic	cap (50 & 100 mg); tab (100 mg)
Enalapril	Vasotec (MSD)	antihypertensive	tab (2.5, 5, 10, & 20 mg)
Enalapril + HCTZ	Vaseretic (MSD)		
Erythromycin	E-Mycin (Boots) Erythrocin (Abbott)	broad-spectrum antibiotic	tab (250 & 500 mg); susp
	Ery-Tab (Abbott) ERYC (P-D)		delayed-release tab (250 & 500 mg) enteric-coated pellets in delayed-release cap (250 mg)
	PCE (Abbott)		tab with polymer-coated particles (500 mg)
Erythromycin ethylsuccinate	E.E.S. (Abbott)		pwd for susp.; chewable tab (200 mg); tab (400 mg); liq (200 & 400)
same + acetyl sulfisoxazole	Pediazole (Ross)		granules for susp (200 + 600 mg)
Erythromycin Estolate	Ilosone (Dista)		cap (125 & 250 mg); susp
Erythromycin Stearate	Erythrocin Stearate (Abbott)		film-coated tab (250 & 500 mg)
Estradiol Transdermal	Estraderm (Ciba)	moderate symptoms of menopause	transdermal patches (4 & 8 mg)
Estradiol	Estrace (M-J)	same; treatment of atrophic vaginitis	tab (1 & 2 mg); vag. cream
Estrogen combinations	Demulen (Searle) Ovral (Wyeth) Ovral-28 (Wyeth)	oral contraceptives	tab

(continued)

Generic Name	Tradename & Company	Category or Use	Dosage Forms and Strength
	Triphasil (Wyeth)		
	Nordette (Wyeth)		
	Tri-Levlen (Berlex)		
Estrogens, conjugated	Premarin (Wyeth-Ayerst)	replacement therapy in menopause and post-menopause	tab (0.3, 0.625, 1.25, & 2.5 mg)
Estropipate	Ogen (Abbott)	estrogen replacement	tab (0.625, 1.25, 2.5, & 5 mg)
Ethinyl Estradiol + Desogestrel	Ortho-Cept (Ortho)	oral contraceptives	tab (30 µg + .15 mg)
	Desogen (Organon)		
Ethinyl estradiol + norethindrone (+ 75 mg ferrous fumarate)	Loestrin 21 & Fe (P-D)	monophasic oral contraceptive	tab
	Ovcon 35; 50 (M-J)		tab
Ethinyl Estradiol + Norgestrol	LoOval 28		
Etodolac	Lodine (Wyeth-Ayerst)	NSAID	cap (200, 300, & 400 mg)
Famotidine	Pepcid (MSD)	treatment of peptic ulcers	tab (20 & 40 mg); pwd for susp.; injection
Fenoprofen	Nalfon (Dista)	antirheumatic	cap (200 & 300 mg)
Fluocinonide	Lidex (Syntex)	antipruritic, anti-inflammatory	oint; cream; gel
Fluoxetine	Prozac (Dista)	antidepressant	pulvules (10 & 20 mg); liq.
Flurazepam	Dalmane (Roche)	treat insomnia	cap (15 & 30 mg)
Flurbiprofen	Ansaid (Upjohn)	NSAID	tab (50 & 100 mg)
Fluvastatin	Lescol (Sandoz)	antihyperlipidemic	cap (20 & 40 mg)
Furosemide	Lasix (Hoechst)	diuretic	tab (20, 40, & 80 mg); injection
Gamma benzene hexachloride (Lindane)	Kwell (Reed & Carnick)	ectoparasiticide (kill head & pubic lice)	liquid shampoo
Gemfibrozil	Lopid (P-D)	antihyperlipidemic	cap (300 mg); tab (600 mg)
Gentamicin	Garamycin (Schering)	broad-spectrum antibiotic	oint; cream; ophth. sol & oint; injection
Glipizide	Glucotrol (Roerig)	antihyperglycemic	tab (5 & 10 mg)
Glyburide	Micronase (Upjohn)	antidiabetic	tab (1.25, 2.5, & 5 mg)
	DiaBeta (Hoechst)		
Granisetron	Kytril (SK-B)	prevent nausea & vomiting during chemotherapy	tab (1 mg)
Guanfacine	Tenex (Robins)	antihypertensive	tab (1 mg)
Haloperidol	Haldol (McNeil)	antipsychotic	tab (1, 2, 5, & 10 mg); liq; injection
Hydrochlorthiazide	Esidrix (Ciba)	diuretic, antihypertensive	tab (25 & 50 mg)
	HydroDIURIL (MSD)		

(continued)

Generic Name	Tradename & Company	Category or Use	Dosage Forms and Strength
Hydrocodone bitartrate + APAP + generic	Vicodin (Knoll) Lortab (Russ) Lorcet Plus (UAD)	narcotic analgesic; antitussive [C III]	tab = 5 mg + 500 mg ES = 7.5 mg + 750 mg APAP tab = 2.5 mg + 500 mg APAP liq. = 2.5 mg + 120 mg APAP
Hydrocortisone + polymyxin & neomycin	Cortisporin (B-W)	antibacterial; anti-inflammatory	otic sol; topical oint
Hydroxyzine HCl	Atarax (Roerig)	antianxiety agent	tab (10, 25, 50, & 100 mg); injection
Hydroxyzine pamoate	Vistaril (Pfizer)	same	cap (25, 50, & 100 mg)
Ibuprofen	Motrin (Upjohn) Rufen (Boots)	NSAID	tab (400, 600, & 800 mg)
Indapamide	Lozol (Rorer)	antihypertensive & diuretic	tab (2.5 mg)
Indomethacin	Indocin (MSD)	anti-inflammatory	cap (25 & 50 mg); SR (75 mg); susp; suppository
Insulin	Humulin (Lilly) Novolin (Novo Nordisk)	control of diabetes	N, 50/50, R, 70/30 70/30
Ipratropium Br	Atrovent (Boehringer)	bronchodilator	inhalation aerosol
Isosorbide dinitrate	Isordil (Wyeth) Sorbitrate (ICI Pharma)	treatment of angina pectoris	oral tab (5 & 10 mg); sublingual tab (2.5 & 5 mg); chewable tab (5 mg-Sorbitrate) Isordil Tembids 40 mg cap & tab; Titradose 5, 10, 20, 30 & 40 mg); chewable tab (10 mg) tab (200 mg); susp (100 mg/5 mL); cream
Isradipine	DynaCirc (Sandoz)	calcium channel blocker	cap (2.5 & 5 mg)
Itraconazole	Sporanox (Janssen)	antifungal	cap (100 mg)
Ketoconazole	Nizoral (Janssen)	antifungal	tab (200 mg); susp (100 mg/5 mL); cream
Ketoprofen	Orudis Oruvail (Wyeth-Ayerst) & generic	NSAID	cap (25, 50, & 75 mg) sustained-release cap (100, 150, & 200 mg)
Ketorolac	Toradol (Syntex) Acular (Allergan)	NSAID	tab (10 mg)
Labetalol	Normodyne (Schering)	antihypertensive	tab (100, 200, & 300 mg); injection
Levothyroxine	Synthroid (Boots)	management of thyroid	tab (0.025 to 0.3 mg)
Lisinopril	Prinivil (MSD) Zestrill (Zeneca)	antihypertensive	tab (2.5, 5, 10, 20, & 40 mg)
Lithium carbonate	Eskalith (SK-B)	treat manic depression	cap (300 mg); controlled release (450 mg)
Lomefloxacin HCl	Maxaquin (Searle)	fluoroquinolone antibiotic	tab (400 mg)
Loperamide	Imodium (Janssen)	antidiarrheal	cap (2 mg)

(continued)

Generic Name	Tradename & Company	Category or Use	Dosage Forms and Strength
Loracarbef	Lorabid (Lilly)	cephalosporin	cap (200 & 500 mg); susp
Loratadine	Claritin (Schering)	antihistamine (long-acting)	tab (10 mg)
	Claritin-D		5 mg + 120 mg pseudoephedrine
Lorazepam	Ativan (Wyeth)	antianxiety agent [C IV]	tab (1, 2, & 5 mg); injection
Lovastatin	Mevacor (MSD)	antihyperlipidemic agent	tab (20 & 40 mg)
Meclizine	Antivert (Roerig)	antiemetic	tab (12.5 & 25 mg)
Medroxyprogesterone	Provera (Upjohn) Cycrin (ESI)	estrogen replacement	tab (2.5, 5, & 10 mg)
Mefenamic acid	Ponstel (P-D)	NSAID	kapseal (250 mg)
Metaproterenol	Alupent (Boehringer)	bronchodilator	tab (10 & 20 mg); syrup; inhalation aerosol
Methyldopa	Aldomet (MSD)	antihypertensive	tab (125, 250, & 500 mg)
Methyldopa + HCTZ	Aldoril 15 or 25 (MSD) Aldoril D30 or D50	same	tab (250 mg + either 15 or 25 mg HCTZ) tab (500 mg + either 30 or 50 mg HCTZ)
Methylphenidate	Ritalin (Ciba)	cortical stimulant	tab (5, 10, 20 mg); SR 20 mg
Methylprednisolone	Medrol (Upjohn)	anti-inflammatory	tab (2, 4, 8, 16, 24, & 32 mg); topical 0.25 & 1%; inj (20, 40, & 80 mg)
Metoclopramide	Reglan (Robins)	antinauseant (esp. cancer chemotherapy); stimulate GI tract motility	tab (10 mg); syrup; injection (10 mg/2 mL)
Metoprolol	Lopressor (Geigy)	antihypertensive (adrenergic-blocking agent)	tab (50 & 100 mg)
	Toprol XL (Astra)		extended-release (50, 100, & 200 mg)
Metronidazole	Flagyl (Searle)	trichomonacide	oral tab (250 mg); vag. tab (500 mg); injection
Miconazole nitrate	Monistat 7	treatment of vulvovaginal candidiasis	cream (2%); vag. supp (200 mg)
	Monistat 3 (Ortho)		vag. supp (100 mg)
Minoxidil	Rogaine (Upjohn)	stimulate growth of hair	sol (20 mg/mL)
Misoprostol	Cytotec (Searle)	prevent stomach ulcers due to NSAIDs	tab (100 & 200 µg)
Mometasone furoate	Elocon (Schering)	topical corticosteroid	oint; cream; lotion (all 0.1%)
Mupirocin	Bactroban (SK-B)	treatment of impetigo	2% oint
Nabumetone	Relafen (SK-B)	NSAID	tab (500 & 750 mg)
Nadolol	Corgard (Princeton)	antihypertensive, treatment of angina	tab (40, 80, 120, & 160 mg)
Naproxen	Naprosyn (Syntex) Naprelan (W-A)	antirheumatic	tab (250, 375, & 500 mg); susp; controlled-release (375 & 500 mg)

(continued)

Generic Name	Tradename & Company	Category or Use	Dosage Forms and Strength
Naproxen sodium	Anaprox (Syntex)	same	tab (275 mg); Anaprox DS tab (550 mg)
Nedocromil sodium	Tilade (Fisons)	anti-inflammatory	respiratory inhaler
Neomycin, polymyxin B, & bacitracin	Neosporin (B-W)	antibiotic combination	topical oint; ophthal. oint.
Nicotine polacrilex	Nicorette (Lakeside)	smoker's aid	chewing pieces (2 mg)
Nifedipine	Procardia (Pfizer) Procardia XL	calcium channel blocker	capsule (10 mg); XL = extended-release (30, 60, & 90 mg)
Nitrofurantoin macrocrystals	Macrodantin (Norwich Eaton)	urinary tract antibacterial	cap (25, 50, & 100 mg)
Nitroglycerin	Nitroglycerin (Lilly) Nitro-Bid (Marion) Nitrostat (P-D) Transderm-Nitro (Summit) Nitro-Dur II (Key)	treatment of angina	sublingual tab (0.15, 0.3, 0.4, & 0.6 mg) cap (2.5 mg); prolonged-release (6.5 mg); oint (2%) regular & SR (2.5, 6.5, & 9 mg) patches oint (2%); inject; patches
Nizatidine	Axid (Lilly)	treatment of duodenal ulcers	cap (150 & 300 mg)
Norfloxacin	Noroxin v(MSD)	broad-spectrum antibacterial	tab (400 mg)
Norgestrel + ethinyl estradiol pilpak	Ovral Lo/Ovral (Wyeth)	oral contraceptive	tab (0.5 + 0.05 mg) tab (0.3 + 0.03 mg)
Norethindrone acetate	Norlestrin (P-D)	same	tab (1 & 2.5 mg)
same + ethinyl estradiol	Ortho-Novum (Ortho) Ortho-Novum 7/7/7 (Ortho)	same	tab (0.5 mg + 35 µg)
Norethindrone + mestranol	Norinyl 1/50 (Syntex) Tri-Norinyl (Syntex)	same	tab (1 mg + 0.05 mg)
Nortriptyline HCl	Pamelor (Sandoz)	antidepressant	cap (10, 25, 50, & 75 mg)
Nystatin	Mycostatin (Squibb)	antifungal	oral tab (500,000 units); vag. tab (100,000 units)
Ofloxacin	Floxin (Ortho)	fluoroquinolone antibiotic	tab (200, 300, & 400 mg); injection
Omeprazole	Prilosec (MSD)	short-term treatment of active duodenal ulcers	sustained-release cap (20 mg)
Ondansetron	Zofran (Glaxo)	antiemetic	injection (2 mg/mL)
Oxaprozin	Daypro (Searle)	NSAID for osteoporosis & rheumatoid arthritis	tab (600 mg)
Oxazepam	Serax (Wyeth)	antianxiety; antispasmodic	cap (10, 15, & 30 mg); tab (15 mg)
Oxycodone HCl + O. terephthalate + ASA	Percodan (DuPont)	analgesic; antipyretic	tab
Oxycodone HCl + acetaminophen	Percocet-5 (DuPont) Tylox (McNeil)	same	tab

(continued)

Generic Name	Tradename & Company	Category or Use	Dosage Forms and Strength
Paroxetine	Paxil	antidepressant	tab (20 & 30 mg)
Penicillin V potassium (Potassium phenoxymethyl penicillin)	Beepen VK (SK-B) Betapen-VK (Apothecon) Ledercillin VK (Lederle) Pen-Vee K (Wyeth) V-Cillin K (Lilly) Veetids (Apothecon)	antibiotic for gram-positive microorganisms	tab and susp of various strengths (usually 125, 250, & 500 mg, which are equivalent to 200,000, 400,000 & 800,000 units, respectively)
Pentoxifylline	Trental (Hoechst)	treatment of intermittent claudication	tab (400 mg)
Perphenazine + amitriptyline	Triavil (MSD) Etrafon Schering)	tranquilizer, antidepressant	tab (2 + 10; 2 + 25; 4 + 10; 4 + 25 mg)
Phenylephrine HCl, PPA, & guaifenesin	Entex (Norwich) Entex LA	decongestant; expectorant	tab (LA formula does not have phenylephrine)
Phenylephrine + PPA, phentoloxamine, & chlorpheniramine	Naldecon (Bristol)	nasal decongestant	tab; syrup
Phenytoin	Dilantin (P-D)	anticonvulsant	cap (30 & 100 mg); susp; infatabs (50 mg)
Piroxicam	Feldene (Pfizer)	NSAID	cap (10 & 20 mg)
Polymyxin B, neomycin, gramicidin, & hydrocortisone	Cortisporin (B-W)	broad-spectrum antibiotic	cream
Potassium bicarbonate & citrate	K-Lyte (Bristol)	potassium supplement	effervescent tab (25 mEq of potassium per tablet)
Potassium chloride	K-Tab v(Abbott) Klotrix (M-J) Slow-K (Summit) Micro-K (Robins) Klor-Con (Upsher-Smith) K-Dur (Key)	same	tab (4 to 10 mEq of potassium per tablet) wax matrix tab (8 mEq) pwd (20 & 25 mEq); tab (8 & 10 mEq) controlled-release tab (10 & 20 mEq)
Pravastatin sodium	Pravachol (Squibb)	antihyperlipidemic	tab (10 & 20 mg)
Prazepam	Centrax (P-D)	antianxiety	cap (5, 10, & 20 mg); tab (10 mg)
Prazosin	Minipress (Pfizer)	antihypertensive	cap (1, 2, & 5 mg)
Same + polythiazide	Minizide (Pfizer)		cap (same + 0.5 mg)
Prednisone	Deltasone (Upjohn)	glucorticoid	tab (2.5, 5, 10, 20, & 50 mg)
Probucol	Lorelco (Merrell-Dow)	antihyperlipidemic agent	tab (250 & 500 mg)
Procainamide HCl	Pronestyl (Princeton)	treat premature ventricular contractions	cap (250 & 500 mg); filmlok tab (250, 375, & 500 mg)

(continued)

Generic Name	Tradename & Company	Category or Use	Dosage Forms and Strength
	Procan SR (P-D)		sustained-release (250, 500 & 750 mg)
Prochlorperazine	Compazine (SK-B)	antianxiety; antiemetic	tab (5, 10, 25 mg); spansule (10, 15, 30, & 75 mg); supp (2.5, 5, & 25 mg)
Promethazine HCl	Phenergan (Wyeth)	antihistamine; antiemetic	tab (12.5 & 25 mg); supp (25 & 50 mg)
Propafenone	Rythmol (Knoll)	antiarrhythmic	tab (150 & 300 mg)
Propranolol HCl	Inderal (Wyeth-Ayerst)	treat angina, arrhythmias, etc.	tab (10, 20, 40, 60, & 80 mg); LA cap (80, 120, & 160 mg)
Propoxyphene napsylate + acetaminophen	Darvocet-N (Lilly) Propacet (Lemmon)	analgesic	tab (50 & 100 mg with 325 or 650 mg APAP)
Quinapril HCl	Accupril	antihypertensive (ACE inhibitor)	tab (5, 10, 20, & 40 mg)
Ramipril	Altace (Hoechst)	antihypertensive (ACE inhibitor)	cap (1.25, 2.5, 5, & 10 mg)
Ranitidine HCl	Zantac (Glaxo)	H_2 antagonist	tab (150 & 300 mg); syrup (150 mg/10 mL); injection (25 mg/mL)
Selegiline	Eldepryl (Somerset)	antiparkinson	tab (5 mg)
Simvastatin	Zocor (Merck)	antihyperlipidemic agent	tab (5, 10, 20, & 40 mg)
Spironolactone	Aldactone (Searle)	antihypertensive; K-sparing diuretic	tab (25 mg)
Spironolactone + HCTZ	Aldactazide (Searle)	antihypertensive	tab (25 + 25 or 50 + 50 mg)
Sucralfate	Carafate (Marion)	treat peptic ulcers	tab (1 g)
Sulfonamide	Bleph-10 (Allergan)	ophthalmic antibacterial	ophth sol (10%)
	Sulamyd (Schering)		ophth sol (10% & 30%)
Sulindac	Clinoril (MSD)	antiarthritic	tab (150 & 200 mg)
Sumatriptan	Imitrex (Cerenex)	treatment of migraine	s.q. injection (12 mg/mL) in unit-of-use syringe
Tamoxifen	Nolvadex (ICI Pharma)	antiestrogen	tab (10 mg)
Temazepam	Restoril (Sandoz)	sedative/hypnotic	cap (15 & 30 mg)
Terazosin	Hytrin (Abbott)	antihypertensive	tab (1, 2, 5, & 10 mg)
Terbutaline	Bricanyl (Marion Merrill Dow) Brethine (Geigy)	bronchodilator	tab (2.5 & 5 mg)
Terconazole	Terazol (Ortho)	vaginal antifungal (candidiasis only)	Terazol 7 cream; Terazol 3 supp
Terfenadine	Seldane (Merrell)	treat seasonal rhinitis	tab (60 mg)
Tetracycline HCl	Achromycin V (Lederle) Robitet (Robins)	broad-spectrum antibiotic	cap (250 & 500 mg); susp

(continued)

Generic Name	Tradename & Company	Category or Use	Dosage Forms and Strength
Tetracycline phosphate	Sumycin (Squibb)	broad-spectrum antibiotic	cap (250 & 500 mg); susp
Theophylline	Elixophyllin (Forest)	treat bronchial asthma and reversible bronchospasms	elixir (80 mg/15 mL)
	Slo-Phyllin (R-PR)		cap (125 & 250 mg)
	Slo-bid (R-PR)	(contains anhydrous theophylline)	cap (50, 100, 200, & 300 mg)
	Theo-Dur (Key)		sustained-action tab (100, 200, 300 & 450 mg); sprinkle
Thioridazine HCl	Mellaril (Sandoz)	tranquilizer	tab (10, 25, 50, 100, 150, & 200 mg)
Thiothixene	Navane (Roerig)	antipsychotic	cap (1, 2, 5, 10, & 20 mg); liq concentrate 5 mg/mL
Timolol maleate	Timoptic (MSD)	treat glaucoma	ophth sol (0.25 & 0.5%)
	Blocadren (MSD)	antihypertensive	tab (5, 10, & 20 mg)
Tramadol	Ultram (Ortho-McNeil)	central analgesic	tab (50 mg)
Torsemide	Demadex (Boehringer)	loop diuretic	tab (5, 10, & 20 mg)
Tretinoin	Retin-A (Ortho)	treat acne vulgaris	cream; gel; liq
Triamcinolone acetonide	Kenalog (Squibb)	anti-inflammatory	cream; oint; topical aerosol
	Azmacort (R-PR)	treatment of asthma	inhalation aerosol
Triamterene + HCTZ	Dyazide (SK-B)	antihypertensive; diuretic	cap (50 + 25 mg)
	Maxzide (Lederle)		tab (75 + 50 mg) Maxzide—25 (37.5 + 25 mg)
Triazolam	Halcion (Upjohn)	sedative/hypnotic	tab (0.25 & 0.5 mg)
Trimethobenzamide	Tigan (Beecham)	antiemetic	cap (100 & 200 mg) & supp; injection
Trimethoprim + sulfamethoxazole	Septra (B-W) Bactrim (Roche)	antibacterial (urinary tract infections)	tab (80 + 400 mg); DS = double strength (160 + 800 mg); infusion sol
Valproic acid	Depakote (Abbott)	anitconvulsant	tab (125, 250, & 500 mg)
	Depakene (Abbott)	same	liq
Venlafaxine	Effexor (Wyeth)	antidepressant	tab (25, 37.5, 50, 75, & 100 mg)
Verapamil	Calan (Searle)	treat angina (calcium channel blocker)	tab (40, 80, & 120 mg) SR = 240 mg; injection
	Isoptin (Knoll)		
Warfarin	Coumadin (DuPont)	anticoagulant	tab (2, 2.5, 5, 7.5, & 10 mg)
	Panwarfin (Abbott)		
	Sofarin (Lemmon)		
Zolpidem tartrate	Ambien (Searle)	non-benzodiazepine hypnotic, sedative, tranquilizer	tab (5 & 10 mg)

Trade Names and Generic Names

Trade Name	Generic Name	Trade Name	Generic Name
Accupril	Quinapril	Bentyl	Dicyclomine
Achromycin V	Tetracycline	Betimol	Sumatriptan
Acular	Ketorolac	Biaxin	Clarithromycin
Adalat CC	Nifedipine	Blocadren	Timolol
Adapin	Doxepin	Brethine	Terbutaline
Aldactone	Spironolactone	Bricanyl	Terbutaline
Aldomet	Methyldopa	Bumex	Bumetanide
Aldoril	Methyldopa + HCTZ	Buspar	Buspirone
Altace	Ramipril		
Alupent	Metaproterenol	Calan	Verapamil
Ambien	Zolpidem	Capoten	Captopril
Amcil	Ampicillin	Carafate	Sucralfate
Amitriptyline	Elavil	Cardizem	Diltiazem
Amoxil	Amoxicillin	Cardura	Doxazosin
Anaprox	Naproxen	Catapres	Clonidine
Ansaid	Flurbiprofen	Ceclor	Cefaclor
Antivert	Meclizine	Ceftin	Cefuroxime
Anusol HC	Bismuth subgallate, resorcin, & hydrocortisone	Cefzil	Cefprozil
		Centrax	Prazepam
		Cipro	Ciprofloxacin
Aspirin with codeine	Empirin with codeine	Claritin	Loratadine
Atarax	Hydroxyzine	Cleocin	Clindamycin
Ativan	Lorazepam	Clinoril	Sulindac
Atrovent	Ipratropium	Compazine	Prochlorperazine
Augmentin	Amoxicillin + clavulanate K	Cogentin	Benztropine
		Corgard	Nadolol
Axid	Nizatidine	Cortisporin	Polymyxin B, neomycin, bacitracin, & hydrocortisone
Azmacort	Triamcinolone acetonide		
Bactroban	Mupirocin	Coumadin	Warfarin
Bactrim	Trimethoprim + sulfamethoxazole	Cycrin	Medroxyprogesterone
		Cytotec	Misoprostol
Beconase	Beclomethasone diproprionate	Dalmane	Flurazepam
Beepen VK	Potassium phenoxymethyl penicillin	Darvocet N	Propoxyphene + acetaminophen
		Daypro	Oxaprozin

Trade Name	Generic Name	Trade Name	Generic Name
Deltasone	Prednisone	Halcion	Triazolam
Demadex	Torsemide	Haldol	Haloperidol
Demulen	Estrogens	Hismanal	Astemizole
Depakene	Valproic acid	Humulin	Insulin
Depakote	Valproic acid	Hydergine	Ergoloid mesylates
Desogen	Ethinyl estradiol	HydroDIURIL	Hydrochlorothiazide
DiaBeta	Glyburide	Hygroton	Chlorthalidone
Diabinese	Chlorpropamide	Hytrin	Terazosin
Dilacor XR	Diltiazem		
Dilantin	Phenytoin	Ilosone	Erythromycin estolate
Dimetapp	Brompheniramine maleate	Imitrex	Sumatriptan
		Imodium	Loperamide
Dobutrex	Dobutamine	Inderal	Propranolol
Dopastat	Dopamine	Indocin	Indomethacin
Duricef	Cefadroxil	Intal	Cromolyn
Dyazide	Triamterene + HCTZ	Intropin	Dopamine
DynaCirc	Isradipine	Isoptin	Verapamil
		Isordil	Isosorbide dinitrate
Elavil	Amitriptyline		
Eldepryl	Selegiline	K-Dur	Potassium chloride
Elixophyllin	Theophylline	K-Lyte	Potassium bicarbonate & citrate
Elocon	Mometasone		
E-Mycin	Erythromycin	K-Tab	Potassium chloride
Entex	Phenylephrine, PPA, & guaifenesin	Keflex	Cephalexin
		Kenalog	Triamcinolone acetonide
Ery-Tab	Erythromycin	Klonopin	Clonazepam
ERYC	Erythromycin	Klor-Con	Potassium chloride
Erythrocin EES	Erythromycin	Kwell	Gamma benzene hexachloride
Entex	Phenylephrine, PPA, & guaifenesin		
		Kytrel	Granisetron
Esidrex	Hydrochlorthiazide		
Eskalith	Lithium carbonate	Lanoxin	Digoxin
Estrace	Estradiol	Larotid	Amoxicillin
Estraderm	Estradiol	Lasix	Furosemide
		Lescol	Fluvastatin
Feldene	Piroxicam	Levoxyl	Levothyroxine
Fioricet	Butalbital, APAP, & caffeine	Lidex	Fluocinonide
		Lodine	Etodolac
Fiorinal	Butalbital + ASA + caffeine	Loestrin-Fe	Ethinyl estradiol + iron
		Lomotil	Diphenoxylate + atropine
Flagyl	Metronidazole	Lo-Ovral 28	Ethinyl estradiol + norgestrel
Flexeril	Cyclobenzaprine		
Floxin	Ofloxacin	Lopid	Gemfibrozil
		Lopressor	Metoprolol
Garamycin	Gentamicin	Lorabid	Lorcarbef
Glucotrol	Glipizide	Lortab	Hydrocodone + APAP
Glynase	Glyburide	Lorcet Plus	Hydrocodone
Gyne-Lotrimin	Clotrimazole	Lotesin	Benazepril
		Lotrimin	Clotrimazole

Trade Name	Generic Name	Trade Name	Generic Name
Lotrisone	Clotrimazole + betamethasone	Pamelor	Nortriptyline
Lorelco	Probucol	Panwarfin	Warfarin
Lozol	Indapamide	Paxil	Paroxetine
Lortab	Hydrocodone + APAP	PCE	Erythromycin
		Pediazole	Erythromycin ethylsuccinate + sulfisoxazole acetyl
Macrobid	Nitrofurantoin		
Macrodantin	Nitrofurantoin	Pepcid	Famotidine
Maxaquin	Lomefloxacin	Percocet-5	Oxycodone HCl + acetaminophen
Medrol	Methylprednisolone		
Mellaril	Thioridazine	Percodan	Oxycodone HCl + O. terephthalate + ASA
Mevacor	Lovastatin		
Micro-K	Potassium chloride	Peridex	Chlorhexidine gluconate
Micronase	Glyburide	Persantine	Dipyridamole
Minipress	Prazosin	Pen-Vee K	Potassium phenoxy-methyl penicillin
Monistat	Miconazole		
Motrin	Ibuprofen	Phenergan	Promethazine
Mycelex-G	Clotrimazole	Polycillin	Ampicillin
Mycostatin	Nystatin	Polymox	Amoxicillin
		Poly-Vi-Flor	Fluoride + vitamins A, D, C, E, Bs, & niacin, pantothenic & folic acids
Nalfon	Fenoprofen		
Naprosyn	Naproxen		
Nasacort	Triamcinolone		
Nasalcrom	Cromolyn	Ponstel	Mefenamic acid
Neosporin	Neomycin, polymyxin B, & bacitracin	Pravachol	Pravastatin
		Premarin	Conjugated estrogens
Nicorette	Nicotine polacrilex	Prilosec	Omeprazole
Nitrobid	Nitroglycerin	Principen	Ampicillin
Nitrodur II	Nitroglycerin	Prinivil	Lisinopril
Nitrostat	Nitroglycerin	Procan SR	Procainamide
Nizoral	Ketoconazole	Procardia	Nifedipine
Nolvadex	Tamoxifen	Pronestyl	Procainamide
Normodyne	Labetalol	Propine	Dipivefrin
Norinyl	Norethindrone + mestranol	Propulsid	Cisapride
		Proventil	Albuterol
Norlestrin	Norethindrone acetate	Provera	Medroxyprogesterone
Noroxin	Norfloxacin	Prozac	Fluoxetine
Norvasc	Amlodipine		
		Questran	Cholestyramine
Ogen	Estropipate		
Omnipen	Ampicillin	Reglan	Metoclopramide
Ortho-Novum	Norethindrone + ethinyl estradiol	Relafen	Nabumetone
		Restoril	Temazepam
Ortho-Cept	Ethinyl estradiol	Retin-A	Tretinoin
Orudis	Ketoprofen	Ritalin	Methylphenidate
Orvail	Ketoprofen	Rogaine	Minoxidil
Ovcon	Ethinyl estradiol + norethindrone	Robitet	Tetracycline
		Roxicet	Oxycodone
Ovral	Ethinyl estradiol + norgestrel	Rufen	Ibuprofen

Trade Name	Generic Name	Trade Name	Generic Name
Rythmol	Propafenone	Tussionex	Hydrocodone and chlorpheniramine polistirexes
Seldane	Terfenadine		
Septra	Trimethoprim + sulfamethoxazole	Tylenol	Acetaminophen
		Tylox	Acetaminophen + oxycodone HCl
Serax	Oxazepam		
Serevent	Salmeterol		
Sinemet	Carbidopa + levodopa	Ultimox	Ampicillin
Sinequan	Doxepin	Ultram	Tramadol
Slo-bid	Theophylline anhydrous		
Slow-K	Potassium chloride	Valium	Diazepam
Slo-Phyllin	Theophylline	Valrelease	Diazepam
Sofarin	Warfarin	Vanceril	Beclomethasone dipropionate
Soma	Carisoprodol		
Sorbitrate	Isosorbide dinitrate	Vancenase	Beclomethasone dipropionate
Sporanox	Itraconazole		
Sulamyd	Sulfonamide	Vasotec	Enalapril
Sumycin	Tetracycline	Vaseretic	Enalapril + HCTZ
Suprax	Cefixime	V-Cillin K	Potassium phenoxymethyl penicillin
Synthroid	Levothyroxine		
Tagamet	Cimetidine	Veetids	Potassium phenoxymethyl penicillin
Tavist	Clemastine		
Tegretol	Carbamazepine		
Tenormin	Atenolol	Ventolin	Albuterol
Terazol	Terconazole	Verelan	Verapamil
Theo-Dur	Theophylline	Vibramycin	Doxycycline
Tigan	Trimethobenzamide	Vicodin	APAP + hydrocodone
Tilade	Nedocromil	Vistaril	Hydroxyzine pamoate
Timoptic	Timolol	Voltaren	Diclofenac
Topex	Benzoyl peroxide		
Toprol	Metoprolol	Wymox	Amoxicillin
Toradol	Ketorolac		
Totacillin	Ampicillin	Xanax	Alprazolam
Toprol XL	Metoprolol		
Transderm-Nitro	Nitroglycerin	Zantac	Ranitidine
Tranxene	Clorazepate	Zinacef	Cefuroxime
Trental	Pentoxifylline	Zestril	Lisinopril
Triavil	Perphenazine + amitriptyline	Zithromax	Azithromycin
		Zocor	Simvastatin
Tri-Levlen	Estrogen combination	Zofran	Ondansetron
Trimox	Amoxicillin	Zoloft	Sertraline
Tri-Norinyl	Norethindrone + mestranol	Zovirax	Acyclovir
		Zyloprim	Allopurinol
Triphasil	Ethinyl estradiol + levonorgestrel		
Tri-Vi-Flor	Fluoride + vitamins A, D, & C		